Genetic Testing for Alzheimer Disease

Recent and Related Titles in Gerontology

John D. Arras, ed., *Bringing the Hospital Home: Ethical and Social Implications of High-Tech Home Care*

Robert H. Binstock, Leighton E. Cluff, and Otto von Mering, eds., *The Future of Long-Term Care: Social and Policy Issues*

Robert H. Binstock, Stephen G. Post, and Peter J. Whitehouse, eds., *Dementia and Aging: Ethics, Values, and Policy Choices*

Tom Hickey, Marjorie A. Speers, and Thomas R. Prohaska, eds., *Public Health and Aging*

Robert B. Hudson, ed., *The Future of Age-Based Public Policy*

Laurence B. McCullough and Nancy L. Wilson, eds., *Long-Term Care Decisions: Ethical and Conceptual Dimensions*

Harry R. Moody, *Ethics in an Aging Society*

Stephen G. Post, *The Moral Challenge of Alzheimer Disease*

ROBERT H. BINSTOCK, Consulting Editor in Gerontology

Genetic Testing for Alzheimer Disease

Ethical and Clinical Issues

EDITED BY STEPHEN G. POST, PH.D., &
PETER J. WHITEHOUSE, M.D., PH.D.

The Johns Hopkins University Press
Baltimore and London

©1998 The Johns Hopkins University Press
All rights reserved. Published 1998
Printed in the United States of America
on acid-free paper

9 8 7 6 5 4 3 2 1

The Johns Hopkins University Press
2715 North Charles Street
Baltimore, Maryland 21218-4363
The Johns Hopkins Press Ltd., London
www.press.jhu.edu

Library of Congress Cataloging-in-
Publication Data will be found at
the end of this book.
A catalog record for this book is
available from the British Library.

ISBN 0-8018-5840-2

Contents

Acknowledgments   vii
List of Contributors   ix

1. Introduction: Genetics and the Moral Future of Dementia Care
   Stephen G. Post, Peter J. Whitehouse, and Arthur B. Zinn   1

PART ONE: The Genetics of Alzheimer Disease

2. The Chromosome 1 Type of Familial Alzheimer Disease
   Thomas D. Bird   17

3. Molecular Genetics of Early-Onset Alzheimer Disease Linked to Chromosome 14 and Chromosome 21
   Peter H. St. George-Hyslop   25

4. A New Paradigm for Clinical Evaluations of Dementia: Alzheimer Disease and Apolipoprotein E Genotypes
   Allen D. Roses   37

5. Therapeutic Interventions in Alzheimer Disease: Implications of Genetic Advances
   Peter J. Whitehouse   65

6. Some Questions Arising in the Commercial Development of Genetic Tests for Alzheimer Disease
   Robert Mullan Cook-Deegan   84

PART TWO: Ethical Aspects

7. Genetic Testing and Counseling for Early-Onset Autosomal-Dominant Alzheimer Disease
   Harry Karlinsky   103

8. Implications of Genetic Susceptibility Testing with Apolipoprotein E
   Kimberly A. Quaid   118

9. Prenatal Genetic Testing for Alzheimer Disease
   Bonnie Steinbock 140

PART THREE: Social Issues

10. Genetics and Long-Term-Care Insurance: Ethical and Policy Issues
    Robert H. Binstock and Thomas H. Murray 155

11. The Ethical Implications of Alzheimer Disease Risk Testing for Other Clinical Uses of APOE Genotyping
    Eric T. Juengst 177

12. Justice, Rights, and Alzheimer Disease Genetics
    Leonard Fleck 190

13. Managed Care Issues in Genetic Testing for Alzheimer Disease
    Steven Miles 209

PART FOUR: Educational Issues

14. Education for a Too-Hopeful Public
    Stephen G. Post 225

15. Alzheimer Genetics and the Primary Care Physician
    Greg A. Sachs 239

16. Culture and Values at the Intersection of Science and Suffering: Encountering Ethics, Genetics, and Alzheimer Disease
    Atwood D. Gaines 256

    Index 275

Acknowledgments

This project was sponsored and funded by the Ethical, Legal, and Social Implications Research Program of the National Human Genome Research Institute of the National Institutes of Health (RO1 HG01092-01A1, "Ethics, Genetics, and Alzheimer Disease," Stephen G. Post, Ph.D., principal investigator, Peter J. Whitehouse, M.D., Ph.D., Thomas H. Murray, Ph.D., Arthur B. Zinn, M.D., Ph.D., coinvestigators).

We are also grateful to the Center for Biomedical Ethics, School of Medicine, Case Western Reserve University, the Cleveland Area Chapter of the Alzheimer's Association, and the Alzheimer Center of University Hospitals of Cleveland, which is supported by a National Institute on Aging Alzheimer Disease Research Center grant.

The Alzheimer's Disease and Related Disorders Association provided travel grants to Dr. Post. Special thanks to the Ethics Advisory Panel of the National Alzheimer's Association, which took an active interest in this project, drew from a dialogue with us, and facilitated Dr. Post's national tour of over forty annual meetings of Alzheimer's Association chapters across the United States between 1995 and 1998 to lead workshops on ethics and genetics.

Thanks as well to Wendy Harris, medical editor with the Johns Hopkins University Press, who helped at every stage of book production.

Contributors

Robert H. Binstock, Ph.D., is professor of aging, health, and society at Case Western Reserve University. A former president of the Gerontological Society of America, he served as director of the White House Task Force on Older Americans under Lyndon B. Johnson and has been chair and a member of a number of advisory panels to the federal, state, and local governments and to foundations. He has published some 150 articles and book chapters dealing with politics and policies on aging. Among his nineteen books are *The Future of Long-Term Care: Social and Policy Issues* (coauthored) and four editions of *Handbook of Aging and the Social Sciences*.

Thomas D. Bird, M.D., is director of the University of Washington Neurogenetics Clinic and a member of the executive board of the University of Washington's Alzheimer's Disease Research Center. He has spent more than twenty years investigating the genetic factors underlying inherited forms of neuropathy, ataxia, spinal cord degeneration, movement disorders, dementia, and Alzheimer disease. He received the 1992 Wartenberg Award from the American Academy of Neurology for excellence in clinical research and shared the 1995 Metropolitan Life Foundation Award for Alzheimer Disease Research.

Robert Mullan Cook-Deegan, M.D., is director of the National Cancer Policy Board. In his previous work at the congressional Office of Technology Assessment, he directed the project "Losing a Million Minds: Confronting the Tragedy of Alzheimer's Disease and Other Dementias." His book, *The Gene Wars: Science, Politics, and the Human Genome,* chronicles the genesis of the human genome project. Dr. Cook-Deegan chairs the Royalty Fund Advisory Committee for the Alzheimer's Association and Section X (Societal Impacts of Science and Engineering) for the American Association for the Advancement of Science.

x Contributors

Leonard Fleck, Ph.D., is professor in the philosophy department and the Center for Ethics and Humanities in the Life Sciences at Michigan State University. He has published over seventy articles and book chapters on a range of issues in health care ethics and health policy. He is currently working on a book tentatively titled *Just Caring: The Moral and Political Challenges of Health Reform and Health Care Rationing*. He is coinvestigator on the three-year project, "Genome Technology and Reproduction: Values and Public Policy," funded by the National Human Genome Research Institute of the National Institutes of Health.

Atwood D. Gaines, Ph.D., M.P.H., is professor of anthropology, biomedical ethics, psychiatry, and nursing at Case Western Reserve University. He has published numerous articles and edited books, including *Ethnopsychiatry: The Cultural Construction of Professional and Folk Psychiatries*. His current research is in the areas of the cultural studies of science, bioethics, and social identity (ethnic, gender) and medicine.

Eric T. Juengst, Ph.D., is associate professor of biomedical ethics at Case Western Reserve University School of Medicine. He was the first chief of the Ethical, Legal, and Social Implications Research Program of the Center for Human Genome Research (later to become the National Human Genome Institute) at the National Institutes of Health and currently serves on the National Ethics Committee of the March of Dimes and on the Committee on Human Genome Diversity of the National Research Council. His research interests and publications have focused on conceptual and ethical issues raised by advances in genetics and biotechnology.

Harry Karlinsky, M.D., is director of psychiatry at the University of British Columbia. His research activities have been directed toward the study of Alzheimer disease and, more recently, health care and information technology. In addition to publishing papers, he has been coeditor of two books related to Alzheimer disease (*Alzheimer's Disease Research: Ethical and Legal Issues* and *Alzheimer Disease, Down Syndrome, and Their Relationship*) and is principal author of a CD-ROM entitled "The Clinical Diagnosis of Alzheimer's Disease."

Steven Miles, M.D., is associate professor of internal medicine in the Division of Geriatric Medicine, Department of Medicine, and associate faculty for the Center for Bioethics, the Center for Advanced Feminist Studies, and the University Council on Aging at the University of Minnesota. He has published and lectured extensively on end-of-life care, nursing home care, medical education, medical ethics, and health care reform. Dr. Miles is president of the American Association of Bioethics. He is a Soros Foundation faculty scholar for the project Death in America and codirected the Health Priorities Project for the Robert Wood Johnson and Pew Foundations' Health of the Public Program.

Thomas H. Murray, Ph.D., is professor and director of the Center for Biomedical Ethics at Case Western Reserve University School of Medicine. His research interests cover a wide range of ethical issues in medicine and science, including genetics, aging, children, organ donation, and health policy. He is an elected fellow of the Hastings Center and of the Environmental Health Institute. He serves as a member of the U.S. Olympic Committee's Sports Medicine Committee and as a presidential appointee to the National Bioethics Advisory Commission, where he serves as chair of the subcommittee on genetics. He is a member of the Committee on Ethics of the American College of Obstetrics and Gynecology; the Social Issues Committee of the American Society for Human Genetics; and the Ethics Committee of the Human Genome Organization (HUGO). He was a founder of the Working Group on Ethical, Legal, and Social Implications Research Program of the National Institutes of Health's National Human Genome Institute and chair of its Task Force on Genetics and Insurance. He is past president of the Society for Health and Human Values and is on the executive committee of the Association for Practical and Professional Ethics. His most recent book is *The Worth of a Child*.

Stephen G. Post, Ph.D., is associate professor and associate director for educational programs at the Center for Biomedical Ethics, Case Western Reserve University School of Medicine, and holds secondary appointments in the Departments of Philosophy, Religious Studies, and Family Medicine. He is an elected fellow of the Hastings Center. Dr. Post is a member of the Medical and Scientific Advisory Panel of Alzheimer's Disease International (the International Federation of Alzheimer's Disease and Related Disorders Societies), affiliated with the World Health Organization. He serves on the Ethics Advisory Board for the National Alzheimer's Disease and Related Disorders Association and the Alzheimer's Society of Canada National Ethics Task Force. In 1996 Dr. Post received two distinguished Templeton Foundation awards for exemplary writing in religion and the medical sciences and in religion and the behavioral sciences. Dr. Post is associate editor of the five-volume *Encyclopedia of Bioethics* and ethics editor for the journal *Alzheimer Disease and Associated Disorders*. His most recent book is *The Moral Challenge of Alzheimer Disease*.

Kimberly A. Quaid, Ph.D., is clinical associate professor of medical and molecular genetics and psychiatry at Indiana University School of Medicine. She started and directed the predictive testing program in the Department of Medical and Molecular Genetics at Indiana University School of Medicine. She codirects the master's program in genetic counseling and serves as assistant to the director of the Office for Women. Dr. Quaid has written extensively in the area of genetic testing and is an internationally recognized expert in the development of ethical protocols for genetic testing. She is coauthor of a forthcoming book entitled *Early Warning: Cases and Ethical Guidance for Presymptomatic Testing in Genetic Diseases.*

Allen D. Roses, M.D., is chief of neurology and leads the research team at the Joseph and Kathleen Bryan Alzheimer's Disease Research Center at Duke University. He was one of the first clinical neurologists to apply molecular genetic strategies to neurological diseases. During the early years of recombinant DNA research, Dr. Roses initiated several pioneering studies. His laboratory reported chromosomal location for more than fifteen diseases, including familial lateral sclerosis (Lou Gehrig disease), Charcot-Marie-Tooth neuropathy, neurofibromatosis, and tuberous sclerosis. The discovery that the apolipoprotein E gene is involved in Alzheimer disease as a susceptibility factor that lowers the age of onset and increases risk of disease illustrates the success of a multidisciplinary collaborative team directed by Dr. Roses. He has received the Metropolitan Life Foundation Award for Alzheimer Disease Research and the American Academy of Neurology Potamkin Award for Alzheimer's Disease Research, among many other national awards. He is a vice president of the Medical Advisory Committee of the Muscular Dystrophy Association and chair of the Medical and Scientific Advisory Committee of the U.S. Alzheimer's Association. Dr. Roses is a consultant for Athena Neurosciences, which markets the apolipoprotein E gene test for diagnostic purposes, and for Glaxo Wellcome.

Greg A. Sachs, M.D., is associate professor of medicine and assistant director of the MacLean Center for Clinical Medical Ethics at the University of Chicago. His research and writings to date have focused on ethical aspects of care for people with dementia, decision making for end-of-life medical care, and ethical issues in biomedical research involving older human subjects. Dr. Sachs serves on the Ethics Advisory Panel of the National Alzheimer's Association and is vice chair of the American Geriatric Society's Ethics Committee.

Peter H. St. George-Hyslop, M.D., is professor in the Division of Neurology, Department of Medicine, at the University of Toronto. His main interest is in the application of molecular genetic techniques to identify the biochemical pathways leading to Alzheimer degeneration and in applying this knowledge to clinical problems affecting patients with Alzheimer disease. He has been awarded the Francis McNaughton Prize of the Canadian Neurological Society, the Potamkin Award from the American Academy of Neurology, the Metropolitan Life Foundation Award, the gold medal from the Royal College of Physicians, and the Medical Research Council of Canada's Scientist Award, among others.

Bonnie Steinbock, Ph.D., is professor in the Department of Philosophy at the State University of New York, Albany, where she has joint appointments in the Department of Public Policy and the Department of Health Policy, Management, and Behavior in the School of Public Health. She is a fellow of the Hastings Center, a board member of the National Advisory Board on Ethics in Reproduction, and a participant in several collaborative projects in biomedical ethics in the Unites States and Europe. She has published more than forty articles on a variety of topics in biomedical ethics and applied ethics, with an emphasis on reproductive issues. She is the author of *Life before Birth: The Moral and Legal Status of Embryos and Fetuses* and coeditor, with Alastair Nocross, of *Killing and Letting Die* and, with John Arras, of *Ethical Issues in Modern Medicine* (4th ed.). She is currently writing a book on the right to reproduce.

Peter J. Whitehouse, M.D., Ph.D., is professor of neurology at Case Western Reserve University School of Medicine and holds a secondary appointment with the Center for Biomedical Ethics. He wrote the strategic plan to create the Alzheimer Center of University Hospitals of Cleveland and directed the center from 1986 to 1997. His clinical interests are in geriatric and behavioral neurology, with a special interest in dementia; his research interests include molecular biology of Alzheimer disease, drug development, health care systems, and ethics. Dr. Whitehouse was a member of the National Alzheimer's Advisory Panel of the Department of Health and Human Services and of the Food and Drug Administration Advisory Panel on Central Nervous System Drugs. He is also active in many professional associations in neurology, neurosciences, and psychiatry. Dr. Whitehouse was a consultant for Parke-Davis.

Arthur B. Zinn, M.D., Ph.D., is associate professor of genetics and pediatrics at Case Western Reserve University. His special interests include inborn errors of metabolism and inherited neurobiological disorders. He is clinically active in caring for patients and providing genetic counseling for those concerned with adult-onset neurodegenerative diseases, such as Huntington disease and Alzheimer disease.

Genetic Testing for Alzheimer Disease

Introduction

Genetics and the Moral Future of Dementia Care

STEPHEN G. POST, PH.D.,

PETER J. WHITEHOUSE, M.D., PH.D., AND

ARTHUR B. ZINN, M.D., PH.D.

This book is about the clinical, ethical, social, and educational implications of new genetic discoveries in Alzheimer disease (AD) that affect an estimated four million Americans. We seek to clarify these discoveries with regard to their potential for both benefit and harm. Our intent is to contribute to public literacy and critical thinking about AD genetics, especially in the many families of people with AD, although we address this book to professional readers as well.

Public Interest and Public Confusion

There is remarkable interest in AD genetic findings, and this will continue to grow. Unfortunately, as the population continues to age, more individuals will be concerned about their own risks of developing AD. The most rapidly growing segment of our population, those over the age of eighty-five, are also at greatest risk (almost 50%) for the disease. The public interest in AD ethics is therefore growing by leaps and bounds (Post 1995).

Alzheimer disease is the most common form of progressive degenerative dementia. It is characterized clinically by insidious onset and slow progression, with cognitive impairment involving memory, language, and other intellectual skills, and is associated with behavioral disturbances, particularly late in its course, such as agitation, depression, and psychosis. It is characterized neuropathologically by the loss of nerve cells in specific populations of neurons accompanied by neuritic plaques and neurofibrillary tangles. Alzheimer disease is diagnosed by this typical history of progressive intellectual impairment and by the absence of other defined forms of dementia. A standard evaluation usually includes a history, a physical examination with selective blood tests, and neuroimaging to rule out metabolic and structural lesions in the brain that may cause cognitive impairment.

Contrary to what some potential consumers of genetic testing believe, no predictive test for the typical late-onset (after age sixty-five) form of AD exists. Only in a very few early-onset cases (before age fifty-five, and most often in the forties), which constitute fewer than 1 or 2 percent of all AD cases, is predictive genetic testing possible. A predictive test, as we define it, clearly foretells the eventual onset of AD. Thus, when the elderly person comes into the genetic testing clinic and asks for the AD predictive test, the only appropriate response is that this test does not yet exist. If the subject shifts to the possibility of a genetic susceptibility test, the clinician should state that while this test is possible, no professional consensus group recommends it in asymptomatic individuals because the information gained is too vague for any reasonable decision making (see below). He or she might add that in future years, if more susceptibility genes are found, risk analysis in asymptomatic individuals might become more precise and, therefore, in some sense more useful to those who desire it.

Alzheimer disease is a genetically heterogeneous disorder; that is, to date it is associated with one susceptibility (risk) gene and three determinative (disease) genes. While more genes in each category are currently being investigated (e.g., another possible susceptibility gene on chromosome 12), we can already discuss these categories themselves as the two major paradigms. Although late-onset AD (after sixty-five years) has traditionally not been considered an inherited or genetic disease, an apolipoprotein E ϵ4 allele on chromosome 19 (*APOE*, gene; *apoE*, protein) has been identified as conferring susceptibility to its development. But the APOE ϵ4 allele is not in and of itself predictive of AD in asymptomatic individuals (Roses 1996). Predictive genetic testing is possible, however, for the extremely rare early-onset forms of AD. Individuals with or at risk for one of these autosomal-dominant forms of AD have a mutation on chromosome 1 (the presenilin 2 gene, or PS2) or 14 (the presenilin 1 gene, or PS1) or, even more rarely, 21. Only in this context can the word *predictive* be validly applied.

Focus groups with the Cleveland Area Chapter of the Alzheimer's Association and elsewhere around the United States indicate anecdotally that many people in the community of caregivers for patients with AD have confused the predictively powerful PS1 and PS2 findings, which are irrelevant to the usual late-onset form of AD, with the nonpredictive APOE findings. This confusion burdens the AD-affected community with the fear of carrying "the" AD gene.

It is, therefore, possible to speak of a public susceptibility to the genetization of culture and to unfounded genetic determinisms.

Educational efforts for both the public and professionals are needed to emphasize that APOE genotyping is nonpredictive. In 1996, the ADmark ApoE Genetic Test was introduced with a brochure that promoted the test "for greater certainty in differential diagnosis of AD," applicable only to patients already presenting with the symptoms of dementia. Before the company will run the test, the ordering physician must sign a statement attesting that the patient has dementia. This qualification is valid, and it is one with which Allen D. Roses, the discoverer of the APOE susceptibility factor, fully concurs.

Primary caregivers, specialists in dementia care, researchers, ethicists, public policy makers, and, most of all, the affected public should be aware of continuing progress in the genetics of AD. New findings raise vexing considerations regarding the introduction of genetic testing for purposes of disease prediction and susceptibility (risk) analysis in asymptomatic individuals and diagnosis in patients who present with dementia. The introduction of a genetic test may be deemed either appropriate or premature on the basis of the clarity of genetic data, the proven or unproven clinical applicability of the test (for predictive, diagnostic, or therapeutic uses), and the resolution of the ethical and policy aspects of test implementation.

There is an urgency to this educational endeavor because of the large population of patients with AD and their families. For which patients and for what purposes is it clinically and ethically appropriate to introduce genetic testing for AD? How much pressure is being created by financial interests, and how is this affecting researchers? How should consumer demand for such testing be answered? How should the principles of justice apply to payment for testing? How should the principle of confidentiality govern testing? What is the potential for actuarial discrimination against those with an AD-related gene (e.g., in the context of private long-term-care insurance policies)? Is genetic testing for AD more harmful than beneficial for those tested? As primary care providers and others receive requests from relatives of AD patients for "the AD test," how can providers be educated in genetics, and will enough trained genetic counselors be available?

To address these questions, a multidisciplinary National Study Group convened over several years to review emerging information about new genetic tests for AD and to analyze the implications of these tests for patients, families, clinicians, and public policy. This group was funded by the Ethical, Legal, and Social Implications Research Program of the National Human Genome

Research Institute of the National Institutes of Health. The study group, composed of leading AD geneticists, policy experts, and ethicists, has received input from lay focus groups of mildly affected AD patients and family caregivers. The chapters in this book present the work of members of the National Study Group.

The Genetics of Alzheimer Disease

Part One focuses on current and future developments in AD genetics (involving all known genetic loci) and takes up the ongoing debate over the scientific justification for the clinical introduction of these genetic developments for predictive testing (i.e., the clear foretelling of disease), susceptibility testing (i.e., providing a measure of risk analysis), diagnostic testing (i.e., as a diagnostic adjunct in patients already presenting with the symptoms of dementia), or potential therapeutic testing (i.e., antidementia compounds might be more efficacious in some genotypes than in others).

At least five academic groups, including the National Study Group, have developed consensus statements addressing potential uses of genetic testing for AD. Some statements address the single-gene disorders as well as the APOE susceptibility locus, others focus exclusively on APOE. All the groups concur that predictive use of APOE testing in asymptomatic individuals is not recommended at this time, although opinion on its use as a diagnostic adjunct is discordant.

1. The American College of Medical Genetics/American Society of Human Genetics Working Group on ApoE and Alzheimer Disease addressed whether genetic testing is justified for purposes of either prediction or diagnosis. This group concluded that, while APOE ε4 is associated with and is a risk factor for AD, the APOE genotype is neither sensitive nor specific enough for use as a diagnostic or predictive test (Farrer and American College of Medical Genetics 1995).

2. The United Kingdom Alzheimer's Disease Genetics Consortium concluded that the APOE data are "not sufficiently robust to inform predictive, diagnostic or risk assessment" (Lovestone 1995, 4).

3. The Medical and Scientific Advisory Committee of Alzheimer's Disease International expressed concern about the potential for misinforming patients about their risk. It concluded that, apart from the rare families with early-onset (single-gene) AD, "the time for presymptomatic predictive testing for AD in general has not yet arrived" (Brodaty and Medical and Scientific Advisory Committee 1995, 186).

Table 1.1. Genetic Testing for Alzheimer Disease

Criteria	Single-Gene Disorders	APOE e4
Locus	Chromosomes 1, 14, 21	Chromosome 19
Mode of inheritance	Autosomal dominant	Complex
Frequency	Rare	Common
Age of onset	Usually early (before 60 years)	Usually late (after 55 years)
Possible applications of testing		
Symptomatic	Yes	Yes
Presymptomatic	Yes	No
Applicability of testing	Limited	Wide
Commercial potential	Low	High
Interpretability of test results		
Symptomatic	High	Appears high (in some populations)
Presymptomatic	High	Low

Source: Post et al. 1997 (© 1997 American Medical Association).

4. The National Institute on Aging and the Alzheimer's Disease and Related Disorders Association supported a consensus conference in which participants recommended against APOE testing for assessing risk in asymptomatic individuals. This consensus statement leaves to the physician's discretion the diagnostic use of APOE testing as an adjunct to established diagnostic tests (Relkin and National Institute on Aging 1996).

5. The National Study Group statement, sponsored by the National Human Genome Research Institute's Ethical, Legal and Social Implications Research Program, concluded that for the rare autosomal-dominant early-onset families, genetic testing in asymptomatic individuals is feasible. The use of APOE genetic testing as a diagnostic adjunct remains under investigation, while its use in asymptomatic individuals is clearly not recommended. Furthermore, the premature introduction of genetic testing and possible adverse consequences are to be avoided (Post et al. 1997). Table 1.1 presents a summary of genetic testing for AD.

The attention given to the issue of clinical introduction of AD genetic testing indicates clearly the monumental implications of moving to this paradigm. The Alzheimer's Disease and Related Disorders Association Ethics Advisory Panel issued a notice to its constituency that APOE genotyping should not be used in asymptomatic individuals.

In Part One of this book, leading geneticists present summaries of the genetic findings on AD to date. Chapter 2 presents the PS2 gene finding located on chromosome 1. Thomas D. Bird, M.D., is recognized internationally as one of the discoverers of this gene mutation, considered causative of one form of early-onset familial AD, particularly in Volga German families. His chapter clearly articulates the significance and usefulness of the PS2 gene finding and includes a laudatory emphasis on the relevant ethical issues.

Chapter 3 addresses the PS1 gene located on chromosome 14. Peter H. St. George-Hyslop, M.D., is among the major investigators of AD genetics and has done pioneering work on both PS1 and the chromosome 21 mutations. His chapter presents the basic science involved as well as the current state of genetic testing.

Chapter 4 presents a bold advocacy position for the potential benefits of the APOE findings. Allen D. Roses, M.D., one of the most prolific genetic researchers in the AD area, and his colleagues are credited with the discovery of the connection between the APOE ε4 allele and susceptibility to AD in later life. Dr. Roses does not think that APOE testing should be done in asymptomatic individuals because the information it provides is not predictive, although he advocates testing in people already diagnosed with dementia to establish that AD is the cause. However, if additional susceptibility genes are discovered, the capacity to refine susceptibility analysis for at-risk populations may become firmer. This, argues Roses, will identify those persons for whom compounds that prevent or delay the onset of AD would be most appropriate.

In chapter 5, Peter J. Whitehouse, M.D., Ph.D., discusses the new and potential therapeutic advances in the prevention and treatment of AD with an eye toward the implications of genetics. Genotyping would be of benefit if linked to available or future therapies, but this appears to be a ways off. Whitehouse also briefly considers the use of APOE genotyping in combination with standard phenotypic measures in the differential diagnosis of patients with dementia. His position, in contrast to that of Roses, is more critical of such current application, in part because the relative values of different components of the diagnostic evaluation are unclear (Geldmacher and Whitehouse 1996). He contends that more research and educational efforts are needed to clarify the current debate about the clinical validity of APOE testing.

One cautionary response suggests that while the APOE ε4 allele "increases the probability that a demented individual has AD, in most instances the association is not strong enough to significantly alter the procurement of other differential diagnostic tests" (Bird 1995, 3). To clarify further the role of APOE testing for diagnostic purposes, APOE genotyping is being studied on autopsied patients who had been followed clinically for probable AD. The diagnostic applications of APOE testing are therefore under debate, both scientifically and with respect to potential cost savings.

In chapter 6, Robert Mullan Cook-Deegan, M.D., provides a comprehensive and timely update on the potential for commercial development of AD genetic testing, on conflict of interest and patents held by scientists, and on likely future scenarios at the interface of huge profits and genetic science.

Ethical Aspects

Part Two takes up ethical aspects of genetic testing for AD. Issues related to predictive testing for autosomal-dominant forms of AD are similar to those pertaining to other autosomal-dominant neurodegenerative diseases, such as Huntington disease. Genetic counseling is an integral component of predictive testing programs and should clarify the potential benefits and burdens of testing outcomes on the counselee's affective state, family members, current life circumstances, and future planning; explain that the individual can refuse the test result if he or she has second thoughts about disclosure of such knowledge after the test is performed; and provide a plan for posttest follow-up. Modifications of established counseling protocols for Huntington disease are being used to conduct predictive testing for early-onset autosomal-dominant forms of AD.

In chapter 7, Harry Karlinsky, M.D., addresses the various ethical issues of relevance. His wealth of personal experience with early-onset families makes this chapter highly engaging. As part of ongoing research studies, argues Karlinsky, all centers that test individuals belonging to early-onset families are obligated to adhere to formal informed consent, provide pretest and posttest counseling by trained professionals, maintain strict confidentiality, and establish the predictive value of the testing.

The issues surrounding the use of APOE alleles in genetic counseling for AD are more complicated than those concerning the use of single-gene mutations. While the genetic information provided by the APOE ε4 genotype may be valuable, it is not easily used for providing genetic counseling to the individual patient. This may be especially true in specific ethnic groups wherein the association between APOE genotype and AD has been less well defined. Genetic counselors are particularly concerned that nonpredictive test results may be used inappropriately by clients in making important life planning decisions.

In chapter 8, Kimberly A. Quaid, Ph.D., a national leader in genetic counseling and ethics, discusses her experience with supplying information that provides little clear data for purposes of decision making and that inevitably causes anxiety. This chapter presents the existential reflections of a counselor as to the benefits of some genetic knowledge and of AD genotyping in particular.

Based on our discussion with focus groups of AD caregivers and mildly demented individuals, it seems that creating unnecessary anxiety would be the major concern in APOE genetic testing; that is, individuals who discover that they have at least one copy of the ε4 allele may falsely attribute normal forgetfulness to the onset of AD and may make significant life-altering decisions based on such misinterpretation of risk. This anxiety has been well documented in autobiographical accounts of the early stages of AD.

In chapter 9, Bonnie Steinbock, Ph.D., a philosopher whose work concentrates on reproductive technologies, uses AD as a heuristic key to the question of prenatal testing and selective abortion more generally. How much do we wish to fine-tune the lives and life spans of the children we will bring into the world? A risk factor such as APOE that is misunderstood as predictive can be harmful. Furthermore, such testing, if applied prenatally, could result in unnecessary selective abortion, although this has not yet occurred. What is more likely is the prenatal use of PS1 and PS2 testing for the early-onset forms of AD for purposes of selective abortion.

Social Issues

Technology transfer from basic genetic research to commercial use with little outcomes-based research in between should be avoided. The prospect of offering an AD genetic test before there is scientific consensus about its clinical usefulness raises questions about the appropriateness of its use, particularly given the potential for discrimination, adverse psychological effects, and inappropriate life decisions. Should the public perceive that researchers, clinicians, and pharmaceutical companies are making financial gains based on scientifically unsupported claims for the benefits of AD genetic testing, the long-term damage to public trust and, ultimately, to research progress may be serious.

When the APOE Genotype Report was introduced briefly in 1994 (by Genica Pharmaceuticals), Robert N. Butler, editor of *Geriatrics*, urged clinicians to be cautious. He emphasized that the testing was not yet established as diagnostic or predictive, that people should avoid the emotional toll of thinking that their APOE genotype means they are doomed, and that discrimination in employment and insurance was likely (Butler 1994).

A new magnitude of genetic knowledge has emerged at a time when there is increasing public concern about large amounts of personal data stored on computers (Gostin, Turek-Brezina, and Powers 1993). Genetic information is readily encoded electronically, and the ease with which it can be accessed and disseminated poses a threat to privacy.

An important social reason for not testing asymptomatic (in contrast to already demented) individuals for dominant disease-causing mutations or APOE genotype is that employers could reduce their potential health-related costs by discriminating on the basis of test results. Moreover, the growing long-term-care insurance industry may use genetic susceptibility testing. Indeed, a major actuarial leader wrote that genetic information on susceptibility to AD would be of absolute importance to the long-term-care insurance industry and that a refusal to make information available would be fraudulent, despite the U.S. Alzheimer's Disease and Related Disorders Association's recommendation for anonymous genetic testing to ensure confidentiality (Pokorski 1997). The insurance industry asserts this position despite the fact that APOE is not a good predictor of AD. In a nation such as Canada, where long-term care is a public entitlement that does not first require a family to "spend down" into near poverty, as Americans must, to become eligible for public medical assistance, actuarial discrimination is of course not a problem.

In chapter 10, Robert H. Binstock, Ph.D., and Thomas H. Murray, Ph.D., address the broad issues of genetics, actuarial policies, and confidentiality. They then focus on AD and the economic and social implications of actuarial discrimination. This chapter draws the debate over confidentiality of genetic information into the context of AD for the first time.

In chapter 11, Eric T. Juengst, Ph.D., discusses APOE as an example of a gene that has serious implications for two major areas of human disease. When APOE testing is done in the course of a medically indicated evaluation of serum lipid profiles for the management of cardiovascular disease, should the patient be prospectively informed of the supplemental information intrinsic to APOE testing that relates to AD? Should the patient be advised that this testing is unavoidably related to AD risk, that there may be implications for recording these data in the medical record, and that he or she has the option of discussing the AD implications of this testing? These complex issues require the careful consideration Juengst applies to them.

Alzheimer disease diagnostic and predictive genetic testing raise several questions of justice. Who should pay for testing? How might testing fit in various managed care and publicly funded systems that prioritize or "ration" beneficial health care? In a budgeted, managed health care plan, the right to a health care service is a matter of balancing the subscriber's wants with the efficacy of the service, the terms of the contract, and the duty to steward finite resources so the plan equitably serves all members.

In chapter 12, Leonard Fleck, Ph.D., reflects on where genetic testing fits in the prioritizing of health care interventions, especially in the context of managed care. He applies several major philosophical theories of health care justice to analyze the likely response to AD genetic testing.

In chapter 13, Steven Miles, M.D., with his remarkable knowledge of the policies of managed care systems, takes on the question of how genetic data are handled and controlled within such systems.

Educational Issues

Unfortunately, because the public may have unrealistic expectations about some genetic advances, the introduction of genetic testing for asymptomatic individuals may be accepted uncritically. In the focus groups, however, there was significant concern with potential discrimination (even though APOE is not a clear predictor of AD), adverse psychological effects, inappropriate alteration of life decisions, and financial costs. There was also a keen interest in further public education.

In chapter 14, Stephen G. Post, Ph.D., describes some of the cultural forces that contribute to the wider public's sometimes unfounded hopes in the promise of new genetic discoveries. He calls for enhanced critical thinking and scientific literacy to prevent various constituencies (e.g., AD-affected families) from being exploited by genetic technologies of limited value. Post's work with chapters of the Alzheimer's Association across the United States has focused on the grassroots response to these issues (Post 1995).

In chapter 15, Greg A. Sachs, M.D., provides a detailed analysis of the current state of primary care physicians in the United States with respect to genetic knowledge and capacity to interpret genetic data for patients and families. The reader cannot but conclude that an educational crisis is at hand and that tremendous efforts need to be made in this area.

In chapter 16, Atwood D. Gaines, Ph.D., M.P.H., begins to examine how different cultural groups in the United States might interpret genetic information on AD. This anthropological perspective is a vitally important one that needs to be brought to the very forefront of the debate over genetics and education.

Gaines also raises some remarkable questions about AD as a disease category cross-culturally considered.

An Editorial Perspective on the Future

The chapters in this book summarize the state of our knowledge concerning the genetics of AD at a time when the field is rapidly evolving. It is likely that other causative and susceptibility loci will be identified in the future. How this additional information will influence clinical practice with regard to diagnostics and therapeutics is unclear. The purpose of this book is to present the issues clearly so that these discoveries can be added to a conceptual framework that will guide fruitful community dialogue and policy making. There is much exciting science to celebrate and much fruitful discussion to be had concerning the clinical implications of this work.

One can look outside the field of AD to see a revolution in molecular medicine involving other diseases as well. A similar process is occurring with regard to the genetic basis of breast cancer. Large-scale studies (Couch et al. 1997; Healy 1997; Krainer et al. 1997; Struewing et al. 1997) suggest that the initial risk estimates associated with causative loci were overstated. According to the commentary accompanying one of these studies, BRCA genetic testing is not yet appropriate in everyday clinical practice because its use violates a common-sense rule of medicine: Don't order a test if you have insufficient information to know how to interpret the results. This advice could as well be applied to AD and other disorders in which we are too quick to celebrate the power of science and too slow to be concerned about the impact of premature and imprecise knowledge on the lives of patients and families.

While we cannot predict the future, there is little doubt that AD will be better understood genetically as time goes on. It is to be hoped that the PS1 and PS2 genes, which clearly cause AD, will enable researchers to elaborate the molecular basis of the disease, leading to a cure or treatment that will prevent or delay onset. Surely there could be no more important scientific pursuit or goal, for demographics have made AD one of the leading public health problems in developed nations.

We expect that other genetic lesions will be identified in AD patients in the future. Some autosomal-dominant families clearly exist in which the specific disease locus has not been identified. Roses and colleagues have reported initial research on a possible additional susceptibility loci on chromosome 12. Perhaps by the time this book is published, these data will have been presented in a full format. Roses is raising the concern that the power of these markers, when combined with APOE, may make it possible to assess the risks of pre-symptomatic individuals with greater precision than with APOE alone. One imagines that some of the ethical dilemmas raised by APOE will be increased as the number of genetic markers for this disease increases. The problem of who will have access to this information, particularly as it relates to insurance companies and eligibility for health care, will only grow.

As we presaged above, considerable additional work has been conducted since the chapters in this book were finished. More than forty mutations have been described in presenilin 1 genes, interest in possible mutations on chromosome 12 continues, and as many as eight additional susceptibility loci have been claimed (Peter St. George-Hyslop, personal communication). In addition, a large-scale study of APOE testing, conducted at the National Institute on Aging Alzheimer Disease Centers on autopsy-proven cases of dementia, was recently reported (Mayeux et al. 1997). Although diagnostic specificity was increased by the use of APOE, the nonrepresentative nature of the sample and the continuing concerns about the different risks in different populations of patients still has not convinced most experts that routine use of this test clinically is appropriate. The Health Care Financing Administration has refused to reimburse for APOE testing. Moreover, the Institute of Medicine has recently reviewed such testing as part of a larger project on genes and behavior and is not likely in the final report to be positive about its current use clinically.

References

Alzheimer's Disease and Related Disorders Association. 1995. Caution urged with Alzheimer gene testing. Chicago: Alzheimer's Disease and Related Disorders Association.
Bird, T. D. 1995. Apolipoprotein E genotyping in the diagnosis of Alzheimer's disease: A cautionary view. *Annals of Neurology* 38:2–4.
Brodaty, H., and Medical and Scientific Advisory Committee of Alzheimer's Disease International. 1995. *Alzheimer Disease and Associated Disorders* 9:182–87.
Butler, R. N. 1994. ApoE—New risk factor for Alzheimer's: Potential is real for abuse of genetic testing for susceptibility to dementia. *Geriatrics* 49:10–11.
Couch, F. J., DeShano, M. L., Blackwood, M. A., Calzone, K., Stopfer, J., Campeau, L., Ganguly, A., Rebbeck, T., and Weber, B. L. 1997. BRCA1 mutations in women attending clinics that evaluate the risk of breast cancer. *New England Journal of Medicine* 335:1409–15.
Farrer, L. A., and American College of Medical Genetics/American Society of Human Genetics Working Group on ApoE and Alzheimer Disease. 1995. Statement on the use of apolipoprotein E testing for Alzheimer disease. *JAMA* 274:1627–29.
Geldmacher, D. S., and Whitehouse, P. J. 1996. Evaluation of dementia. *New England Journal of Medicine* 335:330–36.

Gostin, L., Turek-Brezina, J., and Powers, M. 1993. Privacy and security of personal information in a new health care system. *JAMA* 270:2487–93.

Healy, B. 1997. BRCA gene: Bookmarking, fortunetelling, and medical care. *New England Journal of Medicine* 336:1448–49.

Krainer, M., Silva-Arrieta, S., Fitzgerald, M. G., Shimada, A., Ishioka, C., Kanamaru, R., MacDonald, D. J., Unsal, H., Finkelstein, D. M., Bowcock, A., Isselbacher, K. J., and Haber, D. A. 1997. Differential contributions of BRCA1 and BRCA2 to early-onset breast cancer. *New England Journal of Medicine* 336:1416–21.

Lovestone, S., with U.K. Alzheimer's Disease Genetics Consortium. 1995. The genetics of Alzheimer's disease: New opportunities and new challenges. *International Journal of Geriatric Psychiatry* 10:1–7.

Mayeux, R., Saunders, A. M., Shea, S., et al. 1998. Utility of the Apolipoprotein E Genotype in the Diagnosis of Alzheimer's Disease. *New England Journal of Medicine* 338:506–11.

Pokorski, R. J. 1997. Insurance underwriting in the genetic era. *American Journal of Human Genetics* 60:205–16.

Post, S. G. 1995. *The moral challenge of Alzheimer disease*. Baltimore: Johns Hopkins University Press.

Post, S. G., Whitehouse, P. J., Binstock, R. H., Bird, T. D., Eckert, S. K., Farrer, L. A., Fleck, L. M., Gaines, A. D., Juengst, E. T., Karlinsky, H., Miles, S., Murray, T. H., Quaid, K. A., Relkin, N. R., Roses, A. D., St. George-Hyslop, P. H., Sachs, G. A., Steinbock, B., Truschke, E. F., and Zinn, A. B. 1997. The clinical introduction of genetic testing for Alzheimer disease: An ethical perspective. *JAMA* 277:832–36.

Relkin, N. R., and National Institute on Aging/Alzheimer's Association Working Group. 1996. Apolipoprotein E genotyping in Alzheimer's disease. *Lancet* 347:1091–95.

Roses, A. D. 1996. Apolipoprotein E alleles as risk factors in Alzheimer's disease. *Annual Review of Medicine* 47:387–400.

Struewing, J. P., Hartge, P., Wacholder, S., Baker, S. M., Berlin, M., McAdams, M., Timmerman, M. M., Brody, L. C., Tucker, M. A. 1997. The risk of cancer associated with specific mutations of BRCA1 and BRCA2 among Ashkenazi Jews. *New England Journal of Medicine* 336:1401–7.

PART ONE

The Genetics of Alzheimer Disease

The Chromosome 1 Type of Familial Alzheimer Disease

THOMAS D. BIRD, M.D.

Genes on four different chromosomes—1, 14, 19, and 21—are involved in the pathogenesis of Alzheimer disease (AD). This chapter discusses the chromosome 1 gene, also known as presenilin 2 (PS2).

Background

The chromosome 1 form of familial Alzheimer disease (FAD) was first discovered in a group of families with AD whose ethnic background is Volga German (Bird et al. 1988). In 1763, during the reign of Catherine the Great, several thousand persons migrated from central Europe to the Volga River region of Russia. These individuals originated in the states of Hesse and Palatine, which subsequently became parts of modern Germany. A slightly later migrating group from these same states settled in the area of Odessa, north of the Black Sea, and became known as Black Sea Germans. Between 1880 and 1920 large numbers of these Volga and Black Sea Germans migrated to the Great Plains of the United States and then to the West Coast. They preferred a rural life and were primarily wheat and sugar beet farmers.

In 1988 Bird and colleagues described the occurrence of typical early-onset FAD in several kindreds of Volga German background who had originated from the same two villages in Russia (including three families reported by Cook, Ward, and Austin 1979). They presented the hypothesis that these families probably represented the genetic founder effect, meaning they were likely to have the same genetic disease, which had been inherited from a single unknown ancestor (Bird et al. 1988).

Genetic linkage studies of these Volga German families excluded linkage to the FAD regions on chromosomes 21 and 14 (Schellenberg et al. 1988; Schellen-

Table 2.1. Clinical Comparison of Families with Presenilin 1 (PS1) and Presenilin 2 (PS2) Mutations

	PS1[a] (chromosome 14)	PS2[b] (chromosome 1)
Age of onset		
Mean	44.8 ± 4.8	54.8 ± 8.4
Range	30–55	40–75
Age at death		
Mean	52.6 ± 5.7	65.9 ± 10.2
Range	39–65	43–88
Duration of disease		
Mean	7.6 ± 3.2	11.3 ± 4.6
Range	2–17	5–23

Source: Data from Bird et al. 1996.
[a] Seven families with different PS1 mutations ($n = 57$–77).
[b] Seven Volga German families with a PS2 (N141I) mutation ($n = 34$–46).

berg et al. 1992). In 1995 Levy-Lahad and colleagues showed that the disease in the Volga German kindreds was linked to markers on the long arm of chromosome 1 (Levy-Lahad, Wijsman, et al. 1995). The presenilin 1 gene (PS1) had been simultaneously discovered on chromosome 14 (Sherrington et al. 1995). A homologous gene (PS2) was found on chromosome 1, and a mutation in this gene was discovered by Levy-Lahad and colleagues in most of the Volga German families (Levy-Lahad, Wasco, et al. 1995).

The PS2 gene is composed of twelve exons, two of which are noncoding (Levy-Lahad et al. 1996). This gene codes for a protein that is likely to have seven or eight transmembrane domains, although the exact number of these domains is uncertain. Presenilin 2 is predicted to encode a 448 amino acid protein that is 67 percent identical to PS1. The greatest identity (84%) is within the hydrophobic transmembrane domains. The PS1 and PS2 proteins seem to be localized to the endoplasmic reticulum and Golgi complex (Kovacs et al. 1996). A single mutation in PS1 (N141I) occurred in seven of the Volga German pedigrees, consistent with the hypothesized founder effect. This mutation produces a single amino acid substitution in the second transmembrane domain. An additional PS2 mutation has been found in an Italian FAD family (Rogaev et al. 1995).

Clinical features of PS2 mutations have been reported primarily in the Volga Germans (Bird et al. 1988; Bird et al. 1989; Bird et al. 1996). In these Volga

German kindreds the mean age of onset is 54.8 ± 8.4 years (see table 2.1). Mean duration of disease is 11.3 ± 4.6 years, and mean age at death is about 66 years. It is noteworthy that the PS2 mutation families tend to have a later age of onset and longer duration than the PS1 (chromosome 14) families (see table 2.1). Clinically, the families with PS1 mutations seem to have a more aggressive disease than those with PS2 mutations (Lampe et al. 1994). The Volga German PS2 families also show a remarkably wide variation in age of onset, ranging from 40 to 75 years, even though all individuals carry the identical point mutation. This indicates that other genetic and environmental factors must influence the age of onset.

There have also been a few cases of nonpenetrance over the age of eighty in PS2 mutation families (Bird et al. 1996; Sherrington et al. 1996). Such an example is indicated in individual II-2 in the pedigree illustrated in figure 2.1. Thus, although penetrance is high in PS2 families (over 95%), it may not be complete, at least to over age eighty.

The discovery of the PS2 mutation also allowed for a more accurate genetic analysis of the Volga German kindreds. For example, in figure 2.2, indi-

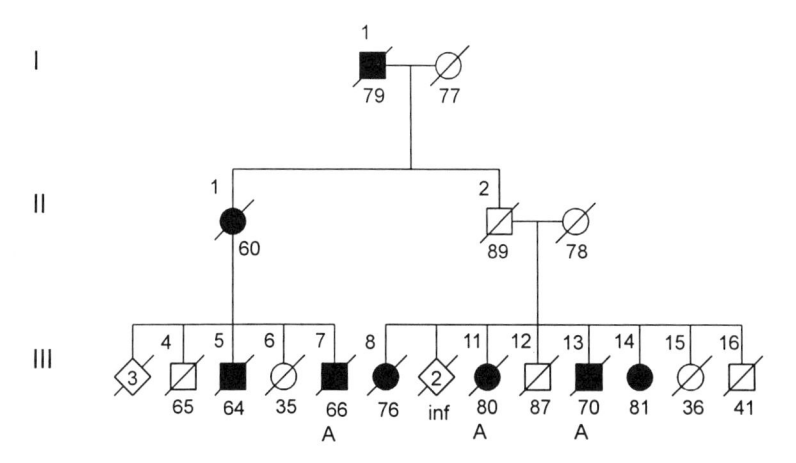

Figure 2.1. Pedigree of a Volga German family with a presenilin 2 mutation. Persons affected with dementia are shown in black, and age at death or present age is shown under the symbol. Note that individual II-2 died at age 89 without clinical dementia. However, the fact that he had affected children and an affected sibling makes it highly likely that he represents nonpenetrance of the PS2 mutation. (A = autopsied.)

vidual IV-2 was discovered to have dementia but did not carry the PS2 mutation. It had been noted that this person had an age of onset (sixty-seven years) that was more than two standard deviations greater than the mean for this kindred and was also found to have an APOE4 genotype of $\epsilon4/\epsilon4$. Thus, this person represents a phenocopy of "sporadic" AD occurring in a family with a PS2 mutation. Furthermore, two of the original Volga German kindreds and all of the Black Sea FAD kindreds were found not to contain the N141I mutation in PS2 (Levy-Lahad, Wasco, et al. 1995). Many of the affected individuals in these families appear to have the more common form of APOE4-related late-onset AD.

Neuropathological studies of the brains in several individuals with dementia from the Volga German families have shown all the microscopic characteristics of classic AD. This includes $A\beta$ amyloid containing neuritic plaques, tau-positive neurofibrillary tangles with paired helical filaments, and amyloid angiopathy (Bird et al. 1989). The $A\beta$ 1–42 form of amyloid predominants in the Volga German brains (Mann et al. 1997). $A\beta$ 1–42 is elevated in the plasma of persons with PS2 mutations and is produced in excess by skin fibroblast cultures of these same individuals (Scheuner et al. 1996). These findings indicate that the PS2 and APP proteins are probably functionally related. Presenilin 2 gene (PS2) may be involved in the intracellular trafficking of APP (amyloid precursor protein). Understanding the normal functioning of these proteins and how mutations in them result in neuronal death and clinical dementia represents an important new area of neurobiology research.

Ethical and Sociological Aspects

The identification of the PS2 gene and mutations in the Volga German families raised some interesting and important ethical and sociological issues, four of which are mentioned here.

1. Following the recognition of FAD in families who belonged to a larger ethnic group called Germans from Russia, it became apparent that efforts should be made not to stigmatize this group. That is, the individuals involved, their families, and the American Historical Society of Germans from Russia (AHSGR) were concerned that the term "Volga German" would become negatively associated in the public mind with dementia. This issue was directly and continuously addressed by our research group. We made it clear in all public forums and publications that we had no evidence for an increased prevalence of AD in the general German-Russian population. Rather, this was a single

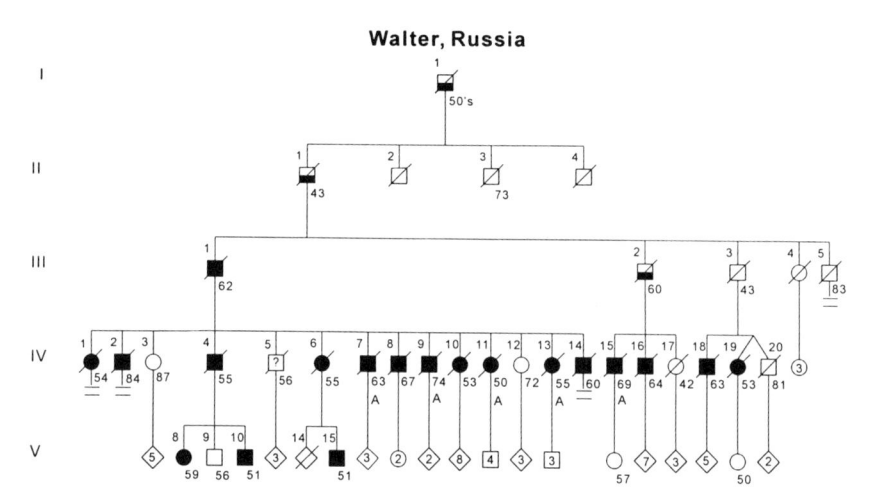

Figure 2.2. Pedigree of another large Volga German family with a presenilin 2 (PS2) mutation. Persons affected with dementia are shown in black, and age at death or present age is shown under the symbol. Individual IV-2 had onset of dementia at age 67 and died at age 84. He did not carry the PS2 mutation present in his other relatives, and his APOE genotype was ε4/ε4; thus, he represents a phenocopy of AD occurring in a PS2 kindred. Half-shaded symbols indicate probable dementia.

gene in a small number of families who were all distantly related. The principle investigator (Thomas D. Bird) met with the AHSGR, made presentations to their annual meetings, published explanations of the FAD phenomena in their quarterly journal, and maintained an active liaison with their board members (Bird 1991, 1995). The emphasis was on research, discovery, and understanding of AD with an effort to "destigmatize" the disease. This strategy has been highly successful, and the society strongly supported the FAD research programs.

2. The discovery of a specific gene mutation for FAD raised questions of how to inform the families, what to tell them, and whether or not to offer DNA testing. The answers to these questions are still evolving. Our developing approach has taken the following lines. We informed the AHSGR membership of our scientific finding. We are in the process of informing each individual family about the discovery of a specific FAD mutation in their relatives. Our research laboratory will provide DNA testing on blood samples from persons at risk for the disease. The testing of such individuals will be entirely voluntary. The testing process will be done in the context of formal professional genetic coun-

seling. The precedent and protocol for this process is the experience with DNA testing in Huntington disease and other autosomal-dominant neurogenetic disorders (Quaid 1992; Bennett, Bird, and Teri 1993).

3. Detailed and informed genetic counseling will be very important in PS2 FAD families. A critical question will be, what are the personal implications of carrying a PS2 mutation? If a PS2 mutation carrier is asymptomatic, what will be the impact of that knowledge on emotional status, interpersonal relationships, plans for the future, employment, and ability to obtain insurance? Such questions are not limited to FAD but are common to the burgeoning population of individuals undergoing DNA testing for genetic disorders (Bird and Bennett 1995). Furthermore, the wide range in age of onset and specifically the frequent late age of onset associated with PS2 mutations as well as the apparent incomplete penetrance must be explained carefully to these families. A positive test for a PS2 mutation does not indicate the age of onset of symptoms, the severity and duration of symptoms, or whether the mutation carrier will be an example of nonpenetrance. Also, even in families with known mutations, the occurrence of clinical dementia does not always indicate the presence of a mutation. In the family in figure 2.2, genetic counseling of offspring of persons such as IV-2 (who does not carry the mutation) would be very different from that of his siblings with the mutation. These can be subtle and difficult concepts for the families to understand and represent major challenges to conscientious genetic counseling.

4. Finally, it seems evident that PS2 mutations are a very rare cause of FAD. To date, only the seven Volga German families and an Italian kindred have been discovered to have PS2 mutations. This makes PS2 FAD an orphan disease, and private laboratories are unlikely to test for PS2 mutations on a commercial basis. On the other hand, it is clear that PS2 mutations can result in late-onset AD (e.g., over the age of sixty-five or seventy) and could play some role in the more common form of late-onset AD in the general population. This last possibility is speculative, and the issue of readily available testing for rare genetic disorders requires further study.

References

Bennett, R. L., Bird, T. D., and Teri, L. 1993. Offering predictive testing for Huntington disease in a medical genetics clinic: Practical applications. *Journal of Genetic Counseling* 2:123–37.

Bird, T. D. 1991. Evaluating family histories and traditions for evidence of medical illness using Alzheimer's disease as a model. *American Historical Society of Germans from Russia Journal* (fall): 49–54.

———. 1995. Update on the Seattle Alzheimer's disease research project. *American Historical Society of Germans from Russia Journal* (fall): 3-4.

Bird, T. D., and Bennett, R. L. 1995. Why do DNA testing?: Practical and ethical implications of new neurogenetic tests. *Annals of Neurology* 38:141-46.

Bird, T. D., Lampe, T. H., Nemens, E. J., Miner, G. D., Sumi, S. M., and Schellenberg, G. D. 1988. Familial Alzheimer's disease in American descendants of the Volga Germans: Probable genetic founder effect. *Annals of Neurology* 23:25-31.

Bird, T. D., Levy-Lahad, E., Poorkaj, P., Sharma, V., Nemens, E., Lahad, A., Lampe, T. H., and Schellenberg, G. D. 1996. Wide range in age of onset for chromosome 1-related familial Alzheimer's disease. *Annals of Neurology* 40:932-36.

Bird, T. D., Sumi, S. M., Nemens, E. J., Nochlin, D., Schellenberg, G., Lampe, T. H., Sadovnick, A., Chui, H., Miner, G. W., and Tinklenberg, J. 1989. Phenotypic heterogeneity in familial Alzheimer's disease: A study of twenty-four kindreds. *Annals of Neurology* 25:12-25.

Cook, R. H., Ward, B. E., and Austin, J. H. 1979. Studies in aging of the brain. Part 4, Familial Alzheimer disease: Relation to transmissible dementia, aneuploidy, and microtubular defects. *Neurology* 29:1402-12.

Kovacs, D. M., Fausett, H. J., Page, K. J., Kim, T.-W., Moir, R. D., Merrimam, D. E., Hollister, R. D., Hallmark, O. G., Mancini, R., Felsenstein, K. M., Hyman, B. T., Tanzi, R. E., and Wasco, W. 1996. Alzheimer-associated presenilins 1 and 2: Neuronal expression in brain and localization to intracellular membranes in mammalian cells. *Nature Medicine* 2:224-29.

Lampe, T. H., Bird, T. D., Nochlin, D., Nemens, E., Risse, S. C., Sumi, S. M., Koerker, R., Leaird, B., Wier, M., and Raskind, M. A. 1994. Phenotype of chromosome 14-linked familial Alzheimer's disease in a large kindred. *Annals of Neurology* 36:368-78.

Levy-Lahad, E., Poorkaj, P., Wang, K., Hui, Y., Oshima, J., Mulligan, J., and Schellenberg, G. D. 1996. Genomic structure and expression of STM2, the chromosome 1 familial Alzheimer disease gene. *Genomics* 34:198-204.

Levy-Lahad, E., Wasco, W., Poorkaj, P., Romano, E. M., Oshima, J., Pettingell, W. H., Yu, C., Jondro, P. D., Schmidt, S. D., Wang, K., Crowley, A. C., Fu, Y.-H., Guenette, S. Y., Galas, D., Nemens, E., Wijsman, E. M., Bird, T. D., Schellenberg, G. D., and Tanzi, R. E. 1995. Candidate gene for the chromosome 1 familial Alzheimer's disease locus. *Science* 269:973-77.

Levy-Lahad, E., Wijsman, E. M., Nemens, E., Anderson, L., Goddard, K. A. B., Wever, J. L., Bird, T. D., and Schellenberg, G. D. 1995. A familial Alzheimer's disease locus on chromosome 1. *Science* 269:970-73.

Mann, D., Iwatsubo, T., Nochlin, D., Sumi, S. M., Levy-Lahad, E., and Bird, T. D. 1997. Amyloid Aβ deposition in chromosome 1-linked Alzheimer's disease: The Volga German families. *Annals of Neurology* 41:52-57.

Quaid, K. 1992. Presymptomatic testing for Huntington disease: Recommendations for counseling. *Journal of Genetic Counseling* 1:277-302.

Rogaev, E. I., Sherrington, R., Rogaeva, E. A., Levesque, G., Ikeda, M., Liang, Y., Chi, H., Lin, C., Holman, K., Tsuda, T., Mar, L., Sorbi, S., Nacmias, B., Piacentini, S., Amaducci, L.,

Chumakov, I., Cohen. D., Lannfelt, L., Fraser, P. E., Rommens, J. M., and St. George-Hyslop, P. H. 1995. Familial Alzheimer's disease in kindreds with missense mutations in a gene on chromosome 1 related to the Alzheimer's disease type 3 gene. *Nature* 376:776–78.

Schellenberg, G. D., Bird, T. D., Wijsman, E. M., Moore, D. K., Boehnke, M., Bryant, E. M., Lampe, T. H., Nochlin, D., Sumi, S. M., Deeb, S. S., Beyreuther, K., and Martin, G. M. 1988. Absence of linkage of chromosome 21q21 markers to familial Alzheimer's disease. *Science* 141:1507–10.

Schellenberg, G. D., Bird, T. D., Wijsman, E. M., Or, H. T., Anderson, L., Nemens, E., White, J. A., Bonnycastle, L., Wever, J. L., Alonso, E., Potter, H., Heston, L. L., and Martin, G. M. 1992. Genetic linkage evidence for a familial Alzheimer disease locus on chromosome 14. *Science* 258:668–71.

Scheuner, D., Eckman, C., Jensen, M., Song, X., Citron, M., Suzuki, N., Bird, T. D., Hardy, J., Hutton, M., Kukull, W., Larson, E., Levy-Lahad, E., Viitanen, M., Peskind, E., Poorkaj, P., Schellenberg, T., Tanzi, R., Wasco, W., Lannfelt, L., Selkoe, D., and Younkin, S. 1996. Secreted amyloid β-protein similar to that in the senile plaques of Alzheimer's disease is increased *in vivo* by the presenilin 1 and 2 and APP mutations linked to familial Alzheimer's disease. *Nature Medicine* 2:864–70.

Sherrington, R., Froelich, S., Sorbi, S., Campion, D., Chi, H., Rogaeva, E. A., Levesque, G., Rogaev, E. I., Lin, C., Liang, Y., Ikeda, M., Mar, L., Brice, A., Agid, Y., Percy, M. E., Clerget-Darpoux, F., Piacentini, S., Marcon, G., Nacmias, B., Amaducci, L., Frebourg, T., Lannfelt, L., Rommens, J. M., and St. George-Hyslop, P. H. 1996. Alzheimer's disease associated with mutations in presenilin 2 is rare and variably penetrant. *Human Molecular Genetics* 5:985–88.

Sherrington, R., Rogaev, E. I., Liang, Y., Rogaeva, E. A., Levesque, G., Ikeda, M., Chi, H., Lin, C., Li, G., Holman, K., Tsuda, T., Mar, L., Foncin, J. F., Bruni, A. C., Montesi, M. P., Sorbi, S., Rainero, I., Pinessi, L., Nee, L., Chumakov, I., Pollen, D., Brookes, A., Sanseau, P., Polinsky, R. J., Wasco, W., Dasilva, H. A. R., Haines, J. L., Pericak-Vance, M. A., Tanzi, R. E., Roses, A. D., Fraser, P. E., Rommens, J. M., and St. George-Hyslop, P. H. 1995. Cloning of a gene bearing missense mutations in early-onset familial Alzheimer's disease. *Nature* 375:754–60.

PETER H. ST. GEORGE-
HYSLOP, M.D.

Molecular Genetics of Early-Onset Alzheimer Disease Linked to Chromosome 14 and Chromosome 21

The etiology of Alzheimer disease (AD) is complex. A number of genetic epidemiological studies have clearly indicated that genetic factors play a role in a significant, but as yet unknown, proportion of cases of AD. In the majority of cases in which there is familial aggregation of disease, the mode of inheritance is usually unclear. Such familial aggregates could represent incompletely penetrant autosomal-dominant single-gene disorders, a multigenic trait, or mixtures of genetic and environmental factors. In a small proportion of cases (probably fewer than 10% of all cases of AD), the pattern of inheritance over multiple generations with equal affectation of male and female offspring and with approximately 50 percent of first-degree relatives developing disease is compatible with a single-gene disorder transmitted as an age-dependent autosomal-dominant trait. Genetic linkage studies on this type of AD have led to the identification of at least three separate disease genes unambiguously associated with inherited early-onset autosomal-dominant AD. A fourth locus, apolipoprotein E (APOE), has been associated with late-onset AD in which the $\epsilon 4$ allele shows a dose-dependent inverse relationship to the age of onset and is increased in frequency in subjects with late-onset AD.

While some forms of AD arise from the inheritance of specific genetic risk factors, several complexities render the use of genetic testing in subjects with AD potentially problematic. The complexities of the relationship between the $\epsilon 4$ allele of APOE and late-onset AD and between the presenilin 2 gene (PS2) and AD is dealt with in other chapters. The current chapter addresses the biology and practical considerations related to genetic testing for mutations in the βAPP and in the presenilin 1 gene (PS1).

The Biology of the Amyloid Precursor Protein Mutations on Chromosome 21

The beta amyloid precursor protein gene (βAPP) was implicated as a potential locus for Alzheimer-associated mutations on the basis of several intersecting lines of evidence. First, subjects with trisomy 21 (Down syndrome) almost invariably develop at least the neuropathological changes of AD by the age of forty years, implying a special relationship between the genetic material on chromosome 21 and AD pathology (Mann, Yates, and Marcyniuk 1984; Mann et al. 1989). Second, a 40-42 amino acid proteolytic peptide derivative of the full-length βAPP protein called the amyloid β-peptide (Aβ) is a major constituent of the senile plaque in patients with AD (Goldgaber, Lerman, and McBride 1987; Kang et al. 1987). Third, genetic linkage studies have shown provisional evidence for linkage of a locus associated with early-onset AD in a subset of pedigrees in the region of chromosome 21 containing the βAPP gene (Goate et al. 1989; St. George-Hyslop et al. 1987).

Finally, other missense mutations in the βAPP gene had already been identified in another illness characterized by excessive intracerebral deposition of Aβ peptide (Levy et al. 1990). To date, sequencing analyses have demonstrated mutations in at least three different codon positions that are reasonably clearly associated with AD. These include the double missense mutation of Lys670Asn/Met671Leu and the Ala692Gly and Val717Ile/Phe/Gly missense mutations (Goate et al. 1991; Hendricks, van Duijn, and Cras 1992; Karlinsky et al. 1992; Mullan, Crawford, and Axelman 1992; Murrell et al. 1991). Several other missense mutations, such as Ala713Val/Thr, Glu693Gly, and Gln665Asp, have been described in individual patients with AD. However, these other mutations have not yet been proven to segregate with disease in these families, and it therefore remains to be determined whether these mutations are simply innocent polymorphisms or missense mutations with incomplete penetrance.

The majority of patients affected with the βAPP missense mutations clearly associated with AD have had onset of their disease before the age of sixty-five years and display a fairly stereotypical clinical and neuropathological phenotype, which is difficult to distinguish from sporadic cases of AD other than by its early age of onset, somewhat shorter disease duration, and obvious autosomal-dominant pattern of inheritance (Karlinsky et al. 1992). It appears that all of the pathogenic βAPP mutations affect βAPP protein processing and result in the production of excess quantities of Aβ peptides with a particular predilection to increasing the amount of longer Aβ isoforms such as Aβ_{1-42} or Aβ_{x-42} (Cai, Golde, and Younkin 1992; Citron et al. 1992; Haass et al. 1994; Shoji et al. 1992; Susuki et al. 1994; Tamaoka et al. 1994; Younkin, Cai, and Golde 1993). It is thought that these high levels of Aβ peptide production promote the accumulation of Aβ peptides, which in turn are thought to have a neurotoxic effect, although the exact mechanisms of this neurotoxicity have not yet been fully defined.

The clinical phenotype associated with βAPP mutations appears to be nearly completely penetrant (i.e., nearly everyone who inherits one of these missense mutations will ultimately develop the disease phenotype). Furthermore, as far as is known today, the majority of cases have had onset of symptoms between the ages of forty and sixty-five years of age. However, it has been shown that the age of onset for the Val717Ile missense mutations is significantly modified by the genotype at the APOE gene (Nacmias et al. 1995; St. George-Hyslop et al. 1994). For instance, several subjects with APOE genotype containing at least one ϵ4 allele have an earlier age of onset than subjects who possess no ϵ4 alleles (Nacmias et al. 1995; St. George-Hyslop et al. 1994). Furthermore, it seems that subjects with Val717Ile missense mutations who have the ϵ2 allele at APOE have a much later age of onset. Indeed, one subject with the APOE ϵ2 genotype has survived to more than two standard deviations beyond the mean age of onset in that family without symptoms of AD (St. George-Hyslop et al. 1994).

Practical Considerations for Genetic Testing and Counseling in Pedigrees with βAPP Mutations

Although the frequency of βAPP mutations is so low that routine screening is probably not cost effective, once a pedigree has been uncovered that segregates a missense mutation in the βAPP gene, it is possible to consider various forms of genetic testing. In symptomatic individuals with a clinical and laboratory phenotype that is compatible with a clinical diagnosis of AD and that do not suggest alternative diagnostic possibilities, the presence of a βAPP missense mutation would serve to confirm the diagnosis very strongly. At a more complicated level, currently asymptomatic relatives can be considered for presymptomatic testing. The tenets of this presymptomatic testing have to be based on the observations above. Specifically, the decision to test has to take into consideration a number of facts: that the majority of gene carriers will develop the disease by age sixty-five years; that very few of the gene carriers will develop disease before the age of forty years; that the age of onset and possibly also the final lifetime risk for development of AD (at least in carriers of the Val717Ile mutation) might be modifiable by other factors such as the genotype at APOE; and that the disease phenotype, like that of the other autosomal-dominant dementing disease, Huntington disease (HD), is associated with severe and progressive cognitive impairment.

Our pragmatic approach, therefore, has been to enroll asymptomatic family members in the same genetic counseling program that has been used by several Canadian centers for members of the HD family (Meissen et al. 1991). This is appropriate because many of the considerations are identical between the two diseases in terms of inheritance, age of onset, societal stigma, and need for long-term follow-up care.

Our experience with counseling of pedigrees with Val717Ile mutation in the βAPP gene at the University of Toronto has been with the TOR3 pedigree described by Karlinsky and colleagues (1992). After the initial missense mutation was discovered in affected pedigree members, we notified other members of the family through an unaffected family member who had previously agreed to be the family contact. The family spokesperson was advised simply that our molecular genetic studies had uncovered the presence of a missense mutation in the βAPP gene present in affected members of the family. The family was advised through this spokesperson that should individual family members wish to know their own genetic status they could do so by enrolling in a genetic counseling program that had been previously set up throughout Canada to handle similar issues for members of HD pedigrees.

The basic requirements for entry into this program would be that the at-risk family member would attend the clinic and undergo precounseling neurological and clinical assessments as well as the appropriate psychological assessments. Following this, the patient would then enter into a precounseling phase during which he or she would be advised of the nature of the tests to be given as well as the various outcomes that could arise. Subsequently, a sample of blood would be taken and submitted for testing in a quality-controlled lab certified by the Province of Ontario or other provinces where the subjects lived. These results would be confirmed by comparison with any results obtained from previously acquired research samples. Finally, the patient would be brought back for further counseling, for administration of the test results, and then posttesting follow-up. Several family members indicated a general interest and asked for information.

Upon hearing the nature of the information that could be provided to them and realizing that this information could effect both positive and negative results (e.g., adverse effects on obtaining long-term health insurance) and that there was no effective treatment at the moment, most family members elected not to proceed further. However, three patients entered into the initial formal pretesting protocol. Two of these patients dropped out after receiving the specific pretesting information. A third family member, who had a low a priori risk of being a gene carrier (i.e., was an offspring of an elderly asymptomatic at-risk family member), proceeded through the testing program, received the results, and has continued to enjoy good psychological and physical health.

The Biology of the Presenilin Genes

Recently, two homologous genes, PS1 on chromosome 14 and PS2 on chromosome 1, were found to be the site of missense mutations associated with early-onset forms of autosomal-dominant familial AD (Levy-Lahad et al. 1995; Rogaev et al. 1995; Sherrington et al. 1995). The first of these genes, PS1, was isolated by a positional cloning strategy from the chromosome 14q24.3 region, which had been identified by genetic linkage studies as the chromosomal region associated with the AD3 subtype of early-onset familial AD (Sherrington et al. 1995). Subsequently, the homologous gene, PS2, was identified by virtue of the fact that an expressed sequenced tagged site (EST) in the nucleotide-sequenced databases was noticed to have significant similarities to the sequence of the PS1 gene (Levy-Lahad et al. 1995; Rogaev et al. 1995). Both the PS1 gene and the PS2 gene are predicted to encode multispanning transmembrane proteins.

Although the precise model for the structural organization of these proteins has not yet been experimentally defined, theoretical considerations suggest that both proteins may contain seven transmembrane domains (as few as five and as many as ten transmembrane domains can be inferred, depending on the exact model and parameters used). Both proteins contain acidically charged residues at the N-terminus and in an exposed domain between the putative transmembrane domain six (TM6) and transmembrane domain seven (TM7). Both genes are expressed in multiple tissues, including the brain. Both genes show some evidence for alternate splicing of the messenger RNA transcript (Rogaev et al. 1995; Rogaev et al. 1997; Sherrington et al. 1996). The function of the presenilins is not yet known, but the strong structural and amino acid sequence similarities between PS1 and PS2 strongly argues that they have overlapping biochemical activities.

Some preliminary studies have suggested that the presenilins may have an effect in signal transduction mechanisms, in protein and membrane trafficking, or in cellular mechanisms related to apoptosis. The hypothesis that the presenilins may have activities in signal transduction is largely derived from the fact that the *Caenohabitis elegans* homologue, sel-12, has a suppressor effect upon intercellular signaling pathways mediated by the Notch/lin-12 genes (Levitan and Greenwald 1995). The alternative hypothesis that the presenilins are involved in membrane and protein trafficking derives from the observation that another *Caenohabitis elegans* homologue, spe-4, appears to be involved in membrane and protein trafficking within the fibrous body/membranous organelle of *Caenohabitis elegans* spermatocytes (L'Hernault and Arduengo 1992). Further support for this hypothesis is derived from preliminary observations suggesting that fibroblasts from subjects with PS1 or PS2 mutations have an abnormality in the processing of βAPP protein (Scheuner et al. 1995).

The analysis of mutations in the PS1 and PS2 genes has led to the discovery of at least twenty-five different missense mutations in the PS1 gene and two mutations in the PS2 gene (Alzheimer's Disease Collaborative Group 1991; Campion et al. 1995; Cruts, Martin, and Van Broeckhoven 1995; Rogaev et al. 1995; Sato et al. 1997; Sherrington et al. 1995; Sherrington et al. 1996; Van Broeckhoven 1995). The clinical features associated with the PS2 mutations are discussed in further detail in the previous chapter. Suffice it to say here that mutations in PS2 are rare and are associated with a highly variable age of onset (for instance, the age of onset may vary within the same family by at least forty years) (Sherrington et al. 1996). Mutations in the PS1 gene, on the other hand, appear to be relatively more common, accounting for up to 50 percent of all cases of early-onset familial AD. Presenilin 1 mutations are associated with a particularly aggressive form of early-onset AD where the age of onset varies from thirty to sixty-five years of age, with the majority of cases having their onset before fifty years of age. Within families, the age of onset tends to have a very narrow range (typically five to ten years). The disease phenotype in families segregating PS1 mutations also appears to be nearly fully penetrant because to date, only a single instance has been found of a bona fide PS1 mutation carrier surviving to eighty years of age without developing symptoms of AD and yet transmitting the disease to an offspring (Tabira 1995).

Like mutations in the βAPP gene, the clinical and pathological phenotypes associated with mutations in the PS1 gene are essentially indistinguishable from the disease phenotypes observed in sporadic cases, excepting, of course, the obvious inheritability and very early age of onset (Foncin et al. 1985; Frommelt et al. 1991; Goudsmit et al. 1981; Nee et al. 1983; Pollen 1993; Pollen, Selkoe, and St. George-Hyslop 1997).

Practical Considerations for Genetics Testing in Pedigrees with Presenilin 1 Mutations

As with mutations in the βAPP gene, the strong similarities between the PS1 form of AD and HD allow for a direct transfer of the clinical genetic testing programs and genetic counseling systems from the HD experience to counseling in members with pedigrees with PS1 mutations. Thus, the stereotypical nature of the clinical phenotype, the reliable and predictable occurrence of disease in mutation carriers, and the narrow age-of-onset range allows quite specific and useful information to be imparted to family members who enroll in genetic counseling programs. Again, in the absence of treatments that will prevent or abort the disease process, our current experience in genetic counseling has largely been toward the provision of general information to family members using the mechanisms described above for the βAPP gene. To date, several members of these early-onset pedigrees segregating missense mutations in the PS1 gene have been enrolled in our genetic counseling programs.

Although the number of subjects who have completed the counseling program and on whom follow-up has been done is too small to make scientifically rigorous conclusions, one particular case is worth noting because it illustrates the powerful emotive forces underlying requests for genetic information. A member of one of the large pedigrees reported by Sherrington and colleagues, whose parent had died with familial early-onset AD caused by a missense mutation in PS1, called our research laboratories within a few weeks of publication of the initial report of missense mutations in the PS1 gene. At that time, no diagnostic testing facilities had been initiated, although we had already made preliminary preparations for requests for counseling. In the initial discussions with this at-risk family member, it was pointed out that the laboratory procedures have not yet been standardized for the detection of mutations other than on a research basis and that in the absence of a treatment very careful consideration of the potential risks and negative side effects of this information should be carefully considered before embarking upon diagnostic testing procedures. Over the next six to eight weeks, the at-risk family member kept in contact with the research laboratories, but it became clear that the uncertainty as to the at-risk family member's genetic status was becoming an all-consuming concern, abrogating both enjoyment of life and useful societal function by this family member. As a consequence, it was decided that the genetic counseling procedures should be embarked upon using the research laboratory as the diagnostic testing facility.

The genetic counseling and testing procedures were followed out in the manner described above, and the test results were ultimately provided to the family member at risk. The act of providing this information had an almost immediate calming effect on the at-risk family member, apparently allowing the family member to set the issue aside and get on with other issues at hand. This observation was particularly enlightening since it clearly illustrates that sometimes an ongoing, unresolved ambiguity over a family member's genetic status may, in and of itself, be more debilitating than even the provision of information that a family member is carrying a potential disease-causing mutation.

A Final Comment

It is obvious from the above that the technical capabilities now exist for both symptomatic and presymptomatic testing of families segregating single-gene autosomal-dominant forms of familial AD. The scientific and factual issues upon which that information should be based are relatively straightforward for the PS1 and βAPP genes. Both genes are associated with an early-onset form of AD, have a narrow range of age of onset within a given family, are virtually fully penetrant, and for all intents and purposes can be considered as a single-gene autosomal-dominant trait with age-dependent penetrance.

The major difference with respect to HD, in terms of genetic counseling, is that there is a small chance that some carriers of mutations in the βAPP or PS1 genes may not develop symptoms until very late in life. In the case of the βAPP Val717Ile mutation, some of this variability in age of onset can be ascribed to transinteracting genotypes at the APOE gene on chromosome 19.

This variability in age of onset, together with the possibility that some mutation carriers may not develop the disease at all, allows the counselor to provide a small ray of hope for asymptomatic family members who are found to carry missense mutations. This small ray of hope can be transmitted in two ways. First, it can be conveyed to the family member via the improbable event that the asymptomatic family member being counseled is one of the few family members who will carry a mutation and not develop disease until very late in life. Second, it can be more realistically conveyed by pointing out that the existence of even a small number of incompletely penetrant cases argues that the genetic program is not immutable and that there is, therefore, hope that a treatment can be devised that will block the deleterious effect of the mutations in the presenilin and βAPP genes.

The other major difference with respect to HD is that asymptomatic members of pedigrees with familial AD who are found not to carry mutations in the PS1, PS2, or βAPP genes are not immune to other forms of AD. In contrast, HD is a disorder with a single etiology, and thus a normal genotype at the HD gene locus virtually precludes the development of HD later in life.

References

Alzheimer's Disease Collaborative Group. 1991. The structure of the presenilin 1 gene and the identification of six mutations in early onset AD pedigrees. *Nature Genetics* 11:219–22.

Cai, X. D., Golde, T. E., and Younkin, S. G. 1992. Release of excess amyloid beta protein from a mutant beta protein precursor. *Science* 259:514–16.

Campion, D., Flaman, J.-M., Brice, A., Hannequin, D., Dubois, B., Martin, C., Moreau, V., Charbonnier, F., Didierjean, O., Tardieu, S., Mallet, J., Bellis, M., Clerget-Darpoux, C., Agid, Y., and Frebourg, T. 1995. Mutations of the presenilin-1 gene in families with early onset Alzheimer's disease. *Human Molecular Genetics* 4:2373–77.

Citron, M., Oltersdorf, T., Haass, C., McConlogue, C., Hung, A. Y., Seubert, P., Vigo-Pelfrey, C., Lieberburg, I., and Selkoe, D. J. 1992. Mutation of the β-amyloid precursor protein in familial Alzheimer's disease increases β-protein production. *Nature* 360:672–74.

Cruts, M., Martin, J.-J., and Van Broeckhoven, C. 1995. Molecular genetic analysis of familial early-onset Alzheimer's disease linked to chromosome 14q24.3. *Human Molecular Genetics* 4:2363–71.

Foncin, J.-F., Salmon, D., Supino-Viterbo, V., Feldman, R. G., Macchi, G., Mariotti, P., Scopetta, C., Caruso, G., and Bruni, A. C. 1985. Alzheimer's presenile dementia transmitted in an extended kindred. *Review of Neurology* (Paris) 141:194–202.

Frommelt, P., Schnabel, R., Kuhne, W., Nee, L. E., and Polinsky, R. J. 1991. Familial Alzheimer disease: A large multigenerational German kindred. *Alzheimer Disease and Associated Disorders* 5:36–43.

Goate, A. M., Chartier-Harlin, M.-C., Mullan, M., Brown, J., Crawford, F., Fidani, L., Guiffra, L., Haynes, A., and Hardy, J. A. 1991. Segregation of a missense mutation in the amyloid precursor protein gene with familial Alzheimer disease. *Nature* 349:704–6.

Goate, A., Haynes, A. R., Owen, M. J., Farrall, M., James, L. A., Lai, L. Y., Mullan, M., Rossor, M., and Hardy, J. 1989. Predisposing locus for Alzheimer disease on chromosome 21. *Lancet* 1:352–55.

Goldgaber, D., Lerman, M. I., and McBride, O. W. 1987. Characterization and chromosomal localization of a cDNA encoding brain amyloid of Alzheimer's disease. *Science* 235:877–80.

Goudsmit, J., White, B. J., Weitkamp, L. R., Keats, B. J., Morrow, C. H., and Gadjusek, D. C. 1981. Familial Alzheimer's disease in two kindreds of the same geographic origin: A clinical and genetic study. *Journal of Neurological Sciences* 49:78–89.

Haass, C., Hung, A. Y., Selkoe, D. J., and Teplow, D. B. 1994. Mutations associated with a locus for familial Alzheimer's disease result in alternative processing of amyloid β-protein precursor. *Journal of Biological Chemistry* 269:17741–48.

Hendricks, M., van Duijn, C. M., and Cras, P. 1992. Presenile dementia and cerebral hemorrhage linked to a mutation at codon 692 of the β-amyloid precursor protein gene. *Nature Genetics* 1:218–21.

Kang, J., Lemaire, H. G., Unterbeck, A., Salbaum, J. M., Masters, C. L., Multhap, G., Beyreuther, K., and Muller-Hill, B. 1987. The precursor of Alzheimer disease amyloid A4 protein resembles a cell surface receptor. *Nature* 325:733–36.

Karlinsky, H., Vaula, G., Haines, J. L., Ridgley, J., Bergeron, C., Mortilla, M., Tupler, R., Percy, M., Robitaille, Y., Crapper-MacLachlan, D. R., and St. George-Hyslop, P. 1992. Molecular and prospective phenotypic characterization of a pedigree with familial Alzheimer disease and a missense mutation in codon 717 of the β-amyloid precursor protein (APP) gene. *Neurology* 42:1445–53.

Levitan, D., and Greenwald, I. 1995. Facilitation of lin-12–mediated signalling by sel-12, a *Caenohabitis elegans* S182 Alzheimer's disease gene. *Nature* 377:351–54.

Levy, E., Carman, M. D., Fernandez-Madrid, I. J., Power, M. D., Lieberburg, I., Sjoerd, G., van Duinen, S. G., Bots, G., Luyendijk, W., and Frangione, B. 1990. Mutation of the Alzheimer's disease amyloid gene in hereditary cerebral hemorrhage: Dutch type. *Science* 248:1124–26.

Levy-Lahad, E., Wijsman, E. M., Nemens, E., Anderson, L., Goddard, K. A., Wever, J. L., Bird, T. D., and Schellenberg, G. D. 1995. A familial Alzheimer's disease locus on chromosome 1. *Science* 269:970–73.

L'Hernault, S. W. L., and Arduengo, P. M. 1992. Mutation of a putative sperm membrane protein in *Caenohabitis elegans* prevents sperm differentiation but not its associated meiotic divisions. *Journal of Cell Biology* 119:55–69.

Mann, D. M., Brown, A., Prinja, D., Davies, C. A., Landen, M., Masters, C. L., and Beyreuther, K. 1989. An analysis of the morphology of senile plaques in Down's syndrome patients of different ages using immunocytochemical and lectin histochemical techniques. *Neuropathology and Applied Neurobiology* 15:317–29.

Mann, D. M. A., Yates, P. O., and Marcyniuk, B. 1984. Alzheimer's presenile dementia, senile dementia of the Alzheimer type, and Down's syndrome in middle age form a continuum of pathologic changes. *Neuropathology and Applied Neurobiology* 10:188–207.

Meissen, G. J., Mastromauro, C. A., Kiely, D. K., McNamara, D. S., and Myers, R. H. 1991. Understanding the decision to take the predictive test for Huntington disease. *American Journal of Medical Genetics* 39:404–10.

Mullan, M. J., Crawford, F., and Axelman, K. 1992. A pathogenic mutation for probable Alzheimer's disease in the APP gene at the N-terminus of β-amyloid. *Nature Genetics* 1:345–47.

Murrell, J., Farlow, M., Ghetti, B., and Benson, M. D. 1991. A mutation in the amyloid precursor protein associated with hereditary Alzheimer's disease. *Science* 254:97–99.

Nacmias, B., Latteraga, S., Tulen, P., Piacentini, S., Bracco, L., Amaducci, L., and Sorbi, S.

1995. APOE genotype and familial Alzheimer's disease: A possible influence on age-of-onset in APP717Val-Ile-mutated families. *Neuroscience Letters* 183:1–3.

Nee, L., Polinsky, R. J., Eldridge, R., Weingartner, H., Smallberg, S., and Ebert, M. 1983. A family with histologically confirmed Alzheimer disease. *Archives of Neurology* 40:203–8.

Pollen, D. 1993. *Hannah's heirs: The quest for the genetic origins of Alzheimer's disease.* Oxford: Oxford University Press.

Pollen, D., Selkoe, D. J., and St. George-Hyslop, P. H. 1997. Comparison of the phenotypes of a pedigree linked to chromosome 14 and a pedigree with a missense mutation in codon 717 of APP. *Neurology* (in press).

Rogaev, E. I., Sherrington, R., Rogaeva, E. A., Levesque, G., Ikeda, M., Liang, Y., Chi, H., Lin, C., Holman, K., Tsuda, T., Mar, L., Sorbi, S., Nacmias, B., Piacentini, S., Amaducci, L., Chumakov, I., Cohen, D., Lannfelt, L., Fraser, P. E., Rommens, J. M., and St. George-Hyslop, P. 1995. Familial Alzheimer's disease in kindreds with missense mutations in a novel gene on chromosome 1 related to the Alzheimer's disease type 3 gene. *Nature* 376:775–78.

Rogaev, E. I., Sherrington, R., Wu, C., Levesque, G., Liang, Y., Rogaeva, E. A., Chi, H., Ikeda, M., Holman, K., Lin, C., Lukiw, W. J., de Jong, P. J., Fraser, P. E., Rommens, J. M., and St. George-Hyslop, P. H. 1997. Analysis of the 5' sequence, genomic structure, and alternative splicing of the presenilin 1 gene associated with early onset Alzheimer's disease. *Genomics* 40:415–26.

Sato, S., Kamino, K., Miki, T., Doi, A., Li, K., St. George Hyslop, P., Ogihara, T., and Sakaki, Y. 1997. Splicing mutation of presenilin 1 gene for early onset familial Alzheimer's disease. *Human Mutation* (in press).

Scheuner, D., Bird, T., Citron, M., Lannfelt, L., Schellenberg, G., Selkoe, D., Viitanen, M., and Younkin, S. G. 1995. Fibroblasts from carriers of familial AD linked to chromosome 14 show increased Aβ production. *Society of Neurosciences Abstracts* 21:1500.

Sherrington, R., Froelich, S., Sorbi, S., Campion, D., Chi, H., Rogaeva, E. A., Levesque, G., Rogaev, E. I., Lin, C., Liang, Y., Ikeda, M., Mar, L., Brice, A., Agid, Y., Percy, M. E., Clerget-Darpoux, F., Karlinsky, H., Piacentini, S., Marcon, G., Nacmias, B., Amaducci, L., Frebourg, T., Lannfelt, L., Rommens, J. M., and St. George-Hyslop, P. H. 1996. Alzheimer's disease associated with mutations in presenilin-2 are rare and variably penetrant. *Human Molecular Genetics* 5:985–88.

Sherrington, R., Rogaev, E., Liang, Y., Rogaeva, E., Levesque, G., Ikeda, M., Chi, H., Lin, C., Holman, K., Tsuda, T., Mar, L., Fraser, P., Rommens, J. M., and St. George-Hyslop, P. H. 1995. Cloning of a gene bearing missense mutations in early onset familial Alzheimer's disease. *Nature* 375:754–60.

Shoji, M., Golde, T., Ghiso, J., Chung, T., Estus, S., Shaffer, L., Cai, X.-D., McKay, D., Frangione, B., and Younkin, S. 1992. Production of the Alzheimer amyloid β protein by normal proteolytic processing. *Science* 258:126–29.

St. George-Hyslop, P. H., Tanzi, R. E., Polinsky, R. J., Haines, J. L., Nee, L., Watkins, P. C., Myers, R. H., Conneally, P. M., and Gusella, J. F. 1987. The genetic defect causing familial Alzheimer disease maps on chromosome 21. *Science* 235:885–89.

St. George-Hyslop, P. H., Tsuda, T., Crapper-MacLachlan, D., Karlinsky, H., Pollen, D., and Lippa, C. 1994. Alzheimer's disease and possible gene interaction. *Science* 263:536–37.

Susuki, N., Cheung, T. T., Cai, X.-D., Odaka, A., Otvos, L., Eckman, C., Golde, T., and Younkin, S. G. 1994. An increased percentage of long amyloid β protein secreted by familial amyloid β protein precursor (βAPP717) mutants. *Science* 264:1336–40.

Tabira, T. 1995. Presentation at symposium on Molecular Mechanisms of Genetic Neurologic Diseases. November. Niigata University, Niigata, Japan.

Tamaoka, A., Odaka, A., Ishibashi, Y., Usami, M., Sahara, N., Suzuki, N., Nukina, N., Mizusawa, H., Shoji, S., Kanazawa, I., and Mori, H. 1994. APP717 missense mutation affects the ratio of amyloid β protein species (Aβ1-42/43 and Aβ1-40) in familial Alzheimer's disease brain. *Journal of Biological Chemistry* 269:32721–24.

Van Broeckhoven, C. 1995. Presenilins and Alzheimer disease. *Nature Genetics* 11:230–32.

Younkin, S. G., Cai, X.-D., and Golde, T. 1993. Release of excess amyloid beta protein from a mutant amyloid beta protein precursor. *Science* 259:514–16.

4 A New Paradigm for Clinical Evaluations of Dementia

Alzheimer Disease and Apolipoprotein E Genotypes

ALLEN D. ROSES, M.D.

For many years, clinical evaluation of cognitively impaired patients consisted in ruling out uncommon reversible causes of dementia. Now, with the discovery of apolipoprotein polymorphisms as the major susceptibility factors for Alzheimer disease (AD) and its age-of-onset distribution, it is possible to diagnose AD with higher accuracy. To be able to "rule in" AD early in the diagnostic process can allow streamlined and focused diagnostic workups and provide accurately defined patient groups for therapeutic trials. The paradigm for the application of susceptibility-gene data to clinical medicine has developed rapidly and provides a framework for the use of future susceptibility-gene discoveries for other common, complex diseases.

Background

Alzheimer disease is the major cause of dementia in the United States, with an estimated prevalence of three million to four million patients (Roses and Pericak-Vance 1995). The clinical phenotype of AD has been defined by convention, and most clinicians use the NINDS-ADRDA (National Institute of Neurological Disease and Stroke/Alzheimer's Disease and Related Disorders Association) criteria to classify patients (McKhann et al. 1984) (see table 4.1). The definition was made to be broad and inclusive to encompass, in practice, virtually all AD patients as well as many patients with other diseases but the same clinical presentation. Thus, 10–20 percent of patients in most autopsy-confirmed series have other pathologically defined causes of the phenotype (e.g., non-AD) (Galasko et al. 1994). A useful diagnostic test for AD would provide early and accurate differential diagnosis with a high positive predictive value.

Table 4.1. Criteria for Clinical Diagnosis of Alzheimer Disease

Criteria for the clinical diagnosis of probable Alzheimer disease are
- Dementia established by clinical examination; documented by the Folstein Mini-Mental test, Blessed Dementia Scale, or some similar examination; and confirmed by neuropsychological tests
- Deficits in two or more areas of cognition
- Progressive worsening of memory and other cognitive functions
- No disturbance of consciousness
- Onset between ages 40 and 90, most often after 65
- Absence of systemic disorders or other brain diseases that in and of themselves could account for the progressive deficits in memory and cognition

Factors supporting diagnosis of probable Alzheimer disease
- Progressive deterioration of specific cognitive functions, such as language (aphasia), motor skills (apraxia), or perception (agnosia)
- Impaired activities of daily living and altered patterns of behavior
- Family history of similar disorders, particularly if confirmed neuropathologically
- Laboratory results normal lumbar puncture as evaluated by standard techniques
- Laboratory results of normal pattern or nonspecific changes in electroencephalograph, such as increased slow-wave activity
- Evidence of cerebral atrophy on computed tomography with progression documented by serial observations

Other clinical features consistent with the diagnosis of probable Alzheimer disease, after exclusion of causes of dementia other than Alzheimer disease
- Plateaus in the course of progression of the illness
- Associated symptoms of depression, insomnia, incontinence, delusion, illusion, hallucination, catastrophic verbal/emotional/physical outburst, sexual disorder, and weight loss
- Other neurologic abnormalities in some patients, especially with more advanced disease and including motor signs such as increased muscle tone, myoclonus, or gait disorder
- Seizures, in advanced disease
- Computed tomography normal for age

Features that make the diagnosis of probable Alzheimer disease uncertain or unlikely
- Sudden, apoplectic onset
- Focal neurologic findings, such as hemiparesis, sensory loss, visual field

deficits, or incoordination early in the course of the illness
- Seizures or gait disturbances at the onset or very early in the course of the illness

Clinical diagnosis of possible Alzheimer disease
- May be made on the basis of the dementia syndrome, in the absence of other neurologic, psychiatric, or systemic disorders sufficient to cause dementia, and in the presence of variations in the onset, presentation, or clinical course
- May be made in the presence of a second systemic or brain disorder sufficient to produce dementia, which is not considered to be the cause of the dementia
- Should be used in research studies when a single, gradually progressive severe cognitive deficit is identified in the absence of other identifiable cause

Criteria for a diagnosis of definite Alzheimer disease
- The clinical criteria for probable Alzheimer disease
- Histopathologic evidence obtained from a biopsy or autopsy

Classification of Alzheimer disease for research purposes should specify features that may differentiate subtypes of the disorder, such as
- Familial occurrence
- Onset before age 65
- Presence of trisomy 21
- Coexistence of other relevant conditions, such as Parkinson disease

---

Alzheimer disease is still classified by clinical phenotypic criteria, but the classification includes several genetic forms of the disease (Roses and Pericak-Vance 1996). Because the phenotypic criteria, including neuropathology, cannot be established during life, all clinical series also contain a variable and indistinguishable group of non-AD patients. Thus, to define an accurate diagnostic test, the data must be correlated with autopsy-confirmed definitive diagnoses. It is, therefore, not possible to define specificity (a negative test in non-AD patients) or predictive value for any diagnostic test without pathological confirmation (Elston and Johnson 1994).

The inability to distinguish within any AD clinical series the 10–20 percent who are not AD patients has an impact on diagnostic testing and interpretations of epidemiological data, clinical trials, and basic research (Saunders et al. 1996). The clinical criteria for AD include between 300,000 and 800,000 patients in the United States who appear to have clinical AD but will have a different diagnosis at autopsy. Non-AD dementia is itself a highly significant medical problem.

Table 4.2. Genetic Classification of the Alzheimer Diseases

Type	Chromosome	Gene
The Alzheimer diseases		
Early-onset familial, autosomal dominant (AD1)	21	APP
Late-onset familial and sporadic susceptibility gene (AD2)	19	APOE associated
Early-onset familial, autosomal dominant (AD3)	14	presenilin 1
Early-onset familial, autosomal dominant (Volga German founder and other) (AD4)	1	presenilin 2
Other late-onset susceptibility genes	Several reported, none yet confirmed	
Other autosomal-dominant mutations	Several large families unlinked to known loci	
Defined pathological disease, Alzheimer-like clinical presentation		
Pick disease	—	—
Subcortical gliosis	—	—
Frontal lobe degeneration	—	—
Diffuse cortical Lewy-body disease	—	—
Lewy-body disease with amyloid plaques	—	
Progressive supranuclear palsy	—	—
Cerebrovascular disease with multiple infarcts	—	—
Associated with other hereditary disorders		
Congophilic angiopathy	—	—
Cerebral hemorrhage of Dutch type	—	—

The neuropathological criteria for AD were also defined by committee to contain a number of neuritic plaques in specified neuroanatomical locations in the brain (Khachaturian 1985). These definitions have been modified during the past decade but are still somewhat arbitrary and the source of continued discussion and development (Mirra et al. 1991). It is frequently stated that "all AD patients have plaques that contain amyloid (by definition), therefore amyloid causes AD" — a syllogism (Selkoe 1994, 439). However, it is well documented that normal, cognitively intact individuals may also have sufficient plaques in their brains to meet neuropathological criteria for AD (Polvikoski et al. 1995; Terry 1994). Thus, even the end-stage pathological criteria for AD are not 100 percent predictive without the clinical disease, because the neuropathology can be observed in nondemented individuals who died from other causes.

Genetic research has provided the clearest definitions of heterogeneity for the field of AD. Three known autosomal-dominant loci cause the AD phenotype when mutations are present (Roses 1996b) (see table 4.2). Although each mutation is important to understanding the basic pathobiology of AD, all of these mutations are rare, accounting for much less than 0.1 percent of the incident or prevalent AD cases.

In contrast, the first susceptibility locus for a common, complex disease to

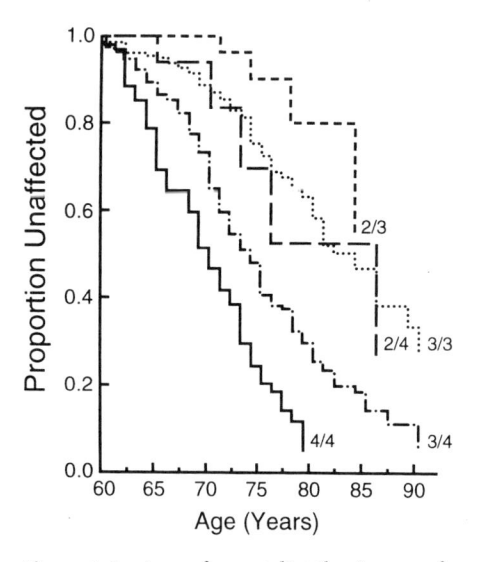

Figure 4.1. Age-of-onset distribution as a function of inherited autosomal-dominant forms of Alzheimer disease and apolipoprotein (APOE) genotypes. The figure represents the proportion of each genotype remaining unaffected as a function of age. The data for APOE are derived from Corder et al. (1994). The median age of onset for APOE ε4/ε4 is less than 70 years, whereas that for APOE ε2/ε3 is greater than 90 years. Each genotype represents a different proportion of the population. Amyloid precursor protein (APP) mutations and presenilin 1 mutations are rare and uncommon, respectively. APOE ε4ε/4 represents approximately 2 percent of the population; ε3/ε4, 21 percent; ε3/ε3, 60 percent; ε2/ε3, 11 percent; and ε2/ε4, 5 percent. APOE ε2/ε2 is not shown because it represents less than 0.5 percent, and there was only a single control with that genotype.

be identified by positional candidate strategies was apolipoprotein E (*APOE,* gene; *apoE,* protein), and APOE accounts for 40–60 percent of the prevalent cases (Roses 1996; Roses and Devlin 1995). Common polymorphisms at the APOE locus are associated with varing risks and age-of-onset distributions of familial and sporadic late-onset AD (Corder et al. 1993; Corder et al. 1994; Roses et al. 1994) (see figure 4.1). The definition of susceptibility genotypes has provided a new paradigm for the clinical genetic community, but one that was more functionally familiar to the epidemiology community. The diagnostic and predictive applications of APOE in AD have led to contradictory published statements and opinions appearing in widely read journals (Bird 1995; Breitner 1996; American College of Medical Genetics 1995; Relkin and National Institute on Aging 1996; Roses 1995a; Seshadri, Drachman, and Lippa 1995). As the data have become more clear and as additional susceptibility loci are defined, AD will continue to provide a prototype for the application of common susceptibility genes for other medical diseases that are currently under investigation, including diabetes, osteoarthritis, Parkinson disease, and cancer.

History

Most AD patients had been considered sporadic AD, occurring in isolation, without a well-defined pattern of inheritance. In fact, only a decade ago there was little support for proposals to determine the genetic susceptibility of the common form of late-onset AD. Thus, when a rare form of AD was linked to chromosome 21 (in four families, whose AD was later demonstrated to be linked to chromosome 14), the use of late-onset AD families to exclude this AD linkage was not considered valid because the disease was not "genetic" (Pericak-Vance et al. 1988; St. George-Hyslop et al. 1987). After the publication of linkage on the long arm of chromosome 19 in 1991, there again was little enthusiasm (Pericak-Vance et al. 1991). In a 1994 review, Lander and Schork stated that the chromosome 19 linkage "was dismissed by many observers" (Lander and Schork 1994). The clear association of specific alleles at the APOE locus with increased risk and earlier onset of AD was similarly met with skepticism (Marx 1993; Saunders, Schmader, et al. 1993; Saunders, Strittmatter, et al. 1993; Strittmatter et al. 1993). The initial response of many prominent AD genetic researchers was linkage disequilibrium, premature public announcements of nonconfirmations at international meetings, and frequent disparaging and sometimes personally hostile quotations in the lay press.

However, because many practicing clinicians who treated large series of AD patients had APOE genotyping available to them locally, letters confirming the increased APOE ε4 association with AD started to appear in the *Lancet* and other journals regularly in the year after publication (Amouyel et al. 1993; Anwar et al. 1993; Borgaonkar et al. 1993; Czech et al. 1993; Alzheimer's Disease Collaborative Group 1993; Houlden et al. 1994; Lucotte and Aouizerate 1995; Mayeux et al. 1993; Noguchi, Murakami, and Yamada 1993; Payami et al. 1993; Poirier et al. 1993; Rebeck et al. 1993; Saunders, Schmader, et al. 1993; Saunders, Strittmatter, et al. 1993; Strittmatter et al. 1993; Ueda et al. 1993). Many of the major AD centers were relatively late in evaluating APOE data in their series. To date, there are more than 150 published confirmations of the increased allele frequency of APOE ε4 in AD series. There are no published nonconfirmations in any general AD series with more than thirty patients and proper controls. One published nonconfirmation in an elderly Swedish population led to subsequent confirmation after more patients were studied (Basun et al. 1995; Lannfelt et al. 1994). Another nonconfirmation in a Seattle HMO that had been referred to during discussions at several major AD meetings was withdrawn by private circulation of a fax communication to participants in an Adler Foundation conference.

Thus, the history of the APOE association with AD has been colorful. Now, with the consideration of diagnostic and predictive applications, there has been another blossoming of statements and pronouncements concerning the "problem" of applying APOE genotype information (Bird 1995; Breitner 1996; American College of Medical Genetics 1995; Relkin and National Institute on Aging 1996; Roses 1995a; Seshadri, Drachman, and Lippa 1995). Some of the published statements themselves have become controversial, containing somewhat selected and inaccurately interpreted information (see below).

Using a susceptibility locus as a diagnostic adjunct, however, raises its own problems. The experience of the genetics community has been primarily with diseases that are inherited as straightforward mutation with high penetrance (Martin 1993). With relatively severe childhood diseases, the emphasis has been on genetic counseling, early identification of carriers, and prenatal diagnosis. With later-onset diseases, such as Huntington disease (HD), a standardized rather stringent set of criteria was generally adopted, prescribing psychiatric assessment and counseling for individuals who sought diagnostic information. Other rare late-onset severe diseases, like familial amyotrophic lateral sclerosis (ALS) or the rare autosomal-dominant mutations in AD, have generally followed similar protocols. Late-onset AD, so-called sporadic AD, however, represents a quantitatively different problem. For example, there are tens of thousands of patients with and between 100,000 and 200,000 individuals at risk for HD. There are hundreds of individuals at risk for familial ALS or rare AD mutations. In common AD, there are millions of patients and approximately 30 percent of the population who carry at least one copy of the disease-associated allele.

Paternalistic attitudes have led to the nihilistic suggestion that an accurate diagnosis may be unnecessary (American College of Medical Genetics 1995). Unfortunately, some of the suggested public policies have come from genetic experts or other sources unfamiliar with the detailed medical problems of AD patients and their caregivers. A schism exists between part of the genetics community and some of the AD community, brought on by different attitudes toward patients and their needs. Within organized AD patient-advocacy groups there are strong pressures for accurate and early diagnosis and prediction, acknowledging the social and legal problems that may accompany such information (see Alzheimer's Association website: http://www.alz.org). Patients with early dementia generally want to play a major role in determining their own affairs and planning with their families. Formal polls by AD advocacy groups consistently show that most patients and their families want accurate diagnosis as well as available effective treatments.

Genetics of APOE

Every person inherits two APOE alleles, one from each parent. There are three common variations or polymorphisms of the APOE gene in humans. The most common variation is the ε3 form, which contains a single cysteine amino acid at position 112 (of 299 amino acids); its proportion in the Caucasian population of European descent is approximately 78 percent. The next most common variation is the ε4 form, which differs from ε3 by the placement of an arginine rather than a cysteine at position 112; its proportion in the population is approximately 15 percent. The least common variation is the ε2 form, which has a cysteine at both position 112 and position 158; its proportion in the population is approximately 7 percent. While the allele frequencies may differ between ethnic and racial groups, the association of inheriting the ε4 variation and the risk of AD has been consistently demonstrated (Maestre et al. 1995; Poirier et al. 1993; Saunders, Schmader, et al. 1993; Saunders, Strittmatter, et al. 1993; Ueki and Kawano 1993).

The distribution of the age of onset of AD can be plotted as a function of APOE genotype (Roses 1994; Roses et al. 1994) (see figure 4.1). While only 2–3 percent of the population carries two alleles for the ε4 form, the risk of AD for individuals with a single ε4 allele is consistently found to be significantly higher than that of individuals without a single ε4 allele (Corder et al. 1993;

Lucotte and Aouizerate 1995). However, onset-distribution curves are related to genotype (figure 4.1). The ε3/ε4 genotype is present in approximately 21 percent of the population. Their risk of AD is less than that of ε4/ε4 subjects but generally higher than that of individuals without an ε4 allele. The risk of individuals with the ε2/ε4 genotype appears to be similar to that of ε3/ε3 homozygotes and may account for much of the residual ε4 risk in the oldest-old populations. The ε2/ε3 genotype is present in 12–14 percent of people, and they have the least risk. The ε2/ε2 genotype represents only 0.5 percent of the population; not enough data are available for illustration (Roses 1995a).

Opposing interactions of different APOE alleles affect the age-of-onset distribution curves. The ε4 allele increases the risk of AD and lowers the age-of-onset distribution, so patients with an ε4 allele, on average, develop AD at an earlier age (Corder et al. 1993; Lucotte and Aouizerate 1995; Yoshizawa et al. 1994). The ε2 allele lowers the risk and increases the age-of-onset distribution (Corder et al. 1994). The median for each genotype in figure 4.1 shows a difference of more than twenty years in the age of onset between individuals with ε4/ε4 and those with ε2/ε3. It is important to stress that these data are collected not from a large-scale epidemiological study but rather from families and case-control groups. These curves cannot be used for accurate prediction for any individual (Roses 1995a).

However, the age-of-onset distributions of different APOE genotypes (shape of the curve) has now been confirmed in several other series, and prospective epidemiological studies are in progress (Lucotte and Aouizerate 1995). The age curves actually begin before the age of sixty years, the age minimum used in the initial studies. In fact, the strongest genetic factor in patients less than sixty years old is ε4, not the very rare early-onset autosomal-dominant mutations (Okuizumi et al. 1994; van Duijn et al. 1994).

Some individuals with the ε3/ε4 genotype can survive one hundred years without developing AD, but it is not possible currently to distinguish which ε3/ε4 individuals will develop AD at age fifty-five years and who will be spared until over one hundred years. However, if a patient is cognitively impaired at age seventy years and has the ε4/ε4 genotype, it is more likely that the autopsy-confirmed diagnosis will be AD than for a similar clinical patient with the ε2/ε3 genotype.

Defining the Clinical Applications of APOE Genotyping

There are two distinctly different applications of APOE genotyping in general clinical practice: prediction in asymptomatic individuals and diagnosis

(Roses 1995a). A third use is in clinical research, including therapeutic trials (Poirier et al. 1995). Prediction refers to attempts to answer unaffected individuals' questions concerning when or whether they might experience the onset of AD. Use in differential diagnosis refers to the use of APOE genotyping in the context of the diagnostic evaluation of a cognitively impaired patient. The prior probabilities (or existing risks) of each of these populations are vastly different (Breitner 1996). Two-thirds of adult dementias are due to AD, and a useful diagnostic test would need to raise the ability to correctly diagnose an individual patient to a level of accuracy of greater than 95 percent. For the general population, the age-dependent risk for most people concerned about predictive testing is unknown and is negligible before age fifty years. The relative risks that could be calculated from epidemiological studies are not yet available, but proper epidemiological studies are currently in progress. By the time they are completed, it might be expected that other confirmed genetic risk factors or susceptibility loci will have been discovered and multifactorial calculations of risk might be possible.

Prediction in Asymptomatic Subjects

All published statements on policy for AD are unanimous in recommending that APOE genotyping not be used for prediction for normal individuals, whether or not they are related to AD patients (American College of Medical Genetics 1995; Relkin and National Institute on Aging 1996; Roses 1995a). The most cogent reason why APOE genotyping should not be used for prediction is that no prospective studies are available that allow one to assess risk properly. The lack of practical usefulness of predictive testing for any individual is usually easily understood by most asymptomatic people seeking risk information. If a fifty-year-old woman has the ε4/ε4 genotype, the currently available range of risk distributions of AD for that genotype span more than forty years (age of onset from fifty to more than ninety years). There is no way to predict whether her disease would start at age fifty-five or not be present at age ninety. Similarly, for ε3/ε4 individuals, who make up more than 20 percent of the population, there is no way to predict whether an individual will develop AD at age fifty-five years or live to one hundred years disease-free.

The age of onset of adult-onset inherited diseases is usually extremely variable, even in patients who carry rare autosomal-dominant inherited mutations (Levy-Lahad, Wasco, et al. 1995; Roses 1994). Contrary to inaccurate but common statements in the literature, autosomal-dominant mutations are not deterministic and are not always associated with 100 percent penetrance (Roses

1996a, 1996b). For example, within the rare families in which the APP717 mutations are associated with an earlier-onset form of AD, there is a wide variation in individuals, onset generally being between thirty-five and sixty-five years of age. In this small group of families there are about thirty mutation carriers in the world who are within or above that age range. Yet there are three individuals from three separate families (not patients) who carry the APP717 mutation who are more than two standard deviations above the mean age of onset yet have no signs or symptoms of disease. Each has the $\epsilon2/\epsilon3$ genotype (Sorbi et al. 1995; St. George-Hyslop et al. 1994). Thus, epistatic interactions between the $\epsilon2/\epsilon3$ genotype and the APP717 mutation affect the clinical phenotype (age of onset) of disease. This should not be surprising, since as a general rule, many adult-onset autosomal-dominant diseases have nonpenetrant mutation carriers, that is, carriers that escape disease. Therefore, even knowing the mutation status of "presymptomatic" family members provides an incomplete basis for accurately predicting the age of onset of any individual at risk.

The situation is more pronounced in the three families with the rare presenilin 2 (PS2) mutation. The age of onset appears to be very variable, with AD onset in the fifties. Yet in two of the three known PS2 families, there are individual patients who did not develop AD until older than age eighty years. The interactions with the APOE locus have not been published yet, but early-onset disease is not determined by the PS2 mutation alone. Finding that an individual in a PS2 family does not carry the mutation covers only part of the risk of late-onset AD, some of which is influenced by APOE genotype.

With susceptibility genes like APOE, the potential use for the prediction of asymptomatic individuals is even more vague. Society has had considerable experience with phenotypic risk factors for common diseases, such as serum cholesterol levels and myocardial infarctions (Wilson et al. 1994). However, after four decades of epidemiological studies, accurate prediction of whether or when a coronary occlusion will occur, even in the presence of an elevated level of serum cholesterol, is impossible. The difference between the general acceptance and public policy for increased relative risk information for cholesterol testing is the ability to apply preventive therapies, including diet, exercise, and cholesterol-lowering agents. In the United States, cholesterol-testing kits are available in local drugstores. At present there is no preventive therapy for AD, so increased relative risk information provides little positive therapeutic value to the individual and opens up the potential for abuse of these data by insurers, employers, or government (Myers et al. 1996). However, once a relatively safe and effective preventive therapy is available, exact information on individual risk will not be needed, and people will decide on treatments based on relative risk estimates and potential side effects of medications — similar to current cholesterol-lowering decisions.

Differential Diagnosis of Cognitively Impaired Patients

The usefulness of APOE genotyping as a diagnostic adjunct in the evaluation of cognitively impaired patients depends on its specificity and sensitivity (Bird 1995). Until now the diagnosis of possible or probable AD was one of exclusion (see table 4.1). Since the diagnosis of definite AD must be confirmed at autopsy (or, rarely, brain biopsy), there has been considerable difficulty in evaluating the sensitivity and specificity of any diagnostic tests during life (Khachaturian 1985; Mirra et al. 1991). When NINDS/ADRDA clinical criteria are used, most Caucasian series contain only 80–90 percent verified AD cases, although the published range is from 40 to 100 percent (American College of Medical Genetics 1995; McKhann et al. 1984; Roses 1996a).

One statement on the use of APOE genotyping pointed out the difficulties in using data from clinical series but incorrectly depicted the diagnosis of AD as "difficult and variable" (American College of Medical Genetics 1995). The diagnostic criteria are actually quite clear and accurate. The problem is that accurate diagnosis is available only after the death of the patient. The proportion of non-AD cases in any group of patients is highly variable between physicians and centers (American College of Medical Genetics 1995; Mayieux and Couderc 1995; Nalbantoglu et al. 1994). Unfortunately, some clinicians and epidemiologists still have difficulty with autopsy confirmation of their clinical diagnoses. Thus, the best way to measure sensitivity and specificity in each clinic would be to study prospectively ascertained probable AD patients who subsequently had autopsy confirmations (Saunders et al. 1996). This allows the direct inclusion of the non-AD patients encountered during the study in a nonselected manner, if the autopsy sample is representative of the clinic experience. Current public policy statements are hampered by the variable estimates of diagnostic accuracy in clinical series. Performing meta-analyses that combine clinical studies in heterogeneous populations with variable APOE allele frequencies serves only to average out the unknown clinical diagnostic variability.

Saunders and colleagues (1996) measured directly the specificity and sensitivity of APOE genotyping in a consecutively ascertained series of sixty-seven probable AD patients cared for at Duke University Medical Center over more than a decade, who were subsequently autopsied. Table 4.3 illustrates the APOE genotypes of the confirmed AD patients and those patients who did not have

Apolipoprotein E Genotypes 49

Table 4.3. Diagnosis of Sporadic Probable AD Confirmed on Autopsy (N = 67)

	ε4/ε4	ε3/ε4	ε2/ε4	ε3/ε3	ε2/ε3	ε2/ε2
AD	11 (5)	29 (9)	3 (1)	14 (2)	0	0
Other	0	0	0	6	4	0

Source: Data from Saunders et al. (1996), 92.

Note: The table presents the results of a study at Duke University Medical Center of 67 individuals clinically diagnosed with dementia, who were subsequently autopsied for Alzheimer disease (AD). The prevalence of definite AD patients in this population of clinically diagnosed probable AD patients is 85%. Sixteen patients also had the secondary pathological diagnosis of Parkinson disease (indicated in parentheses). Three patients had a secondary diagnosis of moderate to severe atherosclerosis, including one ε4/ε4 patient and two ε3/ε4 patients.

Table 4.4. Diagnosis of Definite Alzheimer Disease (AD), with ε4-positive Allele or the ε4/ε4 Genotype as the Tests (N = 67)

	Diagnosis AD	Non-AD	Total
ε4 positive (ε4/ε4 or x/4)	43	0	43
ε4 negative (x/x)	14	10	24
Total	57	10	67

Source: Data from Saunders et al. (1996).

Note: The prevalence of AD in this population was 85%. The sensitivity and specificity of the test were 75% (43/57) and 100% (10/10), respectively. The positive predictive value was 100% (43/43), and the negative predictive value was 42% (10/24).

AD as their autopsy diagnosis. As expected, only 85 percent of the patients were confirmed as having AD.

Table 4.4 illustrates the use of the presence of either at least one ε4 allele or the rarer genotype, ε4/ε4, as the "test." The unexpected results of this study indicate that none of the non-AD patients (14 percent) had an ε4 allele. Thus, the specificity of the ε4 allele was 100 percent in this initial prospectively ascertained series. Two other institutions confirmed very high ε4 specificity in their series (Kakulas and Wilton 1996; Smith et al. 1996).

Itabashi and colleagues (1996) reported the ε4 frequency in an "almost consecutive series" of autopsies (not consecutive dementia patients who came

Table 4.5. Distribution of ε4 Allele in Patients with and without Alzheimer Disease (AD) (N = 156)

	Diagnosis AD	Diagnosis Non-AD	Total
ε4 positive (ε4/ε4) (4/4 or x/4)	112	2	114
ε4 negative (x/x)	27	15	42
Total	139	17	156

Source: Data from Welsh-Bohmer et al. (1996).

Note: The table presents the results of the CERAD Neuropathology Series of 156 patients. The sensitivity and specificity of the test were 81% (112/139) and 88% (15/17), respectively. The positive predictive value was 98% (112/114).

to autopsy) and found, as would be expected, that autopsies from non-AD patients showed the presence of ε4 alleles. Since approximately 30 percent of the population carries an ε4 allele, any series of autopsies from any disease could have an allele frequency of approximately 15 percent. They did not assess the positive predictive value from the appropriate population at risk, that is, a consecutive series of patients suspected of having possible or probable AD who are definitely diagnosed at autopsy. The design of such studies has been suggested by the National Institutes of Health/Department of Energy's Working Group on Ethical, Legal, and Social Implications of Human Genome Research for determining the usefulness of diagnostic tests (http://infonet.welch.jhu.edu/policy/genetics). The positive predictive value pertains to the prospectively ascertained, consecutive clinical series representative of the cognitively impaired patients who would be tested, not a group of autopsies selected by diagnosis. Thus, the data of Itabashi and colleagues have no bearing on the question of positive predictive value for early dementia patients with a clinical diagnosis of possible or probable AD (Itabashi et al. 1996).

Several other prospectively ascertained clinical studies are in progress, including an analysis of the series collected by the Consortium to Establish a Registry for Alzheimer's Disease (CERAD). Table 4.5 illustrates the data from 156 autopsied cases selected prospectively at more than twenty participating CERAD centers (Welsh-Bohmer et al. 1997). In this prospectively collected clinical series, the positive predictive value of carrying an ε4 allele was 98 percent. A cooperative study now in progress of the National Institute on Aging–sponsored Alzheimer disease centers (ADCs) and other specialty clinics includes several thousand patients and is expected to provide accurate specificity and sensitivity measurements with well-defined confidence limits. It appears from initial studies that the positive predictive value of one or more ε4 alleles is high (greater than 94%), well within the range of commonly used, accurate diagnostic tests.

Apolipoprotein E Genotyping as a Useful and Valuable Diagnostic Adjunct

In the context of a cognitively impaired patient who has a nonfocal, normal (and reliable) neurological examination and no known reversible cause, the presence of an ε4/ε4 genotype has a diagnostic accuracy of greater than 99 percent; the ε3/ε4 genotype will probably be greater than 95 percent as more clinical series with autopsy confirmation are analyzed (Saunders et al. 1996). The large study from the ADCs that is in progress will also help determine accurate confidence limits. Thus, the risk of AD in a demented individual over fifty-five years old with the ε4/ε4 or ε3/ε4 genotype goes from a prior probability of approximately 66 percent to a probability conditioned by APOE genotype of greater than 95–99 percent. No other test commonly used to diagnose dementia has been subjected to such a rigorous analysis of positive predictive value, yet many other tests are performed routinely in the United States at a cost of hundreds of millions of dollars per year.

Presymptomatic Research Applications

Metabolic imaging (positron emission tomography, or PET) demonstrated abnormal glucose metabolism in groups of clinically normal individuals who carry the ε4 allele (Small et al. 1995; Reiman et al. 1996). The average age of the subjects was approximately two decades earlier than the median of their expected, APOE genotype-specific, age-of-onset distribution. How young these metabolic changes can be documented still remains to be studied, but it has become quite clear that AD is a slowly developing, insidious metabolic disease that can be predicted in groups of subjects of particular APOE genotypes. Again, accurate prediction, based on PET scans, of when or if disease will develop for any individual is not possible.

An interesting nihilism has developed in some of the recent literature, in which some expert geneticists project a rather paternalistic attitude with respect to the rationale for an accurate diagnosis of AD without currently available effective therapies (American College of Medical Genetics 1995). As practical therapies for either AD or non-AD patients are developed, accurate diagnosis becomes very important. The importance of diagnosis has rarely been raised in the case of other genetic diseases. Certainly, the majority of patients and their families encountered clinically or through the Alzheimer's Association are more comfortable with an accurate diagnosis (see Alzheimer's Association website: http://www.alz.org). Patients and caregivers want accurate information in order to prepare for the predicted course of life events, including the use of coping strategies and external support resources and the involvement of minimally affected patients in their own care and decision making. The use of genetic risk factors in the diagnostic evaluation is similar to other common diagnostic tests for diseases that are usually less than 100 percent specific (Breitner 1996).

When considered in the context of a clinical picture of verifiable cognitive impairment, no known reversible cause for the dementia, and a reliable, nonfocal, or otherwise normal neurological examination, the presence of an ε4 allele would appear to reliably predict the ultimate neuropathological diagnosis of AD in a large number of cognitively impaired patients (66%, or 112 in 156; see table 4.5). Thus, the use of the ε4 allele information adds to diagnostic confidence in two-thirds of the patients ascertained. The absence of the ε4 allele provides no practical diagnostic information for AD but defines a group of patients for which additional diagnostic markers and more extensive diagnostic evaluation are indicated.

An important consideration regarding medical justice is whether it is justifiable *not* to perform APOE genotyping in appropriately cognitively impaired patients when it can provide relatively inexpensive positive predictive value for more than half of the individuals tested. It is important to exercise caution against any current use of APOE genotyping to predict AD in any cognitively intact individual. It is possible to carry an ε4 allele and never develop dementia. Without proper epidemiological data, as exist for other risk factors (such as cholesterol levels for heart disease), it is impossible to provide a quantitative risk estimate. It is not possible to predict at what age any individual will develop AD during a five-decade period of risk. At present, without a safe preventive therapy, potential ethical and legal concerns outweigh any benefits of prediction. However, in the context of a diagnostic evaluation of cognitively impaired patients, carrying an ε4 allele is a useful and relatively inexpensive adjunct in early diagnosis and provides a basis for stratifying patients for the evaluation of other AD diagnostic tests and clinical trials.

Therapeutic Trials

The ultimate promise of AD research is to discover safe preventive therapies and effective treatments. It is widely assumed that candidate compounds will result from hypothesis-driven basic research (Roses 1994; Selkoe 1994). With the discovery of the autosomal mutations and the association with APOE genotypes, new metabolic targets for therapy can be defined (Goate et al. 1991; Levy-Lahad, Wasco, et al. 1995; Rogaev et al. 1995; Roses 1994; Selkoe 1994; Sherrington et al. 1995). All AD therapeutic trials currently suffer from the variable accuracy of diagnosis of the patients in the trial. Patients who are recruited for therapeutic trials may carry the diagnosis of probable AD at the time, but it has been expected that 10–40 percent of such patients would not be autopsy-confirmed years after the trial. In the past, when the diagnosis of probable AD was solely a matter of excluding other etiologies of dementia, this situation was unavoidable.

The recent literature clearly illustrates the potential for misinterpretation of data from therapeutic trials. Poirier and colleagues (1995) suggest that patients from the initial tacrine trials who did not carry an $\epsilon 4$ allele responded better than patients with an $\epsilon 4$ allele. Whether or not the efficacy data are accurate for tacrine (or any other compound) is not the point of this discussion. Data from the two "treatment" groups ($\epsilon 4$ carriers, with clinically diagnosed AD patients, and non-$\epsilon 4$ carriers, with some AD patients and most of the non-AD patients) can now be interpreted more clearly as a consequence of using APOE genotypes for more accurate diagnosis during life (Saunders et al. 1996).

Tables 4.3, 4.4, and 4.5 illustrate typical clinical AD series with pathological confirmation of diagnosis. The non-AD patients were not evenly distributed between the $\epsilon 4$-positive and $\epsilon 4$-negative groups; most were in the $\epsilon 4$-negative group (see figure 4.2). Thus, an alternative explanation of a drug that seems to be effective in the $\epsilon 4$-negative clinical AD group may be that the compound works only in the non-AD patients. A truly effective treatment for AD might be expected to work in both groups, perhaps more effectively in the $\epsilon 4$ carriers since this group is more homogeneous for authentic AD patients. The evidence suggests not that there is a fundamentally different pathogenic mechanism for $\epsilon 4$-positive AD patients compared to $\epsilon 4$-negative AD patients but rather that there is a difference in the distribution of the rate (age) of developing disease (onset) in the population (Roses 1994, 1995). Other dementing diseases (in patients who are not pathologically confirmed as having AD) would not be expected to have the same age-of-onset distribution curves (see figure 4.1).

Thus, one important benefit of APOE genotyping that has not yet been widely perceived or discussed is the accuracy of interpretation of data from therapeutic trials. Patients with early-onset and a rare form of autosomal-dominant AD mutation (such as APP, PS1, or PS2) would be excluded from most clinical trials. However, when non-AD patients make up more than 10–

54   The Genetics of Alzheimer Disease

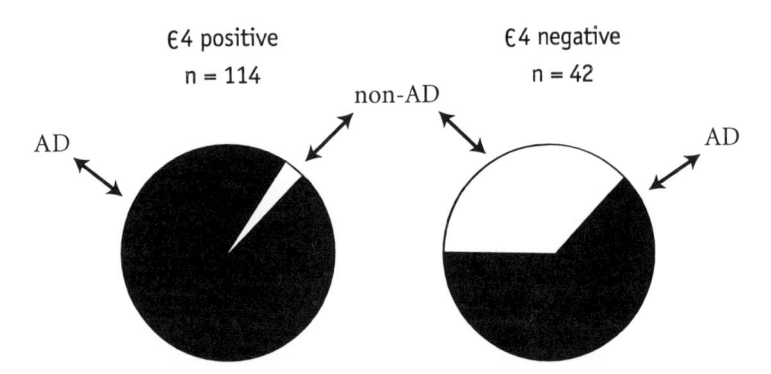

ε4 positive
n = 114

ε4 negative
n = 42

non-AD

AD

AD

Figure 4.2. Example of ε4 distribution between Alzheimer disease (AD) and non-Alzheimer disease patients. The data, from the CERAD study of 156 subjects (Welsh-Bohmer 1996), demonstrate the positive predictive value of ε4 for AD and the concentration of non-AD patients in the ε4 negative group.

40 percent of any clinical trial, it is useful to be able to distribute most of the non-AD patients into a single, identifiable treatment group prospectively, even if that group also includes authentic ε4-negative AD patients (see figure 4.2).

Gene-Environment Interactions

Once a particular susceptibility locus is identified for any disease, it becomes possible to study the myriad of specific environmental effects. With regard to APOE genotypes, there are now several initial studies of APOE genotyping and head injury, intracerebral hemorrhage, and general cardiac bypass anesthesia. The APOE genotype appears to be related to efficient and effective response to environmental stresses.

Epidemiological studies have identified age and head injury as two risk factors for AD. The epidemiologic data of Mayeux and colleagues (1995) suggest that head injury and carrying the ε4 allele are synergistic factors. The risk for AD was reported to be greater by an order of magnitude in the presence of both factors compared with either factor alone. Nicoll, Roberts, and Graham (1995) published a fascinating pathologic study of severely head-injured patients. The criteria for entry into that study included head injury, coma, and death within thirty days. They examined the patients for the appearance of large amounts of cerebral amyloid deposition and divided the patients into two groups: those with and those without heavy deposition of amyloid. The group with heavy amyloid deposition had a very high ε4 allele frequency (0.78) compared with the other group (0.15). The authors concluded from these data that deposition of amyloid was related to the etiology of AD. The data of Nicoll, Roberts, and Graham were reexamined, and it was noted that the group with the heavy amyloid formation had a mean age of fifty-eight years, while the mean age of the other group was twenty-eight years (Roses and Saunders 1995). There were two obvious explanations for this age difference: (1) the older patients without an ε4 allele did not get into accidents and had no head injuries, or (2) older patients without an ε4 allele did not qualify for entry into the study because they did not die.

To test the hypothesis that carrying an ε4 allele is associated with a less effective and less efficient response to brain trauma, Alberts and colleagues (1995) examined death and functional recovery in a consecutive series of patients with spontaneous intracerebral hemorrhage (ICH). As a general rule, approximately 50 percent of patients with ICH die within thirty days of hospital admission. The ε3/ε3 and ε3/ε4 groups had sufficient numbers of ICH patients to compare. The death rate was 70 percent for the ε3/ε4 patients and 30 percent for the ε3/ε3 patients. In the ε3/ε4 patients who survived, the mean neurological functional recovery was in the severely handicapped range. The ε3/ε3 patients recovered more neurological function, to the mildly handicapped but functional range. These data are consistent with the interpretation that carrying an ε4 allele negatively affects clinical response to severe brain injury.

Tardiff and colleagues (1994) examined a series of patients who were scheduled to undergo elective cardiac bypass surgery (Newman et al. 1995). These patients agreed to undergo neuropsychological testing preoperatively and at intervals postoperatively. It is possible to provide quantitative scales for each of the neuropsychological domains. The patients generally functioned normally preoperatively and postoperatively. At six weeks after surgery, although several of the quantitative neuropsychological scales had a normal mean, the standard deviations were much greater than those of the same tests preoperatively. When the APOE genotype data were factored into the analyses, there were statistically significant differences in the recovery of ε4 carriers. The data accounting for the slightly lowered scores, and the increased standard deviations came from the ε4 carriers. Thus, carrying an ε4 allele may negatively affect recovery from anesthesia in coronary bypass. Several additional studies are under way testing the relationship of symptoms after other milder brain stress, such as concussion or anesthesia without coronary bypass.

Research Methodology

Genetic Strategies

The search for susceptibility genes for common complex diseases has become a hot area for genetics in academe and industry (Lander and Schork 1994). Genomics companies have concentrated on high throughput genotyping methods and attempts to corner the clinical resources for particular diseases. The current methods being used have to date resulted in more venture capital investment than discoveries of susceptibility loci. Alzheimer disease is still the only major disease for which positional candidate strategies have resulted in the association of a complex disease with commonly occurring polymorphisms (APOE, in the case of AD). Subsequent studies used the same linkage methods and identified significant linkage of the angiotensinogen-gene locus to essential hypertension (Caulfield et al. 1994). The breast cancer (and other associated cancers) genes BRCA1 and BRCA2 represent mutations that occur in susceptibility loci. Other studies in many common diseases, such as diabetes mellitus, Parkinson disease, multiple sclerosis, and autism, are under way.

The main limitation for any linkage study is the availability of accurately diagnosed patients and families for genetic linkage studies. Two main avenues are being pursued for identifying susceptibility genes. The discovery of the chromosome 19 linkage of AD used multiple large families of complex structure for screening. Affected-relative-pair approaches were used to identify the region of chromosome 19 linkage (Pericak-Vance et al. 1991; Weeks and Lange 1988). Considerable progress has been made refining sib-pair approaches to be able to use more accessible family samples (Lander and Schork 1994).

Methods of rapid genotyping have been developed so that a genomic screen can take weeks instead of years. Genomic biotech companies have been formed to map human disease genes, but the studies require the ability to collect well-characterized patients and DNA samples. The most pressing academic as well as commercial need is the support of clinical studies. Without DNA samples, there is nothing to screen. Every genomic company, despite impressive abilities to perform the mechanics of a full genomic screen rapidly, identifies the shortage of high-quality clinical material and DNA samples as the limiting factor for success.

The literature has been active with reports of other genetic susceptibility associations with AD. Candidate genes have been tested, including antichymotrypsin (ACT), very low density lipoprotein (VLDL), an intronic polymorphism of the PS1 gene, and others (Kamboh et al. 1995; Okuizumi et al. 1995; Wragg, Hutton, and Talbot 1996). To date there have been no consistent confirmations of any of these loci (Haines et al. 1996; Pritchard et al. 1996). An ongoing strategy is to look for additional susceptibility loci in the group of AD families that originally identified the chromosome 19 linkage (Pericak-Vance et al. 1995; Pericak-Vance et al. 1996). Collaborative studies with another large series are under way (Pericak-Vance et al. 1997).

After the Genes Are Discovered

Every week a new mutated gene for a disease is identified in the literature. Although APOE was found almost four years ago, there has been much slower progress in defining susceptibility polymorphisms for complex diseases. Identification of additional susceptibility genes may be reasonably expected during the next few years. What happens after the gene is found?

A major problem in determining the mechanism with which the disease develops is partly scientific and partly organizational (Roses 1996b). There has been a tacit assumption that once a genetic defect was found, there would be instant recognition of the relevant metabolic pathogenesis. Many newly discovered genes were previously unknown, and upon identification it becomes necessary to characterize the protein and its potential functions. Many of the discovery laboratories are skilled in molecular genetics but less so in protein biochemistry and cell biology. The molecular probes and tools may not be readily available or shared, frequently due to commercial considerations. In the academic arena, few support resources are available to take maximal multidisciplinary advantage of new discoveries. If any area has been disappointing, it is the elucidation of disease mechanisms based on the relevant genetic mutations (Roses 1996b).

In the case of APOE, an entirely new insight into the role of apoE in neurobiology has developed, so principles that were assumed from lipid metabolism outside the blood-brain barrier are not necessarily descriptive of the role of apoE in the brain (Roses 1995b). As the anatomy of the human genome is filled in, biochemistry and cell biology will become dominant areas of discovery.

Public Perceptions and Attitudes

The public attitude toward AD can be assessed from documents generated by the Alzheimer's Association. By and large the two major concerns are obvious: (1) a public desire for effective treatments or preventives; and (2) strategies for relief from the horrible plight of patients' families and other caregivers resulting from the long-term morbidity of AD. Patient advocacy groups have taken a more aggressive stand on APOE "testing" than the medical genetics community. There are multiple examples of patient advocates insisting that predictive testing be available, without a clear understanding of the limitations of "testing." The lay press and expert commentators have inconsistently made the distinction between the use of APOE genotyping for predicting normal individuals and its use as an adjunct in the diagnosis of symptomatic patients.

The genetics community has also contributed to the confusion. The highly publicized "Statement on the Use of APOE Testing" in the *Journal of the American Medical Association* made little distinction between use in prediction and diagnosis (American College of Medical Genetics 1995). The statement was incompletely referenced and was unbalanced in the relative weight given to published studies. A consensus conference held in October 1995, which included clinicians, geneticists, lawyers, ethicists, genetic counselors, anthropologists, patient advocacy groups, and other scientific and government observers, provided a broader view (Relkin and National Institute on Aging 1996). As is often the case, the first published statement precluded widespread press coverage of the second — old news to journalists. Experimental data on specificity and sensitivity in large autopsy-confirmed series had yet to be generated, so the diagnostic uncertainty of clinical series was amplified (Saunders et al. 1996). The field of AD gives the outward appearance of uncertainty and conflicting messages.

A patent for APOE genotyping in the diagnosis of AD has been issued to Duke University Medical Center and licensed exclusively to Athena Neurosciences. The use of the test is limited by Athena Neurosciences to patients with cognitive impairment. Although it is impossible to completely control clinical applications by physicians, Athena Neurosciences requires that the ordering physician sign a statement confirming that the sample for testing is from a cognitively impaired patient. The ethical and legal ramifications of abuse would then fall on the physician who inappropriately ordered the test for prediction. Thus, contrary to the inferences in the lay literature, the exclusive licensee provides testing only in the context of the diagnosis of cognitively impaired patients. Recent data on specificity and sensitivity, and studies currently in progress, will provide useful confidence limits for interpretations of APOE genotyping in clinical situations (Saunders et al. 1996).

References

Alberts, M. J., Graffagnino, C., McClenny, C., DeLong, D., Strittmatter, W., Saunders, A. M., and Roses, A. D. 1995. ApoE genotype and survival from intracerebral hemorrhage. *Lancet* 346:575.

Alzheimer's Disease Collaborative Group. 1993. Apolipoprotein E genotype and Alzheimer's disease. *Lancet* 342:737-38.

American College of Medical Genetics/American Society of Human Genetics Working Group on ApoE and Alzheimer Disease. 1995. Statement on use of apolipoprotein E testing for Alzheimer disease. *JAMA* 274:1627-29.

Amouyel, P., Brousseau, T., Fruchart, J. C., and Dallongeville, J. 1993. Apolipoprotein E ε4 allele and Alzheimer's disease. *Lancet* 342:1309.

Anwar, N., Lovestone, S., Cheetham, M. E., Levy, R., and Powell, F. 1993. Apolipoprotein E ε4 allele and Alzheimer's disease. *Lancet* 342:1308-9.

Basun, H., Grut, M., Winblad, B., and Lannfelt, L. 1995. Apolipoprotein ε4 allele and disease progression in patients with late-onset Alzheimer's disease. *Neuroscience Letters* 183:32-34.

Bird, T. D. 1995. Apolipoprotein E genotyping in the diagnosis of Alzheimer's disease: A cautionary view. *Annals of Neurology* 38:2-3.

Borgaonkar, D. S., Schmidt, L. C., Martin, S. E., Edelsohn, L., Growdon, J., and Farrer, L. A. 1993. Linkage of late-onset Alzheimer's disease with apolipoprotein E type 4 on chromosome 19. *Lancet* 342:625.

Breitner, J. C. S. 1996. APOE genotyping and Alzheimer's disease. *Lancet* 347:1184-85.

Caulfield, M., Lavender, P., Farrall, M., Lawson, M., Turner, P., and Clark, A. J. 1994. Linkage of the angiotensinogen gene to essential hypertension. *New England Journal of Medicine* 330:1629-33.

Corder, E. H., Saunders, A. M., Risch, N. J., Strittmatter, W. J., Schmechel, D. E., Gaskell, P. C., Rimmler, J. B., Locke, P. A., Conneally, P. M., and Schmader, K. E. 1994. Protective effect of apolipoprotein E type 2 allele for late onset Alzheimer disease. *Nature Genetics* 7:180-84.

Corder, E. H., Saunders, A. M., Strittmatter, W. J., Schmechel, D. E., Gaskell, P. C., Small, G. W., Roses, A. D., Haines, J. L., and Pericak-Vance, M. A. 1993. Gene dose of apolipoprotein E type 4 allele and the risk of Alzheimer's disease in late onset families. *Science* 261:921-23.

Czech, C., Monning, V., Tienari, P. J., Hartmann, T., Masters, C., and Beyreuther, K. 1993. Apolipoprotein E ε4 allele and Alzheimer's disease. *Lancet* 342:1309.

Elston, R. C., and Johnson, W. D. 1994. *Essentials of biostatistics.* Philadelphia: F. A. Davis.

Galasko, D., Hansen, L. A., Katzman, R., Wiederholt, W., Masliah, E., Terry, R., Hill, L. R., Lessin, P., and Thal, L. J. 1994. Clinical-neuropathological correlations in Alzheimer's disease and related dementias. *Archives of Neurology* 51:888-95.

Goate, A., Chartier-Harlin, M. C., Mullan, M., Brown, J., Crawford, F., Fidani, L., Giuffra, L., Haynes, A., Irving, N., and James, L. 1991. Segregation of a missense mutation in the amyloid precursor protein gene with familial Alzheimer's disease. *Nature* 349:704-6.

Haines, J. L., Pritchard, M. L., Saunders, A. M., Schildkraut, J. M., Growden, J. H., Gaskell, P. C., Farrer, L. A., Auerbach, S. A., Gusella, J. F., Locke, P. A., Rosi, B. L., Yamaoka, L., Small, G. W., Conneally, P. M., Roses, A. D., and Pericak-Vance, M. A. 1996. No genetic effect of alpha(1)-antichymotrypsin in Alzheimer disease. *Genomics* 33:53-56.

Houlden, H., Crook, R., Hardy, J., Roques, P., Collinge, J., and Rossor, M. 1994. Confirmation that familial clustering and age of onset in late onset Alzheimer's disease are determined at the apolipoprotein locus. *Neuroscience Letters* 174:222–24.

Itabashi, S., Arai, H., Higuchi, S., Sasaki, H., and Trojanowska, J. Q. 1996. APOE ε4 allele in Alzheimer's and non-Alzheimer's dementia. *Lancet* 348:960–61.

Kakulas, B. A., and Wilton, S. D. 1996. Apolipoprotein-E genotyping in the diagnosis of Alzheimer's disease in an autopsy-confirmed series. *Lancet* 348:483.

Kamboh, M. I., Sanghera, D. K., Ferrell, D. K., and DeKosky, S. T. 1995. APOE*4-associated Alzheimer's disease risk is modified by alpha 1-antichymotrypsin polymorphism. *Nature Genetics* 10:486–88.

Khachaturian, Z. S. 1985. Diagnosis of Alzheimer's disease. *Archives of Neurology* 42:1097–1105.

Lander, E. S., and Schork, N. J. 1994. Genetic dissection of complex traits. *Science* 265:2037–48. Published erratum appears in *Science* 266:353.

Lannfelt, L., Lilius, L., Nastase, M., Viitanen, M., Fratiglioni, L., Eggertsen, G., Berglund, L., Angelin, B., Linder, J., and Winblad, B. 1994. Lack of association between apolipoprotein E allele ε4 and sporadic Alzheimer's disease. *Neuroscience Letters* 169:175–78.

Levy-Lahad, E., Wasco, W., Poorkaj, P., Romano, D. M. J., Oshima, J., Pettingell, W. H., Yu, C. E., Jondro, P. D., Schmidt, S. D., Kang, K., and Wang, K. 1995. Candidate gene for the chromosome 1 familial Alzheimer's disease locus. *Science* 269:973–77.

Levy-Lahad, E., Wijsman, E. M., Nemens, E., Anderson, L., Goddard, K. A., Wever, J. L., Bird, T. D., and Schellenberg, G. D. 1995. A familial Alzheimer's disease locus on chromosome 1. *Science* 269:970–73.

Lucotte, G., and Aouizerate, A. 1995. Allele doses of apolipoprotein E type ε4 in sporadic late-onset Alzheimer's disease. *American Journal of Medical Genetics* 60:566–69.

Maestre, G., Ottman, R., Stern, Y., Gurland, B., Chun, M., Tang, M. X., Shelanski, M., Tycko, B., and Mayeux, R. 1995. Apolipoprotein E and Alzheimer's disease: Ethnic variation in genotypic risks. *Annals of Neurology* 37:254–59.

Martin, J. B. 1993. Molecular genetics in neurology. *Annals of Neurology* 34:757–73.

Marx, J. 1993. New Alzheimer's theory stirs controversy. *Science* 262:1210–11.

Mayeux, R., Ottman, R., Maestre, G., Ngai, C., Tang, M. X., Ginsberg, H., Chun, M., Tycko, B., and Shelanski, M. 1995. Synergistic effects of traumatic head injury and apolipoprotein ε4 in patients with Alzheimer's disease. *Neurology* 45:555–57.

Mayeux, R., Stern, Y., Ottman, R., Tatemichi, T. K., Tang, M. X., Maestre, G., Ngai, C., Tycko, B., and Ginsberg, H. 1993. The apolipoprotein ε4 allele in patients with Alzheimer's disease. *Annals of Neurology* 34:752–54.

Mayieux, F., and Couderc, R. 1995. Isoform 4 of apolipoprotein E and Alzheimer disease: Specificity and clinical study (in French). *Rev Neurol* (Paris) 151:231–39.

McKhann, G., Drachman, D., Folstein, M., Katzman, R., Price, D., and Stadlan, E. M. 1984. Clinical diagnosis of Alzheimer's disease: Report of the NINDS-ADRDA Work Group under the auspices of Department of Health and Human Services Task Force on Alzheimer's Disease. *Neurology* 34:939–44.

Mirra, S. S., Heyman, A., McKeel, D., Sumi, S. M., Crain, B. J., Brownlee, L. M., Vogel, F. S.,

Hughs, J. P., van Belle, G., Berg, L. 1991. Consortium to Establish a Registry for Alzheimer's Disease (CERAD). Part 2, Standardization of the neuropathologic assessment of Alzheimer's disease. *Neurology* 41:479–86.

Myers, R. H., Schaefer, E. J., Wilson, P. W., D'Agostino, R., Ordovas, J. M., Espino, A., Au, R., White, R. F., Knoefel, J. E., Cobb, J. L., McNulty, K. A., Beiser, A., and Wolf, P. A. 1996. Apolipoprotein E ϵ4 association with dementia in a population-based study: The Framingham study. *Neurology* 46:673–77.

Nalbantoglu, J., Gilfix, B. M., Bertrand, P., Robitaille, Y., and Gauthier, S. 1994. Predictive value of apolipoprotein E genotyping in Alzheimer's disease: Results of an autopsy series and an analysis of several combined studies. *Annals of Neurology* 36:889–95.

Newman, M. F., Croughwell, N. D., Blumenthal, J. A., Lowry, E., White, W. D., Spillane, W., Davis, R. D., Glower, D. D., Smith, L. R., and Mahanna, E. P. 1995. Predictors of cognitive decline after cardiac operation. *Annals of Thoracic Surgery* 59:1326–30.

Nicoll, J. A., Roberts, G. W., and Graham, D. I. 1995. Apolipoprotein E ϵ4 allele is associated with deposition of amyloid beta-protein following head injury. *Nature Medicine* 1:135–37.

Noguchi, S., Murakami, K., and Yamada, N. 1993. Apolipoprotein E genotype and Alzheimer's disease. *Lancet* 342:737.

Okuizumi, K., Onodera, O., Namba, Y., Ikeda, K., Tamamoto, T., Seki, K., Ueka, A., Nanko, S., Tanaka, H., and Takahashi, H. 1995. Genetic association of the very low density lipoprotein (VLDL) receptor gene with sporadic Alzheimer's disease. *Nature Genetics* 11:207–9.

Okuizumi, K., Onodera, O., Tanaka, H., Kobayashi, H., Tsuji, S., Takahashi, H., Oyanagi, K., Seki, K., Tanaka, M., and Naruse, S. 1994. ApoE ϵ4 and early-onset Alzheimer's. *Nature Genetics* 7:10–11.

Payami, H., Kaye, J., Heston, L. L., Bird, T. D., and Schellenberg, G. D. 1993. Apolipoprotein E genotype and Alzheimer's disease. *Lancet* 342:738.

Pericak-Vance, M. A., Bass, M. P., Yamaoka, L. H., Gaskell, P. C., Scott, W. K., Terwedow, H. A., Menold, M. M., Conneally, P. M., Small, G. W., Vance, J. M., Saunders, A. M., Roses, A. D., and Haines, J. L. 1997. Complete genomic screen in late-onset familial Alzheimer disease: Evidence for a new focus on chromosome 12. *JAMA* (in press).

Pericak-Vance, M. A., Bebout, J. L., Gaskell, P. C., Yamaoka, L. H., Hung, W. Y., Alberts, M. J., Walker, A. P., Bartlett, R. J., Haynes, C. A., and Welsh, K. A. 1991. Linkage studies in familial Alzheimer disease: Evidence for chromosome 19 linkage. *American Journal of Human Genetics* 48:1034–50.

Pericak-Vance, M. A., Conneally, P. M., Small, G. W., Saunders, A. M., Yamaoka, L., Gaskell, P. C., Robinson, M., Terminassian, M., Locke, P. A., Pritchard, M., Haynes, C. S., Growdon, J. F., and Gusella, J. F. 1995. The search for additional Alzheimer disease (AD) genes. In *Apolipoprotein E and Alzheimer disease,* ed. A. D. Roses, K. Weisgraber, and Y. Cristen, 180–86. Berlin: Springer-Verlag.

Pericak-Vance, M. A., Johnson, C. C., Rimmler, J. B., Saunders, A. M., Robinson, L. C., D'Hondt, E. G., Jackson, C. E., and Haines, J. L. 1996. Alzheimer's disease and apolipoprotein ϵ4 allele in an Amish population. *Annals of Neurology* 39:700–704.

Pericak-Vance, M. A., Yamaoka, L. H., Haynes, C. S., Speer, M. C., Haines, J. L., Gaskell, P. C., Hung, W. Y., Clark, C. M., Heyman, A. L., and Trofatter, J. A. 1988. Genetic linkage studies in Alzheimer's disease families. *Journal of Experimental Neurology* 102:271-79.

Poirier, J., Davignon, J., Bouthiller, D., Kogan, S., Bertrand, P., and Gauthier, S. 1993. Apolipoprotein E polymorphism and Alzheimer's disease. *Lancet* 342:697-99.

Poirier, J., Delisle, M. C., Quirion, R., Aubert, I., Farlow, M., Lahiri, D., Hui, S., Bertrand, P., Nalbantoglu, J., and Gilfix, B. M. 1995. Apolipoprotein E4 allele as a predictor of cholinergic deficits and treatment outcome in Alzheimer disease. *Proceedings of the National Academy of Sciences* 92:12260-64.

Polvikoski, T., Sulkava, R., Haltia, M., Kainulainen, K., Vuorio, A., Verkkoniemi, A., Niinisto, L., Halonen, P., and Kontula, K. 1995. Apolipoprotein E, dementia, and cortical deposition of beta-amyloid protein. *New England Journal of Medicine* 333:1242-47.

Pritchard, M. L., Saunders, A. M., Gaskell, P. C., Small, G. W., Conneally, P. M., Rosi, B., Yamaoka, L. H., Roses, A. D., Haines, J. L., and Pericak-Vance, M. A. 1996. No association between very low density lipoprotein receptor (VLDL-R) and Alzheimer disease in American Caucasians. *Neuroscience Letters* 209:105-8.

Rebeck, G. W., Reiter, J. S., Strickland, D. K., and Hyman, B. T. 1993. Apolipoprotein E in sporadic Alzheimer's disease: Allelic variation and receptor interactions. *Neuron* 11:575-80.

Reiman, E. M., Caselli, R. J., Yun, L. S., Chen, K., Bandy, D., Minoshima, S., Thibodeau, S. N., and Osborne, D. 1996. Preclinical evidence of Alzheimer's disease in persons homozygous for the ε4 allele for apolipoprotein E. *New England Journal of Medicine* 334:752-58.

Relkin, N. R., and National Institute on Aging/Alzheimer's Association Working Group. 1996. Apolipoprotein E genotyping in Alzheimer's disease. *Lancet* 347:1091-95.

Rogaev, E., Sherrington, R., Rogaeva, E. A., Levesque, G., Ikeda, M., Liang, Y., Chi, H., Lin, C., Holman, K., Tsuda, T., Mar, L., Sorbi, S., Nacmias, B., Piacentini, S., Amaducci, L., Chumakov, I., Cohen, D., Lannfelt, L., Fraser, P. E., Rommens, J. M., and St. George-Hyslop, P. H. 1995. Familial Alzheimer's disease in kindreds with missense mutations in a novel gene on chromosome 1 related to the Alzheimer's disease type 3 gene. *Nature* 376:776-78.

Roses, A. D. 1994. Apolipoprotein E affects the rate of Alzheimer disease expression: Beta-amyloid burden is a secondary consequence dependent on APOE genotype and duration of disease. *Journal of Neuropathology and Experimental Neurology* 53:429-37.

———. 1995a. Apolipoprotein E genotyping in differential diagnosis, not prediction, of Alzheimer's disease. *Annals of Neurology* 38:6-14.

———. 1995b. Perspective: On the metabolism of apolipoprotein E and the Alzheimer diseases. *Journal of Experimental Neurology* 132:149-56.

———. 1996a. Apolipoprotein E alleles as risk factors in Alzheimer disease. *Annual Review of Medicine* 47:387-400.

———. 1996b. From genes to mechanisms to therapies: Lessons to be learned from neurological disorders. *Nature Medicine* 2:267-269.

Roses, A. D., and Devlin, B. 1995. Measuring the genetic contribution of APOE in late onset Alzheimer disease. *American Journal of Human Genetics* 57:A202.

Roses, A. D., and Pericak-Vance, M. A. 1996. Alzheimer's disease and other dementias. In

Emery and Rimoin's principles and practice of medical genetics, ed. D. L. Rimoin, J. M. Connor, and R. E. Pyeritz, 1807–25. New York: Churchill Livingstone Publishing.

Roses, A. D., and Saunders, A. M. 1995. Head injury, amyloid, and Alzheimer's disease. *Nature Medicine* 1:603–4.

Roses, A. D., Strittmatter, W. J., Pericak-Vance, M. A., Corder, E. H., Saunders, A. M., and Schmechel, D. E. 1994. Clinical application of apolipoprotein E genotyping to Alzheimer's disease. *Lancet* 343:1564–65.

Saunders, A. M., Hulette, C., Welsh-Bohmer, K. A., Schmechel, D. E., Cain, B., Burke, J. R., Alberts, M. J., Strittmatter, W. J., Breitner, J. C. S., Rosenberg, C., Scott, S. V., Gaskell, P. C., Pericak-Vance, M. A., and Roses, A. D. 1996. Specificity, sensitivity, and predictive value of apolipoprotein E genotyping in a consecutive autopsy series of sporadic Alzheimer disease. *Lancet* 348:90–93.

Saunders, A. M., Schmader, K., Breitner, J. C., Benson, M. D., Brown, W. T., Goldfarb, L., Goldgaber, D., Manwaring, M. G., Szymanski, M. H., and McCown, N. 1993. Apolipoprotein E ε4 allele distributions in late-onset Alzheimer's disease and in other amyloid-forming diseases. *Lancet* 342:710–11.

Saunders, A. M., Strittmatter, W. J., Schmechel, D., St. George- Hyslop, P. H., Pericak-Vance, M. A., Joo, S. H., Rosi, B. L., Gusella, J. F., Crapper-MacLachlan, D. R., and Alberts, M. J. 1993. Association of apolipoprotein E allele ε4 with late-onset familial and sporadic Alzheimer's disease. *Neurology* 43:1467–72.

Sclkoc, D. J. 1994. Alzheimer's disease: A central role for amyloid. *Journal of Neuropathology and Experimental Neurology* 53:438–47.

Seshadri, S., Drachman, D. A., and Lippa, C. F. 1995. Apolipoprotein E ε4 allele and the lifetime risk of Alzheimer's disease: What physicians know, and what they should know. *Archives of Neurology* 52:1074–79.

Sherrington, R., Rogaev, E. I., Liang, Y., Rogaeva, E. A., Levesque, G., Ikeda, M., Chi, H., Li, G., and Holman, K. 1995. Cloning of a gene bearing missense mutations in early-onset familial Alzheimer's disease. *Nature* 375:754–60.

Small, G. W., Mazziotta, J. C., Collins, M. T., Baxter, L. R., Phelps, M. E., Mandelkern, M. A., Kaplan, A., LaRue, A., Adamson, C. F., and Chang, L. 1995. Apolipoprotein E type 4 allele and cerebral glucose metabolism in relatives at risk for familial Alzheimer disease. *JAMA* 273:942–47.

Smith, A. D., Jobst, K. A., Johnston, C., Joachim, C., and Nagy, Z. 1996. Apolipoprotein-E genotyping in diagnosis of Alzheimer's disease. *Lancet* 348:483–84.

Sorbi, S., Nacmias, B., Forleo, P., Piacentini, S., Latorraca, S., and Amaducci, L. 1995. Epistatic effect of APP717 mutation and apolipoprotein E genotype in familial Alzheimer's disease. *Annals of Neurology* 38:124–27.

St. George-Hyslop, P. H., McLachlan, D. C., Tsuda, T., Rogaev, E., Karlinsky, H., Lippa, C. F., and Pollen, D. 1994. Alzheimer's disease and possible gene interaction. *Science* 263:537.

St. George-Hyslop, P. H., Tanzi, R. E., Polinsky, R. J., Haines, J. L., Nee, L., Watkins, P. C., Myers, R. H., Feldman, R. G., Pollen, D., Drachman, D., et al. 1987. The genetic defect causing familial Alzheimer's disease maps on chromosome 21. *Science* 235:885–90.

Strittmatter, W. J., Saunders, A. M., Schmechel, D., Pericak- Vance, M., Enghild, J., Salvesen,

G. S., and Roses, A. D. 1993. Apolipoprotein E: High-avidity binding to beta-amyloid and increased frequency of type 4 allele in late-onset familial Alzheimer disease. *Proceedings of the National Academy of Sciences* 90:1977–81.

Tardiff, B., Newman, M., Saunders, A., Strittmatter, W., Smith, L. R., Roses, A., and Reves, J. G. 1994. Apolipoprotein E allele frequency in patients with cognitive defects following cardiopulmonary bypass. *Circulation* 90:1–201.

Terry, R. D. 1994. Neuropathological changes in Alzheimer disease. *Progress in Brain Research* 101:383–90.

Ueda, K., Fukushima, H., Masliah, E., Xia, Y., Iwai, A., Yoshimoto, M., Otero, D. A., Kondo, J., Ihara, Y., and Sautoh, T. 1993. Molecular cloning of cDNA encoding an unrecognized component of amyloid in Alzheimer disease. *Proceedings of the National Academy of Sciences* 90:11282–86.

Ueki, A., and Kawano, M. 1993. A high frequency of apolipoprotein E4 isoprotein in Japanese patients with late-onset nonfamilial Alzheimer's disease. *Neuroscience Letters* 163:166–68.

van Duijn, C. M., de Knijff, P., Cruts, M., Wehnert, A., Havekas, L. M., Hofman, A., and Van Broeckhoven, C. 1994. Apolipoprotein E4 allele in a population-based study of early-onset Alzheimer's disease. *Nature Genetics* 7:74–78.

Weeks, D. E., and Lange, K. 1988. The affected-pedigree-member method of linkage analysis. *American Journal of Human Genetics* 42:315–26.

Welsh-Bohmer, K. A., Gearing, M., Saunders, A. M., Roses, A. D., and Mirra, S. 1997. Apolipoprotein E genotypes in a neuropathological series from the Consortium to Establish a Registry for Alzheimer's Disease (CERAD). *Annals of Neurology* (in press).

Wilson, P. W. F., Myers, R. H., Larson, M. G., Ordovas, J. M., Wolf, P. A., and Schaefer, E. J. 1994. Apolipoprotein E alleles, dyslipidemia, and coronary heart disease: The Framingham offspring study. *JAMA* 272:1666–71.

Wragg, M., Hutton, M., and Talbot, C. 1996. Genetic association between intronic polymorphism in presenilin-1 gene and late-onset Alzheimer's disease. *Lancet* 347:509–12.

Yoshizawa, T., Yamakawa-Kobayashi, K., Komatsuzaki, Y., Arinami, T., Oguni, E., Mizusawa, H., Shoji, S., and Hamaguchi, H. 1994. Dose-dependent association of apolipoprotein E allele epsilon 4 with late-onset, sporadic Alzheimer's disease. *Annals of Neurology* 36:656–59.

Therapeutic Interventions in Alzheimer Disease
Implications of Genetic Advances

PETER J. WHITEHOUSE, M.D., PH.D.

Genetic discoveries in Alzheimer disease (AD) have profound implications for improving the quality of life of patients with dementia (Selkoe 1996). Exploration of these opportunities has focused principally on improving predictive and diagnostic testing as a result of the identification of specific genetic lesions and susceptibility factors (Brodaty and Medical and Scientific Advisory Committee 1995; Mayeux and Schupf 1995; National Institute on Aging/Alzheimer's Association Working Group 1996; Post et al. 1997; Roses 1995). Early detection and more accurate diagnosis will have implications for initiating treatment. However, there are other important therapeutic implications of these genetic discoveries for patients affected by AD and related degenerative dementias. This chapter reviews links between genetic advances and potential therapeutic interventions. Such links include the potential use of genetic knowledge to improve diagnosis, predict therapeutic responsiveness, and suggest avenues to develop new drugs. Moreover, to the extent that a genetic test might identify at-risk individuals or those in early stages, the availability of effective therapies influences individuals' decisions to take the test or not.

To understand the implications of the genetic work for research in therapeutics, we first consider a framework for conceptualizing the development of more effective biological interventions, starting with consideration of treatment goals. Second, we specifically explore the implications of genetic work for therapies. For example, can the genotype for apolipoprotein E (APOE) predict responsiveness to currently available therapy, and what are the possibilities based on genetic knowledge for developing potentially more effective disease-course-altering therapies in the future? We conclude by celebrating the power of the genetic knowledge, recognizing that the challenges for successful application in clinical practice are considerable. It is important that we do not create unrealistic expectations for success but at the same time are responsible in maintaining hope.

Therapeutic Goals

At first glance the therapeutic goals in AD and related dementias appear simple, that is, to improve the cognitive impairment from which the patient is suffering. However, as one explores in greater detail what one is trying to accomplish with drug treatment, particularly how to develop clinical trials to demonstrate these effects, the need for more careful exploration of the goals of therapeutic interventions becomes apparent. This recognition led to the establishment of the Therapeutic Goals Project of the Department of Health and Human Services's National Alzheimer's Advisory Board Panel, for example.

This group has developed a conceptual framework that recognizes several broad dimensions to goal setting. First, although we tend to focus on cognitive disability as the principal problem in dementia, the noncognitive or behavioral symptoms are also important. These symptoms include agitation, hallucination, delusions, and affective dysfunction. Thus, drugs may be targeted to improve either cognitive or behavioral symptoms or, potentially, both. Second, we recognize that our goal is not just to improve clinician's ratings of symptoms but also to have a more profound impact on the patient's daily life. We would like interventions that improve activities of daily living and quality of life. The concept of quality of life has been important in the development of drugs in other fields (for example, antihypertensive medications). In AD research today, drug studies include quality-of-life measures, although there are complex conceptual and methodological issues surrounding assessment of quality of life in dementia (Whitehouse and Rabins 1992).

Quality of life includes a number of different objectively assessable aspects, including cognitive and behavioral function, social relationships, and financial status (Lawton 1994). However, quality-of-life assessment also includes a subjective judgment about the subject's personal sense of well-being (Whitehouse 1997). In AD the patients' ability to make judgments about quality of life are often impaired, requiring either observational or caregiver ratings of quality of life to complement self-ratings. Individual patients vary in memory, communication, and judgment skills as well as degree of insight into the nature of their condition (Patterson et al. 1996). Deficits in any of these areas of thinking can create difficulties for patients in assessing their own quality of life.

Quality of life of the caregiver is also affected by the dementing process. Thus, drug and other interventions can have therapeutic goals that focus on caregiver stress and burden. Finally, at the level of social interests we must ask what will be the population benefits and costs of using new medications for patients with dementia. We are increasingly recognizing that health care resources are limited. Thus, we need to decide how much money can be spent on the care of dementia patients and how resources should be distributed among biological and psychosocial interventions across the often long course of the illness. Thus, health economics and specifically pharmacoeconomics are becoming increasingly important when we discuss therapeutic goals in AD.

Pharmacoeconomic studies of dementia are in an early stage of development (Whitehouse n.d.). It is becoming increasingly clear that models developed for acute illnesses of earlier life may not work with chronic progressive diseases like dementia. Traditional approaches such as cost-benefit and cost-utility analysis can be used. In cost-benefit analysis the costs of different interventions are compared with the benefits that they achieve, measured in dollars, often in terms of willingness to pay. In cost-utility analysis, the costs of interventions are compared with outcomes measured in terms of the perceived value of the outcome, as measured, for example, in quality-adjusted life years. In summary, one dimension of our conceptual framework of therapeutic goals is quality of life, which incorporates many of the symptoms and consequences of AD for patients, caregivers, and society.

Another dimension to the scheme for examining therapeutic goals is the severity of disease. We can now identify individuals at high risk for the disease through genetic means; thus, anticipation of the stages of AD can begin with a presymptomatic state. Most attention in research is focused on the patients with mild to moderate dementia who present to our academic centers as outpatients willing to participate in drug studies. At the neglected other end of the spectrum is the severely demented patient who can no longer recognize family members and provide any self-care. An examination of this phase of the disease leads to our consideration of whether AD is in fact terminal and whether the treatments offered during this period of the disease should be focused more on palliative care, perhaps adopting a hospice model (Post and Whitehouse 1998). Overly enthusiastic basic biological scientists and others may draw simplistic conclusions about therapeutic goals if they do not appropriately consider the stage of the disease. For example, do we want to slow the progression of the disease of a severely demented individual?

The stage of disease or severity of disease also correlates often with the site of care. Thus, patients with mild disease are more likely to be at home. Those with moderate disease are likely to participate in community services such as home and day care, and those with more severe dementia are often found in a variety of institutional settings, such as nursing homes or special care units. Therapeutic goals for biological interventions will depend in part on the other services offered in these particular locations of care.

Finally, the conceptual framework for therapeutic goals ought to include some traditional considerations of the nature, duration, and power of the biological interventions. We see medications that can prevent or cure the disease as more powerful than those that provide relief of symptoms. In the field of AD, scientists are conducting biological research, including genetic studies that allow us to conceptualize such profound interventions in the future. In the present, most of the drugs in late stages of clinical development and those that have already been approved around the world are designed to improve symptoms. For the remaining portion of this section on establishing therapeutic goals, we review short-term, intermediate, and long-term prospects for symptomatic and disease-course-altering effects of treatment.

Symptomatic Therapies

The symptoms of AD can be divided into two overlapping groups: cognitive and noncognitive. These categories overlap because phenomena such as attention and arousal and certainly executive functions such as judgment cannot easily be placed into either a cognitive or a noncognitive category (Patterson et al. 1996). However, most drug development has been focused on medications to address intellectual disabilities, primarily memory function. We consider first these cognitive symptoms and then the relatively neglected behavioral symptoms.

Cognition. Around the world a number of medications have been approved to alleviate the cognitive symptoms of older individuals suffering from intellectual decline. We focus exclusively on tacrine and donepezil, the only drugs approved in the United States and elsewhere for the treatment of cognitive symptoms in AD specifically.

Both tacrine (Warner Lambert Parke-Davis) and donepezil (Eisai/Pfizer) are cholinesterase inhibitors designed to increase the amount of acetylcholine in the brains of patients affected by dementia. These drugs were developed using a rational strategy based on an understanding of the cellular and neurochemical abnormalities in the brains of patients with AD that underlie the memory and attention problems (Whitehouse et al. 1982). Loss of cholinergic markers has been correlated with the severity of dementia, and cholinomimetic drugs have been shown to improve cognition in both humans and animals.

While tacrine was being developed, the Food and Drug Administration provided advice to pharmaceutical companies concerning guidelines for approval. In fact, draft FDA guidelines were developed with input from academics, industry, and caregivers (Leber 1990). These guidelines suggest that a drug should improve cognition on an objective psychometric test and have clinically meaningful efficacy. The measure of clinical meaningfulness is perhaps the most difficult and is usually either a clinical global impression of change (i.e., a clinician rates overall whether or not the patient is better) or an activities-of-daily-living scale. It is important to recognize, particularly for those who complain about the approval of tacrine, that the development of guidelines was an open process to which many contributed. The guidelines do not specify, however, how much improvement on either psychometric tests or clinical global scales would be necessary before the drug could be approved, nor do they specify how many patients of those treated with drugs must benefit. More international effort is needed to harmonize proposed regulatory guidelines for approval in different countries (Whitehouse et al. 1997).

Interpretations of the data on tacrine vary, of course. A fairly common view is that perhaps 20 percent of patients show a noticeable positive response to tacrine. Side effects limit the ability of some patients to achieve adequate doses. On average, patients show perhaps a two-point improvement on the Folstein Mini-Mental Scale (scores range from zero to thirty). Thus, some argue that on this scale the drug can lead to the same amount of improvement as the amount of deterioration that would occur in a typical patient in approximately six months of illness. However, it may be unwise to equate such similarities in magnitudes of effect size, because the drug does not delay clinical progression compared with placebo. The clinical global impression of change was also statistically significantly improved on active drug; hence, the drug met the preestablished criteria and was eventually approved.

In clinical practice, considerable controversy exists as to the usefulness of tacrine. My own view is that it is minimally effective in a modest number of patients. Our expectations were probably too high for the first drug approved in modern times for the particularly challenging therapeutic task of improving cognition in a disease in which nerve cells die.

In November 1996, donepezil was approved with the same standards as tacrine and having perhaps approximately the same efficacy but a pharmacology that makes the drug easier for physicians and patients to use. It can be administered once a day rather than four times a day and does not appear to have as many side effects as tacrine. This profile means that the patient can be started on a dose that may prove effective, whereas with tacrine one has to build up the dose slowly, and considerable time elapses before therapeutic doses are achieved.

Numerous other drugs are under development with the same kind of therapeutic target of improvement of cognitive symptoms by enhancing cholinergic mechanisms. Several other cholinesterase inhibitors are under development (a New Drug Application for ENA 713 from Novartis was submitted March 1997), as well as muscarinic cholinergic receptor agonists, which directly stimulate the postsynaptic neurons. The hope is to develop more effective medications that are more focused in their action on the cholinergic systems by stimulating certain specific receptors. It remains to be seen, however, whether these medications can provide a better ratio of symptomatic benefits to side effects.

How effective a drug should be before the FDA approves it and, perhaps more important, how good it should be before a health maintenance organization or a government pays for it are complex questions. It is clear that the regulatory decisions about AD drugs have been made in an open environment and with input from numerous groups.

A retrospective study of patients in a Phase III trial of tacrine has been done (Knopman et al. 1996), which has claimed more-profound effects. In this non-randomized follow-up study, patients who remained on tacrine after the trial was finished entered nursing homes approximately one year later than those who chose not to remain on the drug. However, once again, it is important to recognize that this study did not use a randomized assignment of patients.

Further studies of the effectiveness of both biological and psychosocial treatments for AD are needed using broader consideration of possible outcomes—for example, as milestones in the progression of the disease, such as quality of life and use of health services. Recently, the Alzheimer's Association and the Agency for Health Care Policy and Research (under the Department of Health and Human Services) sponsored a conference that for the first time systematically considered outcomes assessment approaches in AD and compared these techniques to those used in other fields (Whitehouse and Maslow n.d.).

Noncognitive Therapeutic Agents. Until recently, noncognitive or behavioral symptoms have been relatively neglected in academic studies of AD. For years clinicians have used psychoactive medications, such as antidepressants and tranquilizers approved for other conditions, to treat these symptoms in dementia. Only recently have we paid attention to the assessment of these symptoms and developed therapeutic trials to measure the effectiveness of drugs for the behavioral manifestations of dementia. These symptoms are important targets for treatment because they can be disturbing for patients and caregivers alike. New hope exists in this area of concern as well. New-generation antipsychotics such as risperidane, olanzepine, and sertindol offer the promise of efficacy with fewer side effects than current drugs, although adequate studies to justify their use are just now being completed. Moreover, some studies (Kaufer, Cummings, and Christine 1996) suggest that cholinomimetic drugs may improve some of these behavioral symptoms. Since patients with AD who have a family history of depression are more likely to become depressed during the course of their illness (Strauss and Ogrocki 1996), genetic markers for psychiatric symptoms might ultimately guide therapeutic treatments in AD.

Intermediate Goals: Slowing the Progression of Disease

Alzheimer disease is characterized pathologically by dysfunction and eventual death of nerve cells. Drugs designed to improve symptoms by enhancing the function of neurotransmitter function, such as cholinomimetic agents, are not likely to slow the degeneration or death of nerve cells, although claims have been made that they may have effects on cell viability in laboratory situations (Whitehouse and Geldmacher 1994). Thus, we need interventions in the intermediate term that are based on an understanding of the general mechanisms of neuronal death. Eventually, our biological interventions to slow the progression of the neuronal damage should be based on an understanding of the pathogenesis of the disease. It is theoretically possible to enhance the viability of nerve cells generally without necessarily directly altering the specific mechanism of cell death in AD.

A variety of mechanisms have been proposed that may contribute to cell death and neurodegenerative diseases in general, including absence of growth factors or estrogen, the accumulation of oxidative damage through free radical formation, alterations in the adenosine metabolism, inflammatory processes, and intracellular accumulation of calcium (Mattson 1994; McGeer, Schulzer, and McGeer 1996; Rudolphi et al. 1992; Smith et al. 1995). Each of these proposed mechanisms of neuronal death can be studied in a variety of model systems. Epidemiologic studies also provide evidence that patients exposed to certain drugs—nicotine (Lerner et al. 1996), estrogen (Henderson et al. 1995), and anti-inflammatory agents (McGeer, Schulzer, and McGeer 1996)—may have a lower risk of AD. Moreover, some initial therapeutic trials have been conducted with patients to attempt to measure an alteration in disease course based on these approaches. For example, interventricular mouse nerve growth factor (NGF) has been administered to patients in Sweden. Nerve growth factor is a prototype for slowing progression of disease, as in animals it is clear that this protein is important for the viability of cholinergic basal forebrain cells, which die in AD.

Unfortunately, in human beings NGF produces too many side effects to be therapeutically useful (Nordberg 1993). A new drug, propentofylline, submitted for approval in Europe, purports to enhance NGF action to increase adenosine levels locally and may reduce neuronal damage. Moreover, a multicenter study of the free radical scavengers, deprenyl and vitamin E, in the United States showed some evidence of delaying disease progression, although some problems with interpretation exist (Sano et al. 1997). Trials of estrogen are also under way in several countries, including a long-term prospective study to examine whether estrogen slows cognitive deterioration in normal women.

These clinical developments are occurring despite the fact that we have not established a clear consensus on how to demonstrate to a regulatory body that more than a prolonged symptomatic benefit was produced by a drug. Most proposed protocol designs include a phase of withdrawal of an effective medication to see if patients on the medication are left with any residual or long-lasting improvement over a group that had never been on the drug (Leber 1997).

Thus, it is important when discussing attempts to slow progression of the disease that one is explicit about the criteria for a successful outcome. Is the goal to maintain a higher level of cognitive function as measured by an objective psychometric test, to alter the course of the disease, or to delay the appearance of milestones in the disease, such as the transition to a more profound stage of dependency or placement in a nursing home? These criteria refer to slowing the progression of disease at the clinical level, but one could also develop biological markers (e.g., use neuroimaging to measure brain atrophy as a sign of neuronal death) (Rossor et al. n.d.). However, how these biological markers relate to measures of clinical progression is unclear.

Long-Term Approaches: Understanding Pathogenesis

The principal pathological hallmarks of AD associated with neuronal death are neuritic or senile plaques and neurofibrillary tangles (Whitehouse n.d.). Neuritic plaques are extracellular structures in which glial cells and abnormal neurites surround an amorphous core that contains proteins, particularly beta amyloid. The intracellular pathologic features, neurofibrillary tangles, are paired helical filaments composed of proteins, perhaps most importantly abnormally phosphorylated tau, a microtubule-associated protein. Presumably these two pathologic features relate, in ways that are as yet unclear, to the death of nerve cells. Thus, if we are to develop interventions that have more profound effects on the genesis of AD relating to prevention and cure, we must understand more about these pathologic features. As discussed below, genetic clues, particularly clues to the formation of amyloid, are important in this fundamental basic research.

Neuritic Plaques. One of the fundamental observations in understanding the pathogenesis of AD was the identification of the beta amyloid protein at the core of neuritic plaques and the genetic mutations in the amyloid precursor protein on chromosome 21 (see chap. 2, above; Selkoe 1996). Many studies of pathogenesis focus on understanding how this substance is formed and how it does damage to nerve cells. Intense activity has been focused on developing transgenic models to study amyloid processing (Cordell et al. 1996). However, until recently, these model systems have been unable to produce consistent pathology and behavioral abnormalities in animals with these amyloid mutations. A number of processing pathways have been identified, including some involving endolysosomes, that allow the beta amyloid protein to accumulate. The amyloid precursor protein is produced on chromosome 21, and the 42 amino acid portion of that precursor, called beta amyloid, is found in senile plaques. Mutations on chromosome 21 clearly alter amyloid processing (Selkoe 1996; Younkin 1996). Moreover, mutations on chromosomes 14 and 1, affecting presenilins 1 and 2, respectively, may also alter amyloid processing (see chap. 1, above; Selkoe 1996). The mechanism by which amyloid is toxic to nerve cells is the subject of controversy. A number of proteins have been determined to be associated with amyloid and may affect its aggregation, which seems key to toxicity.

Neurofibrillary Tangles. A close association exists between intracellular neurofibrillary tangles and cell death. Neurofibrillary tangles are structures found inside and outside of dead neurons in populations of cells that die in AD. The association of phosphorylated tau with the neurofibrillary tangle appears to be critical (Grundke-Iqbal et al. 1986). Thus, drugs that affect the kinases and phosphatases involved in the phosphorylation and dephoysphorylation of tau and tau-related proteins are the targets for drug development. Tangles are found in different cell populations and in different diseases. Understanding this diversity should provide clues to how tau and tangles are associated and why they damage neurons. The fundamental goal of basic research on neurofibrillary tangles and senile plaques is to understand how these structures form and how they might relate to each other and to neuronal death.

Implications of Genetic Studies

The discussion of the implications of genetic work for therapy falls into three broad questions. First, how useful are genetic markers such as autosomal-dominant notations and APOE in identifying at-risk individuals or those in the early stages of disease? Second, is there any evidence that currently available genetic markers are helpful predictors of responsiveness to the drugs that are currently approved (namely, tacrine) and drugs under development for the treatment of symptoms, (namely, xanomelline [Eli Lilly] and S12024 [Servier])? Finally, what are the implications of knowledge of genetic mutations and heterogeneity for the development of long-term approaches to interventions that will interrupt the pathogenetic mechanisms of AD?

Role of Genetic Markers in Presymptomatic Detection and Diagnosis

Diagnosis and treatment go hand in hand. More precise diagnoses may lead to better understanding of which therapies are effective for what type of dementias or even subtypes of degenerative dementias such as AD. For some time now, the identification of autosomal-dominant mutations has made it possible to offer both presymptomatic and diagnostic genetic testing. In the relatively rare situation of a family with an autosomal-dominant mutation, one can establish with high accuracy whether an individual carries the mutation associated with the disease and can, therefore, allow counseling concerning genetic risk. In the presence of cognitive impairment, the identification of a mutation, particularly if the age of onset is consistent with the rest of the affected family members, suggests that this gene represents the cause of dementia, although other causes of cognitive impairment, some of which may be reversible, could also coexist in these individuals.

The complexities of the use of genetic testing and diagnosis has increased with the discovery of susceptibility locus, APOE. As discussed elsewhere in this book (chap. 4), it is clear that those individuals who are homozygotes for ε4 are more at risk for suffering from AD in the future. Moreover, if they already have symptoms of cognitive impairment, AD is more likely to be the appropriate diagnosis. Numerous studies confirm the association between APOE ε4 and increased risk of AD. This association has led to the commercialization of APOE testing as a diagnostic test. As he identifies in chapter 4, Dr. Roses, the leader of the team who discovered the association between APOE and dementia, has a commercial interest in its application and has been the major proponent for its use.

Whereas there is no question that having an ε4 allele does confer additional risk, the question is how precisely this risk can be defined and how useful it is in different clinical settings. There are major current limitations to its clinical utility. First, many of the studies of association between APOE and diagnosis have been done in populations with patients who have come to autopsy. This is desirable in that one can identify precisely whether AD is the final definitive diagnosis. However, individuals that have an autopsy are relatively rare in the population of patients as a whole. They tend to be Caucasian, middle or upper class, and their progress tends to have been followed at academic centers. Thus, generalizing the risk data from this population to a larger clinical population may be unwise. Preliminary evidence has already been provided that the risk associated with APOE status varies as a function of gender, ethnicity, and age (Farrer 1997). Thus, for an individual patient appearing in the office, one cannot be sure what the increased risk is associated with the presence of an APOE ε4 or, for that matter, the potential protective effects of an APOE ε2 locus.

An additional problem has to do with the availability and quality of genetic counseling. If an individual is found to have an ε4 allele and is accompanied to the clinic by, for example, a son or daughter, one also needs to be aware that the other family members have information available about altered risk due to the genotyping of the subject. Not only do we not know what the additional risks are for the subject and family members, but also it is clear that we do not as yet have adequate methods for genetic counseling, particularly in primary care settings. Physicians themselves may or may not recognize their limitations in incorporating genetic risk information into their clinical decision making (Weinstein and Fineberg 1980a, 1980b).

There may be some circumstances in which APOE testing is now useful, although these have not been clearly established. For example, if one is considering a brain biopsy for a possible vasculitis or an interventricular shunt for a suspected case of normal pressure hydrocephalus, the presence of APOE ε4 homozygosity in the individual being considered for these invasive procedures might diminish the enthusiasm for such diagnostic or therapeutic approaches, given that the likelihood of a final diagnosis of AD would be increased by the gene status.

Thus, although the identification of APOE is an exciting scientific discovery, we do not as yet believe that the commercialization of this technology for clinical use is appropriate. Many complex ethical issues relating to financing of testing and insurance coverage implications are not resolved (Post et al. 1997). Moreover, we simply do not have the risk information in populations of patients who come for routine diagnostic assessment and the wherewithal to interpret these results in a way that is clearly beneficial to patients and families. There is strong pressure from those who benefit financially from the test to implement this in clinical practice. However, it appears that most academic opinion leaders are not using this test in a routine clinical fashion (although many are using it for research), and we would not recommend it for general use by primary care physicians or geriatricians now.

Once additional risk information is available about APOE or perhaps by the identification of other susceptibility loci (Saunders et al. 1997), it may become reasonable to consider the use of these tests in clinical practice. In fact, Roses has implied that such new loci (perhaps on chromosome 12) would make presymptomatic testing reasonable to consider. However, the ethical issues associated with reporting information to presymptomatic individuals concerning their likelihood of suffering from AD later in life, particularly when the information is likely to remain somewhat imprecise, are complex. Although we believe that it is necessary to consider these ethical issues, we currently believe the most pressing issues in genetic susceptibility testing in AD concerns premature commercialization and conflict of interest (chap. 6, below). How can we trust opinions about the power of genetic technology to help affected persons and families when data to support such positions are not fully presented and are hidden by the commercialization process?

Genetic Tests As Predictors of Responsiveness to Symptomatic Drugs

One of the problems with trials of many medications in dementia is that only a certain population of patients appears to respond to the drugs. Intensive efforts have been made to identify which patients are more likely to respond to drugs (e.g., tacrine). Although no prospective trials have been done, retrospective analyses have been conducted on tacrine studies. Poirier and colleagues (1995) examined patients who were participants in a thirty-week tacrine study. The observation was made that APOE ϵ4-negative AD patients showed marked improvement on the psychometric test employed (Alzheimer Disease Assessment Scale), whereas APOE ϵ4 carriers were worse when compared with their baseline. This study was prompted by the observation made by that group of investigators that the loss of cholinergic markers appeared to be greater in the brains of individuals affected by AD who were of APOE ϵ4 type (Poirier et al. 1993). This conclusion was based on only a subsample of patients who completed the double-blind thirty-week clinical trial, however.

An analysis that included more of the individuals has also been conducted (Farlow et al. 1996). Initially, the analysis confirmed the observation that APOE ε4 predicted less responsiveness to tacrine and, interestingly, found that this effect was mainly present in women. The researchers speculated that this may relate to other factors, including coadministration of estrogen, which has been shown to possibly be involved in the pathogenesis of AD and to be protective. Also, different rates of progression occurred between those patients with APOE ε4 and those with APOE ε2 and ε3. Clearly, these preliminary observations deserve further exploration. One should also note, however, that the differences in drug responsiveness in the two genetic groups were relatively small. Another analysis of the same data (Poirier et al. 1996) concluded with a slightly different interpretation that tacrine was effective in patients with and without the ε4 allele, although with slightly different effect sizes. It is not clear that the magnitude of difference predicted by ε4, even if confirmed in subsequent studies, is enough to suggest that physicians should not offer therapy to particular individuals.

Other studies of tacrine and the effects of APOE subtype are being conducted, and we look forward to having further data published soon. Wilcock and colleagues (1995) and MacGowan and colleagues (1995) confirmed that persons with APOE ε4 appear less responsive to tacrine, whereas Ritchie and colleagues (1996) and Lucotte, Oddoze, and Michel (1995) reported the opposite pattern. Other pharmaceutical companies are examining whether APOE subtype affects responsiveness to their drugs. Altstiel and colleagues (1995) claimed that in a study of a novel M1 cholinergic receptor agonist xanomelline, with more than eight hundred subjects enrolled in a Phase II trial, those with the APOE ε4 subtype were less responsive to the M1 agonist. However, an opposite pattern was reported in a multicenter study of S12024 (Amouyel et al. 1995). At one particular dose, an interaction between APOE ε4 and drug effect was detected on both the Mini-Mental State Examination and the clinical global scale. In this situation, however, the presence of APOE ε4 allele predicted better drug responsiveness, a pattern opposite to that reported for xanomelline and most studies of tacrine. Interestingly, some companies are not examining the effect of APOE, perhaps not wishing to reduce the size of the potential sales market by identifying factors that might exclude some individuals from receiving therapy based on a marker that predicts low responsiveness to their drug.

My own view is that these studies are provocative but inconclusive. Not only are they based on relatively small samples examined in retrospect, but also the statistical analysis is often complex because of the many other variables that may affect drug responsiveness. Such subgroup analysis is particularly fraught with difficulty. This conclusion has also been drawn by others with access to more unpublished data (Schneider 1996). Moreover, as stated above, it is not clear that these studies demonstrate effects of significant enough magnitude that they would affect health care provider behavior in treating with these agents.

Implications of Genetic Studies for the Understanding of Pathogenesis

In the long run, genetic studies offer great hope for developing more effective therapies by contributing to an understanding of pathogenesis. As clues to the earliest stages of the onset of AD, genetic mutations can contribute to understanding the mechanisms by which cell death occurs. These forms of therapies could include gene therapy, where genetic material could be inserted into cells to correct for the genetic abnormalities found in certain families with dementia. More likely, however, the genetic information will lead to an understanding of the role of different proteins in pathogenesis and suggest ways to alter action of these proteins through the use of drugs or biological products. The principal means by which genetic studies have contributed to an understanding of pathogenesis has been to understand the formation of the amyloid protein at the core of senile plaques. We are in the early stages of understanding how apoE affects pathogenesis.

Attempts to block amyloid toxicity are being made by preventing the formation of beta amyloid, altering its clearance, or reducing its aggregation (Whitehouse 1997). The identification of mutations in the amyloid precursor protein on chromosome 21 has clearly provided us a clue to the distribution and action of amyloid in the brain. For example, the 42 amino acid form of beta amyloid appears more critical to pathogenesis than the shorter 40 amino acid peptide. However, we do not understand the normal function of the amyloid-processing protein. Is the toxicity of beta amyloid due to excess of the abnormal protein or dysfunction in a normal protein? It seems fairly clear that the formation of the relatively insoluble core is critical, as amyloid appears not to be toxic unless it aggregates. Preventing fibril formation may be a good long-term therapeutic strategy; proteoglycans, metals, and other substances may be targets for drugs, as these substances have been shown in vitro to alter aggregation.

Moreover, as mentioned previously, mutations on chromosomes 1 and 14, affecting the presenilins, may also affect amyloid processing and may offer clues about cell death in AD (see chaps. 2, 3 and 4, above). More energy is being focused on amyloid processing than on any other single therapeutic strategy in the biotechnology industry.

The effect of APOE ε4 genotype on the risk for AD is particularly impressive, given that apoE ε2, ε3, and ε4 differ from each other by one or two amino acids. Thus, it is theoretically possible to understand the mechanism by which ε2 is a protective factor and ε4 is a susceptibility factor for AD and to use this knowledge to develop new therapeutic approaches. Ideally, one might want to transfer the protective effect of ε2 to those not naturally endowed with that particular genotype (chap. 4, above). There are thus major efforts under way to develop interventions based on understanding APOE effects in pathogenesis.

Although such approaches offer tremendous opportunity, the challenges of modifying normal protein functioning with a drug are enormous when the effects of the disease vary through time (i.e., when do critical events occur in AD?) and space (where in the brain, and where in the individual neurons?). One must hope to deliver the right drug to the right place at the right time to have a therapeutic effect and yet avoid disrupting normal protein function and creating unwanted side effects.

Often, therapeutic approaches based on molecular genetic studies create the expectation that we are considering gene therapy. Although it is theoretically possible to correct genetic mutations very early in development of the embryo (or even in germ lines), this is not a currently tractable approach in AD. Making changes in the genetic function of somatic cells is also a daunting task. Most of the current long-term implications of molecular biological studies of AD relate to understanding the proteins produced by abnormal genes and developing drugs that work after the genetic message has been translated into proteins.

Conclusion

There is no question that genetic discoveries offer great promise for better diagnostic and therapeutic approaches in AD. Moreover, research has led to the development of advanced technologies to attempt to convert this genetic knowledge into drug products. The screening of large libraries of genetic material, combined with approaches that allow one to associate a gene with a particular disease and identify neuroanatomical areas in which the gene is expressed, allow the discovery and optimization of lead compounds to be more efficient. Moreover, combinatorial chemistry and high throughput screening of drug candidates allows the creation and testing of diverse groups of potential therapeutic agents. Rapid screening of potential medications for initial effectiveness can be done in model systems such as cell cultures. Combinatorial chemistry allows tens to hundreds of thousands of compounds to be created efficiently at a low cost. Moreover, our understanding of structure-activity relationships (that is, the relationship between the chemical structure of a drug and its effect on the target protein) is increasing. For example, nuclear magnetic resonance can be used to guide the construction of compounds based on how components affect the structure of the target protein, as measured by the electromagnetic signal. Rational drug design based on an understanding on pathogenesis is increasingly becoming not the exception but the rule in industry.

Thus, genomic approaches combined with combinatorial chemistry and efficient screening offer tremendous promise for interventions that go beyond symptomatic treatment to disease-course-altering effects. Yet we must juxtapose the power of the technology with the remarkable challenge of improving human cognitive abilities. Human cognition is enormously complex, and the notion that approaches such as a single transmitter replacement can have profound effects is perhaps simplistic. Moreover, AD occurs in the substrate of the aging brain, where shrinkage and loss of nerve cells is a part of normal aging.

The molecular revolution in medicine creates tremendous expectations in the minds of patients and families affected by this disease. Although these promises are considerable, we must avoid creating false hope by making unrealistic promises about the likelihood of short-term success. Those who claim that in a specified period of time we may be able to delay disease run the risk of appealing more to individuals' fears and hopes than to their rational minds.

We must recognize that AD drugs are being developed at a time of tremendous change in the health care system. We will be asked to demonstrate the effect of drugs not only on cognition but also on function and quality of life. Economic considerations will compel us to compare the value of our biological interventions with that of psychosocial interventions. How many resources can be spent on slowing the progression of disease in older individuals when many children are underinsured and not immunized? If our hopes for biological interventions are to be realized, we must be aware of the changing environment in which our research and clinical practices are being conducted.

References

Altstiel, L., Mohs, R., Marin, D., Lebow, L., Yang, X. P., Greenberg, D., Bodick, N., Offen, W., Cooper, V., and Poirier, J. 1995. ApoE genotype and clinical outcome in Alzheimer's disease. Abstract presented at the International Psychogeriatrics Association conference, Apolipoprotein E et Maladie d'Alzheimer, May 29, Paris.

Amouyel, P., Neuman, E., Dilleman, L., Richard, F., Barrandon, S., Helbecque, N., Malbezin, M., and Guez, D. 1995. Characterization of the apolipoprotein E genotypes in clinical trials on Alzheimer's disease: The 12024 (memory enhancer) European multicentre project. Abstract presented at the International Psychogeriatrics Association conference, Apolipoprotein E et Maladie d'Alzheimer, May 29, Paris.

Brodaty, H., and Medical and Scientific Advisory Committee, Alzheimer's Disease International. 1995. Consensus statement on predictive testing for Alzheimer's disease. *Alzheimer Disease and Associated Disorders* 9:182–87.

Cordell, B., Higgins, L. S., Higaki, J., Zhong, Z., Moran, P. M., and Moser, P. M. 1996. A model of amyloid formation and Alzheimer's disease. *Alzheimer Research* 1:111–16.

Farlow, M. R., Lahiri, D. K., Poirier, J., Davignon, J., Hui, S. 1996. Apolipoprotein E genotype and gender influence response to tacrine therapy. *Annals of New York Academy of Science* 802:101–10.

Farrer, L. A. 1997. Effects of age, gender, and ethnicity on the association between apolipoprotein E genotype and Alzheimer disease. Abstract presented at 41st OHOLO conference, Progress in Alzheimer's and Parkinson's Diseases, May 18–23, Eilat, Israel.

Grundke-Iqbal, I., Iqbal, K., Quinlan, M., Tung, Y. C., Zaidi, M. S., and Wisniewski, H. M. 1986. Microtubule-associated protein tau: A component of Alzheimer paired helical filaments. *Journal of Biological Chemistry* 83:6084–89.

Henderson, A. S., Easteal, S., Jorm, A. F., Mackinnon, A. J., Korten, A. E., Christensen, H., Croft, L., and Jacomb, P. A. 1995. Apolipoprotein E allele ε4, dementia, and cognitive decline in a population sample. *Lancet* 346:1387–90.

Kaufer, D. I., Cummings, J. L., and Christine, D. 1996. Effect of tacrine on behavioral symptoms in Alzheimer's disease: An open-label study. *Journal of Geriatric Psychiatry and Neurology* 9:1–6.

Knopman, D., Schneider, L., Davis, K., Talwalker, S., Smith, F., Hoover, T., Gracon, S., and the Tacrine Study Group. 1996. Long-term tacrine (Cognex) treatment: Effects on nursing home placement and mortality. *American Academy of Neurology* 47:166–77.

Lawton, M. P. 1994. Quality of life in Alzheimer's disease. *Alzheimer Disease and Associated Disorders* 8:138–50.

Leber, P. 1990. Guidelines for the clinical evaluation of antidementia drugs. Paper prepared for the Federal Drug Administration, November 8, Washington, D.C.

———. 1997. Slowing the progression of disease: Regulatory aspects. *Alzheimer Disease and Associated Disorders* (in press).

Lerner, A. J., Koss, E., Gilham, S., Cole, R., Debanne, S., Esteban-Santillan, C., Petot, G. J., Rowland, D. Y., Smyth, K. A., Whitehouse, P. J., and Friedland, R. P. 1996. Estrogen replacement therapy as a protective factor for Alzheimer disease: Interactions with other risk factors. *Society of Neuroscience* 22:15.

Lucotte, G., Oddoze, C., and Michel, B. F. 1995. Apolipoprotein E and response to tacrine in French Alzheimer's disease patients. Abstract presented at the International Psychogeriatrics Association conference, Apolipoprotein E et Maladie d'Alzheimer, May 29, Paris.

MacGowan, S. H., Scott, M., Agg, M., and Wilcock, G. K. 1995. Influence of apolipoprotein E genotype on response to tacrine in male and female patients with Alzheimer's disease. Abstract presented at the International Psychogeriatrics Association conference, Apolipoprotein E et Maladie d'Alzheimer, May 29, Paris.

Mattson, M. P. 1994. Calcium and neuronal injury in Alzheimer's disease: Contributions of beta-amyloid precursor protein mismetabolism, free radicals, and metabolic compromise. *Annals of New York Academy of Science,* n.s., 15:50–76.

Mayeux, R., and Schupf, N. 1995. Apolipoprotein E and Alzheimer's disease: The implications of progress in molecular medicine. *American Journal of Public Health* 85:1280–84.

McGeer, P. L., Schulzer, M., and McGeer, E. G. 1996. Arthritis and anti-inflammatory agents as possible protective factors for Alzheimer's disease: A review of seventeen epidemiologic studies. *Neurology* 47:425–32.

National Institute on Aging/Alzheimer's Association Working Group. 1996. Apolipoprotein E genotyping in Alzheimer's disease. *Lancet* 347:1091–95.

Nordberg, A. 1993. In vivo detection of neurotransmitter changes in Alzheimer's disease. *Annals of New York Academy of Science* 695:27–33.

Patterson, M. B., Mack, J. L., Geldmacher, D. S., and Whitehouse, P. J. 1996. Executive functions and Alzheimer's disease: Problems and prospects. *European Journal of Neurology* 3:5–15.

Poirier, J., Davignon, J., Bouthillier, D., Kogan, S., Bertrand, P., and Gauthier, S. 1993. Apolipoprotein E polymorphism and Alzheimer's disease. *Lancet* 342:697–99.

Poirier, J., Delisle, M. C., Quirion, R., Aubert, I., Farlow, M., Lahiri, D., Hui, S., Bertrand, P., Nalbantoglu, J., Gilfix, B. M., and Gauthier, S. 1995. Apolipoprotein E4 allele as a predictor of cholinergic deficits and treatment outcome in Alzheimer disease. *Professional National Academy of Science, USA* 92:12260–64.

Poirier, J., Knopman, D., Schneider, L., Davis, K., Farlow, M., Gracon, S., Smith, F., and Soon, G. 1996. Long-term tacrine treatment and impact of ApoE, ε4 allele. Paper presented at the *Lancet* conference, Challenge of the Dementias, April 25, Edinburgh.

Post, S. G., and Whitehouse, P. J. 1998. The moral basis for limiting treatment: Hospice and advanced progressive dementia. In *Hospice care for people with advanced progressive dementia,* ed. L. Volicer and A. C. Hurley. New York: Springer, forthcoming.

Post, S. G., Whitehouse, P. J., Binstock, R. H., Bird, T. D., Eckert, S. K., Farrer, L. A., Fleck, L. M., Gaines, A. D., Juengst, E. T., Karlinsky, H., Miles, S., Murray, T. H., Quaid, K. A., Relkin, N. R., Roses, A. D., Sachs, G. A., Steinbock, B., St. George-Hyslop, P. H., Truschke, E. F., and Zinn, A. B. 1997. The clinical introduction of genetic testing for Alzheimer disease: An ethical perspective. *JAMA* 277:832–36.

Ritchie, K., Kotzki, P.-O., Touchon, J., and Cristol, J.-P. 1996. Characteristics of Alzheimer's disease patients with and without ApoE4 allele. *Lancet* 348:960.

Roses, A. D. 1995. Apolipoprotein E genotyping in the differential diagnosis, not prediction, of Alzheimer's disease. *Annals of Neurology* 38:6–14.

Rossor, M. N., Bodick, N., Forette, F., Hadler, D., Harvey, R. J., McKeith, I., Riekkinen, P., Scheltens, P., Shimohama, S., Spiegel, R., Tanaka, S., Thal, L., Urata, Y., and Wilcock, G. n.d. Protocols to demonstrate slowing of disease progression. *Alzheimer Disease and Associated Disorders* (in press).

Rudolphi, K. A., Schubert, P., Parkinson, F. E., and Fredholm, B. B. 1992. Neuroprotective role of adenosine in cerebral ischaemia. *Trends in Pharmacological Science* 13:439–45.

Sano, M., Ernesto, C., Thomas R. G., Klauber, M. R., Schafer, K., Grundman, M., Woodbury, P., Growdon, J., Cotman, C. W., Pfeiffer, E., Schneider, L. S., and Thal, L. J., for the members of the Alzheimer's Disease Cooperative Study. 1997. A controlled trial of selegiline, alpha-tocopherol, or both as treatment for Alzheimer's disease. *New England Journal of Medicine* 336:1216–22.

Saunders, A. M., Welsh-Bohmer, K., Mirra, S., Gearing, M., and Roses, A. D. 1997. Positive predictive value of APOE ∈4 testing for Alzheimer disease. Abstract presented at the 41st OHOLO Conference, Progress in Alzheimer's and Parkinson's Diseases, May 18–23, Eilat, Israel.

Schneider, L. 1996. Unpublished presentation, American College of Neuropsychopharmacology, San Diego, Calif.

Selkoe, D. J. 1996. Amyloid protein and the genetics of Alzheimer's disease. *Journal of Biological Chemistry* 271:18295–98.

Smith, M. A., Sayre, L. M., Monnier, V. M., and Perry, G. 1995. Radical AGEing in Alzheimer's disease. *Trends in Neuroscience* 18:172–76.

Strauss, M. E., and Ogrocki, P. K. 1996. Confirmation of an association between family history of affective disorder and the depressive syndrome in Alzheimer's disease. *American Journal of Psychiatry* 153:1340–42.

Weinstein, M. C., and Fineberg, H. V. 1980. The elements of clinical decision making. In *Clinical decision analysis*, 1–13. Philadelphia: W. B. Saunders.

———. 1980b. The use of diagnostic information to revise probabilities. In *Clinical decision analysis*, 75–130. Philadelphia: W. B. Saunders.

Whitehouse, P. J. 1997. Genesis of Alzheimer's discase. *Neurology* 48 (supp. 7): 1–6.

———. n.d. International Working Group for Harmonization of Dementia Drug Guidelines: A progress report. *Alzheimer Disease and Associated Disorders* (in press).

Whitehouse, P. J., and Geldmacher, D. S. 1994. Pharmacotherapy for Alzheimer's disease. In *Clinics in Geriatric Medicine: Alzheimer's Disease Update* 10:339–50.

Whitehouse, P. J., and Maslow, K. n.d. Are we ready for outcomes research in AD? *Alzheimer Disease and Associated Disorders* (in press).

Whitehouse, P. J., Orgogozo, J.-M., Becker, R. E., Gauthier, S., Pontecorro, M., Erzigkeit, H., Rogers, S., Mohs, R. C., Budick, N., Bruno, G., and Dal-Bianco, P. 1997. Quality of life assessment in dementia drug development. *Alzheimer Disease and Associated Disorders* 11 (supp. 3): 57–61.

Whitehouse, P. J., Price, D. L., Struble, R. G., Clark, A. W., Coyle, J. T., and DeLong, M. R. 1982. Alzheimer's disease and senile dementia: Loss of neurons in the basal forebrain. *Science* 215:1237–39.

Whitehouse, P. J., and Rabins, P. V. 1992. Quality of life and dementia. *Alzheimer Disease and Associated Disorders* 6:135–38.

Wilcock, G. K., MacGowan, S. H., Scott, M., and Dawbarn, D. 1995. Apolipoprotein E genotype and response to tacrine in Alzheimer's disease. Poster presented at the International Psychogeriatrics Association conference, Apolipoprotein E et Maladie d'Alzheimer, May 29, Paris.

Younkin, S. G. 1995. Evidence that A-42 is the real culprit in Alzheimer's disease. *Annals of Neurology* 37:287–88.

Some Questions Arising in the Commercial Development of Genetic Tests for Alzheimer Disease

ROBERT MULLAN COOK-DEEGAN, M.D.

The quest for genes associated with Alzheimer disease (AD) has been driven mainly by the desire to understand a disease whose cause is unknown, pathogenesis mysterious, prevalence high, and impact substantial. Financial questions involving who renders services, develops diagnostic tests, and brings drugs to market have appropriately taken a backseat to research questions, in part because until recently science had relatively little to offer commerce. That is changing, because research is beginning to produce practical results. Discoveries are being turned into goods and services.

Genetic discoveries are only some among many relevant research advances, but they have been especially important in the quest for diagnostics and in focusing research efforts to discover drugs. The genes associated with AD are playing a big role in the debate over optimal diagnostic algorithms for dementia and in directing the search for second- and third-generation therapeutic pharmaceuticals. Questions that arise when private firms begin to interact with publicly funded research have become salient and promise to become ever more prominent as more products and services reach the market.

Changes in Research on the Genetics of Alzheimer Disease over the Past Two Decades

The clinical and pathological descriptions of AD emerged from work done in the first decade of this century. For most of the next five decades, the disease was generally regarded as rare. Theories of causation were so numerous, underdetermined, and speculative that most work remained descriptive rather than probing molecular or physiological events. In the late 1970s, in part motivated by Robert Katzman's editorial (Katzman 1976), AD was again classified with senile dementia (Fox 1989). This led to recognition of much higher prevalence and appreciation of its enormous social toll. Family support groups emerged in the early 1980s, growing into a social movement that recognized that significant progress against the disease depended on much more biomedical research.

This broad public constituency became a persuasive political force, convincing Congress to appropriate funding for research on AD. Federal funding for AD, estimated at $3.9 million in 1976, rose to $54 million a decade later (Office of Technology Assessment 1987) and over $317 million in 1997 (Walkington 1997). The massive increase in resources has changed the qualitative character of research on AD, mainly in ways that were directly intended or clearly foreseeable. The number of investigators has increased manifold. Indeed, because players have proliferated faster than ideas, more investigators are pursuing overlapping or parallel lines of research. The form of AD research was also initially focused on centers, which reward the home institutions with relatively stable, high-prestige programs, in turn attracting attention and support from deans and university presidents. Research on AD has gone from being a neglected outpost to a major front on the battle against disease. Competition for first discovery and other rewards of research success has intensified as the stakes have risen.

Two decades ago, the quest for the genetic origins of AD was a field in dire need of attention. It is now the subject of fractious rivalry, and the pathologies of hypercompetition have begun to appear. In his book on the discovery of Alzheimer-associated genes on chromosomes 1, 14, 19, and 21, Daniel Pollen chronicles violations of confidentiality in manuscript review and suspicious behavior on peer review panels (Pollen 1996), and his portrait captures only a fraction of the skullduggery that forms the grist for the gossip mills of AD research. To date, the competition has been motivated mainly by a quest for scientific recognition. Behind every scientific controversy, however, there is likely to loom a patent battle that lags behind it by several years. Such controversies may well become more frequent as money enters the picture.

Most research progress on AD over the past two decades derives from the strong foundation of federal funding, especially from several institutes within the National Institutes of Health (NIH), augmented by private philanthropies such as the Alzheimer's Association, John Douglas French Foundation, Howard Hughes Medical Institute, Robert Wood Johnson Foundation, and MetLife Foundation (Walkington 1997). The fruits ripening from this large scientific effort include knowledge, technologies, and experts. Public policy has focused on generating knowledge in the hope it will point to technologies that might prevent or treat the disease. Most services have focused on recognizing AD by observing symptoms and ruling out other diagnoses or on dealing with its ravages.

Until the past decade, the mysterious origins of the disease and unmapped pathways toward its expression kept hopes of prevention, cure, or even significant treatment beyond the horizon. During the past decade, that has begun to change, with specific causal hypotheses becoming sufficiently specific and the body of knowledge about the disease sufficient to make advances in diagnosis likely and hopes of better therapy and prevention or delay of onset much more concrete. Genetic research has been a major factor in this change.

Economic Complexity and the Public Good

Specific biochemical markers, genetic tests, and therapeutic drugs are all relatively new. Before such science-based measures were developed, there were no known gold mines in medicine. Public funding for research, along with private philanthropy, was intended to promote the public good by generating information about a dread disease, making the information widely available, and hoping it would be relevant for practical remedies. The public good inherent in the advance of science, however, is subject to intellectual property claims of those who helped create it. That is, information intended for the public good is often not treated as a public good in the economic sense.

The desert of information about AD has grown into a mountain of scientific data, which contains veins of gold and silver, and those veins still to be found are suspected to be more valuable that those already being mined. Mining rights are beginning to matter. The rising prospect of goods and services derived from a base of publicly funded research is probably the most significant change in AD research over the past two decades. Two related but distinct factors have also increased commercial interest in AD genetics: (1) a shift in policy regarding the ownership of intellectual property arising in federally funded research, and (2) a significant influx of private research moneys.

The Bayh-Dole Act

The Bayh-Dole Act of 1980 mandated a consistent policy across all federal agencies supporting research and development, conferring patent rights to nonprofit and small business grantees and contractors. Up to that point, patent policies had been less consistent. In some areas of biomedical research, the federal government had retained patent rights, although in others, such as contract work to develop anticancer drugs, the Bayh-Dole policies were already in effect. Other technology-transfer executive orders and legislation reinforced and broadened the federal pro-patent policies by extending rights to large businesses (by executive order of President Ronald Reagan), giving governmental employees patent incentives (through the Stevenson-Wydler Act of 1980, the Federal Technology Transfer Act of 1986, and other laws) and extending patent incentives to government-owned, contractor-operated national laboratories (the National Competitiveness Technology Transfer Act of 1989). The Bayh-Dole Act and other federal technology-transfer policies gave grantees and contractors strong incentives to patent potentially lucrative inventions (Office of Technology Assessment 1995).

One result has been an extraordinary rise in the number of patent applications arising from federally funded research (Henderson, Jaffe, and Trajtenberg 1997). Although not causally connected, the level of interest in patents among biomedical investigators has risen dramatically in parallel with federal funding for Alzheimer research. Two decades ago, patenting academic biomedical discoveries was relatively rare, and direct attachments between university researchers and private commercial firms were unusual outside clinical testing.

As the practical possibilities of recombinant DNA, cell fusion, and other innovations associated with molecular biology and biotechnology have become apparent, however, norms have shifted dramatically. Patenting a major discovery has become the default pathway, whether in academe or in industry. The main technologies under discussion when the Bayh-Dole Act was passed were nonbiological (e.g., aviation, electronics, computers, communication, space launch vehicles, and weapon systems), but biotechnology was coming into its own as the new policies caught hold (Eisenberg 1996). Some of the norm shift would likely have occurred even without the Bayh-Dole impetus, but the policy shift strongly reinforced changes induced by technological advance.

Research and Development

The rise of research investment by private pharmaceutical firms and the creation of a welter of biotechnology firms also took place in the same period. During the 1980s, several large drug firms recognized that their greatest competitive advantage lay in the discovery of entirely new therapeutic pharmaceuticals (Cockburn and Henderson 1996; Gambardella 1995; Henderson 1994; Henderson and Cockburn 1993). Corporate leaders began to focus much more attention on their R&D strategies, and the level of private pharmaceutical R&D escalated dramatically. The Pharmaceutical Research and Manufacturers Association (PhRMA) surveyed its members to estimate R&D expenditures of $980 million in 1976 in the United States, rising to $3.9 billion in 1986 and $15 billion in 1997 (PhRMA 1997). These figures entail significant multiple counting, which has worsened as research efforts among different firms have become more interdependent.

If a large firm agrees to license a drug discovered in a small firm, for example, the small firm will report its direct R&D expenses, and the large firm will also report its payment to the small firm as an R&D investment (OTA 1993). This double-counting effect, however, does not account for more than a small fraction of the rise in R&D funded by private pharmaceutical firms in the United States. The real level of investment in R&D has risen enormously, increasing more than tenfold in total dollars (sixfold in deflation-adjusted dollars) over the past two decades, with a large increase in funds for research intended to discover new drugs.

The rise in private R&D funding in major pharmaceutical firms is paralleled by the emergence of an entirely new set of firms specializing in translating discoveries from genetics and molecular biology into products and services. Many of these firms are not large enough to be members of the PhRMA, and the level of investment is quite difficult to monitor. The origin of private genomic companies is just one of many examples. Several small biotechnology firms dedicated to genomics started up in 1993–94, and a few existing firms shifted their research efforts to become focused mainly on gene discovery during the same period. It appears that the size of private investments in commercial companies in 1993 was of roughly the same magnitude as federal funding. In 1994 and since, the private investment in genomics has greatly exceeded federal funding (Cohen 1997). While only a small fraction of this investment is directed at AD, such investment indicates a significant shift within biotechnology toward gene discovery and characterization. Alzheimer research has benefited from this shift.

The substantial private R&D investments in established pharmaceutical firms and nascent biotechnology firms derive from two distinctive features of the pharmaceutical sector: a strong dependence on patents and an extraordinary mutualism between academic science and industrial application. Pharmaceutical firms have a significantly longer time horizon for R&D investment than most other high-technology sectors, with product cycles that often extend beyond a decade and returns on investment often not expected for a comparable period. The strength of patent protection is part of the reason such a long time horizon is possible. Corporate directors report that pharmaceuticals are much more patent dependent than electronics, software, transportation, and other sectors (National Academy of Engineering 1992).

Patents are not only stronger in pharmaceuticals but also significantly more likely to arise from academic research. This makes the academic research base exceptionally important to private pharmaceutical R&D, as indicated by surveys of corporate leaders (Mansfield 1995), citations of academic research in pharmaceutical product areas (Narin and Olivastro 1992), and the unusually high number of patents held by academic inventors (Cockburn and Henderson 1997; Narin and Rozek 1988). Only a small fraction of academic research is directly funded by industry; rather, the pharmaceutical industry draws on a large base of research funded by philanthropies and federal agencies, especially the NIH.

The increased scale and scope of Alzheimer research, its focus on genetics, enhanced scientific competition, the availability of private capital for Alzheimer research, and the complex interdependency between federally funded academic research and pharmaceutical R&D have all changed dramatically over the past two decades. These changes raise many questions likely to require explicit attention over the next decade. The remainder of this chapter addresses several such questions.

Commercial Pressures and the Premature Introduction of New Diagnostic and Screening Tests

The premature use of genetic tests has been a major concern in the bioethics of human genetics for well over a decade. It is dealt with in several other chapters of this volume (chaps. 14 and 15, below). Many of the policy statements that followed on the heels of discovering genes for cystic fibrosis, breast and colon cancer, hemochromatosis, Huntington disease, and other conditions were intended to forestall widespread testing and especially population screening.

Attention to potential problems of introducing new tests too quickly predates concern about commercial incentives. In 1983, the President's Commission for the Study of Ethical Problems in Medicine and Biomedical and Behavioral Research released a report on genetic testing and screening (President's Commission 1983). The report devoted a chapter to the possibility that the discovery of a genetic test for cystic fibrosis might overwhelm genetic services. Part of the reason was the high prevalence of the condition, which would lead to more diagnostic tests. More important, however, the commission noted that cystic fibrosis might be sufficiently prevalent that population screening would be practical. The shift from testing those with previously identified risk (family history or symptoms) to population screening would lead to many more tests, more complex interpretation, and greater demands on testing and counseling services. In 1989, the short-lived Biomedical Ethics Advisory Committee decided to focus its first report on questions of genetic testing, including risks of premature use. The committee died before its report was even started, but the mantle was quickly donned by the Working Group on Ethical, Legal, and Social Implications (ELSI) of Human Genome Research sponsored by the National Institutes of Health and the Department of Energy.

In February 1990, the ELSI working group decided to support a research initiative on the introduction of genetic tests, using the newly discovered cystic fibrosis gene as a case example. The National Center for Human Genome Research and other NIH institutes subsequently issued a request for applications. A few years later, several NIH institutes cosponsored a similar initiative to look at the introduction of genetic tests for colon, breast, and ovarian cancers. As these research projects were unfolding, the Institute of Medicine (IOM) released another ELSI-funded report, "Assessing Genetic Risks," in which premature use of genetic tests featured as a major preoccupation (Andrews et al. 1994). The IOM report pointed specifically to potential commercial pressures to introduce genetic tests. Picking up on several recommendations of the IOM report, the ELSI working group and the NIH moved in 1995 to establish a Genetic Testing Task Force (http://www.nchgr.nih.gov/Policy and public_affairs/Communications/Meeting_reports/task-force.html). Several external (mainly academic) advisers have been brought together with representatives from several federal agencies with jurisdiction over research (not only in the sciences but also on health services) and regulations (the Health Care Financing Administration, for clinical laboratories, and the Food and Drug Administration, for services and test kits). That task force proposed a framework for assessing and regulating genetic tests and genetic testing services, including quality control, education, and oversight of genetic testing (http://www.med.jhu.edu/tfgtelsi/).

The increased attention to commercial factors in genetic testing is in part due to the changing climate of biomedical research. Growing attention to industrial relevance pervades all of science and technology but is felt with special force in materials science, molecular biology, computation, and several other fields. In human genetics, the rapid transit from scientific discovery to application became more obvious as many disease-related genes were discovered in the late 1980s and early 1990s. The first major success in AD came with genetic linkage to chromosome 21 in 1987, followed by a series of discoveries discussed elsewhere in this section. In a technical sense, gene discovery is quite close to a diagnostic test, although the sociology of genetic testing differs substantially from academic research involved in gene discovery. Experience with the pilot genetic testing projects on cystic fibrosis and cancer testing has shown, however, that technical capacity will not necessarily induce an overwhelming demand for testing, so the long-held fear of overuse may not be as severe as many had thought.

Other constraints on demand can be found in the business dynamics of genetic testing. The total revenue expected from any test, genetic or otherwise, is simply the product of the price times the number of tests. The price the market will bear depends on several factors, including the strength of patent protection and the availability of other tests to supply similar information of value. The strength of patent protection depends on many factors, including the number of other patents that have been issued for the same gene, protein, or testing method and the scope of their claims. It also depends on whether the infringement of the patent is readily detected and on judgment about how likely courts will be to uphold patent claims. The number of tests depends critically on the prevalence of the condition, the fractional number of cases for which a genetic test may prove relevant, and whether the test is used in widespread population screening, testing those who have increased risk but no symptoms, or only as a diagnostic test following the onset of symptoms. Pricing and volume interact in the economically predictable fashion, with inverse relations between price and volume, but also through many indirect pathways. A high price reduces volume but also provides incentives to infringe on or work around any relevant patents, inducing investment to weaken the monopoly rights.

Alzheimer Disease and the Genetics Market

The incidence and prevalence of AD can set crude ceiling estimates of the maximum market size. The incidence of new cases, on the order of several hundred thousand per year, is a rough proxy for the number of new diagnoses being made. A test used solely for new diagnosis would be perhaps 1.5 to 2 times this figure (leaving room for testing of suspected but unconfirmed AD), suggesting a maximum of roughly a million diagnostic tests per year.

A screening test for the general population might pertain to the oldest twenty million or thirty million Americans, but such a test would have to be sensitive and specific. Population screening is utterly impractical unless a test can simultaneously detect a large number of independent causes of AD for a few dollars or so. The gene discoveries to date either have high predictive power only in families showing Mendelian inheritance or have insufficient sensitivity (i.e., miss too many cases) and specificity (i.e., include too many noncases) for population screening. Unless genetic factors prove more strongly predictive than studies currently suggest, genetic testing would be a poor choice for population screening. Even if genetic tests were a good screen on technical grounds, they would encounter two further constraints: (1) there would have to be a compelling reason to screen, such as a technical means of prevention or treatment; and (2) the cost per test would have to drop by several orders of magnitude.

Technologies for the analysis of DNA are improving quickly. A test that in one pass detects multiple different mutations of several different genes (or their corresponding peptides) may well be technically conceivable in the next half decade. Many forms of multiplex genetic testing of various kinds are being developed. Any such test for AD, however, would confront complex cross-licensing of multiple patents, for reasons discussed below, making it less profitable for any one inventor and turning it into a formidable challenge of business diplomacy. The biggest impediment to widespread genetic testing for AD could be, ironically, the complex patent status, related business dynamics, and the number of players with fingers in the pie rather than the underlying instrumentation and reagents.

The revenue of a diagnostic test equals its price times the number of tests. Both price and volume for future AD genetic testing are highly uncertain, but some parameters can be sketched in outline. Given the patent uncertainties discussed below, strong monopoly pricing is unlikely. An estimate of the price upper limit may be the recent price of roughly $195 charged by Athena Diagnostics for its APOE genotyping (Athena Diagnostics 1996). A test in the $100–200 range is unlikely to be used for all potential diagnoses, but it does suggest the ceiling market size may be $200 million for all AD genetic tests in aggregate, and that is likely optimistic. Markets for screening and treatment prediction are potentially larger. For purposes of comparison, a blockbuster therapeutic drug generates more than $1 billion in annual revenues. The most valuable gene patent to date is the one for Amgen's erythropoietin, with annual drug sales of $1.1 billion (http://www.shareholder.com/visitors/edgarlist.cfm?company=amgh).

A test useful for predicting therapy could significantly expand the market size over one useful only for diagnosis. This is because it would be useful not only for new diagnosis but also for the two million to five million Americans who already have a diagnosis of AD but would have a reason to get tested also. This larger market might be tapped only once, and the bolus effect would dissipate with time, dropping to parallel incidence of new cases. The market might also rise because of the number of tests as well as higher drug price. If genetic subtypes predict response to expensive drugs, the price of a genetic test can be higher because users offset the even greater potential future treatment cost for those who will not benefit. Demand will also be greater because the test has practical significance rather than merely augmenting prognostic and diagnostic accuracy. With many new drugs likely to appear on the scene, the interactions between genetics and treatment could prove important.

In its March 1996 survey of members, the PhRMA reported nine Alzheimer drugs in Phase II testing and ten in Phase III, the final stage before approval (although reaching Phase III does not imply approval). If these drugs do improve treatment, and if they do so selectively for different causes of the disease that map to different genotypes, then the market for testing could expand considerably. At least one pending patent application has been publicly reported for genotyping to predict treatment response, so the patent situation could become more complicated if genotyping before treatment proves useful.

The screening market will emerge only with price drops of several orders of magnitude, and genetic testing to predict treatment response is currently speculative, so the diagnostic market seems a good proxy for AD genetic testing in the near term. A $200 million market, even if carved into small fragments, is large by diagnostic testing standards and sufficient to generate interest among established firms—enough for several niche products that could sustain a few small start-up firms. The commercial factors that figure into decisions about introducing a genetic test go beyond the revenue potential.

Business decisions have to take into account competitors' strategies, the availability of alternative tests, how genetic testing fits into the diagnostic algorithm, control over the use of the technology, and the urgency of generating revenue. Some factors have nothing to do with the technology and much to do with the demands of capital formation and expectations about the rate of return for a given firm or specific project. A large established pharmaceutical firm may not need quick returns on R&D investments if it has ample patient capital and anticipates lower profits on diagnostics compared to therapeutics. Those investing in start-up firms, in contrast, often expect returns of 20 to 40 percent per year or even more and may anticipate payout in a few years. A small firm may get launched with only a patent or two, exclusive licensing rights to others' patents, or a novel business strategy.

The demand for high returns can create immense urgency to generate revenue. A large number of biotech start-up firms have cash sufficient for fewer than three years operation, as their "burn rate" to fund ongoing R&D exceeds revenues. A small firm with a high capital burn rate and low cash reserves is under much more pressure to probe the market than a large firm with lots of cash in reserve. Sources of new capital depend on demonstrated R&D successes, and revenue generated from new product sales is an important index of success. Between a desperate single-patent start-up and an established multinational pharmaceutical giant lie many companies along a continuum of fiscal urgency. The firm offering the APOE typing test, Athena Diagnostics, is a relatively small firm, but it has many tests other than AD to sustain it (including genetic tests for Huntington disease, Charcot-Marie-Tooth disease, fragile X syndrome, and others).

How technical, intellectual property and business factors will play out in genetic testing for AD is terribly murky. Firms of all sizes could be involved, and developments in therapeutics could well interact with diagnostics, causing strong fluctuations in demand. A few tentative observations can nonetheless be hazarded about testing for genes associated with AD to date.

Plausible Commercial Scenarios

Three commercial scenarios appear plausible, associated with (1) the amyloid precursor protein (APP) gene on chromosome 21 and peptide processing related to it, (2) the presenilin genes associated with early-onset familial AD, located by positional cloning on chromosomes 1 and 14, and (3) assessment of genetic risk factor through APOE genotyping on chromosome 19. (There is also some evidence of a risk factor on chromosome 12.) Mutation of the APP gene on chromosome 21 causes a very rare form of familial AD. Chromosome 21 genetics have been extremely important in ferreting out molecular factors involved in the pathogenesis of AD, but as a diagnostic test, the APP mutations are unlikely to prove commercially valuable because the prevalence of familial AD caused by them is quite low. Even if the prevalence were higher, the pursuit of substantial development investments would be fraught with considerable uncertainty. At least twelve different patents pertain to the APP gene or related amyloid processing. A 1987 patent assigned to the University of California by Glenner and colleagues claims use of amyloid peptide and fragments for diagnostic use (U.S. Patent #4666829). A 1990 patent assigned to NIH by Goldgaber and colleagues discloses a partial sequence of the APP gene and claims uses of such fragments as well as the entire gene (U.S. Patent #4912206). A separate patent assigned to Scios Nova covers a transgenic mouse model of AD constructed by inserting the mutated APP gene (U.S. Patent #5387742). At least nine other patents could also prove relevant, most for different mutants or novel uses and all potentially complicating any use for AD (U.S. Patents #5571671, 5547841, 5525714, 5525467, 5455169, 5297562, 5223482, 5218100, 5220013, 5015570).

Rights for these patents have been assigned to the U.S. Department of Health and Human Services, five nonprofit institutions (Harvard College, the

University of California, the Alzheimer's Institute of America, McLean Hospital, and the University of Rochester), and five for-profit firms (Bayer, Innogenetics, Scios Nova, Imperial Chemical Industries, and Molecular Therapeutics). (The number of assignees does not equal the number of patents because some patents are assigned to more than one institution, and both Harvard and Scios Nova hold more than one of the patents.) Any firm hoping to introduce an APP genetic test would face a daunting thicket of claims, raising the prospect of (1) complex cross-licensing, (2) threats of litigation, and (3) risks of inadvertent or deliberate patent infringement, some combination of the two, or all three. The science underlying these patents is wonderful, but the commercial prospects for high profits appear dim, given the low prevalence and uncertain strength of patent protection. There is ample room for surprise, but the likely population prevalence of APP mutations as a cause of AD seems quite low, making genotyping a poor candidate as a screening method. (This does not rule out assays of APP function or processing.) Continuing study of APP dynamics might yet uncover a single powerful diagnostic test or therapeutic drug, but that would likely be the subject of a separate patent, with benefits accruing to the future inventor.

The patent situation for the presenilin genes on chromosomes 1 and 14 could prove similar but could also prove simpler. The prevalence of the relevant forms of familial AD is higher, and the patent positions might (or might not) prove stronger for patent owners. To date, only one relevant patent has been issued, to Schellenberg and colleagues, assigned to the University of Washington. It claims genetic linkage to chromosome 14 (U.S. Patent #5449604). The patent application predated the discovery of the presenilin 1 gene itself, which is presumably the subject of one or more pending applications. No patents have been issued for the presenilin 2 gene on chromosome 1. Since patents remain pending, any guidance is speculative. One can only turn to the scientific history of presenilin gene discoveries (Pollen 1996). The patent story should parallel the science. There may or may not be disputes about who first discovered genetic linkage and who discovered the genes in the legal sense of invention. If multiple overlapping patent applications have been filed, then interference proceedings will be used by the patent office to decide the scope of claims granted to different inventors, according to legal criteria under U.S. law. The final result, with or without interference, could be multiple patents with somewhat different claims, or patents on the presenilin 1 and 2 genes themselves could prove dominant, with meaningful commercial rights held by only one inventor group for each gene on chromosomes 1 and 14.

The prevalence of chromosome 14-associated AD is higher than that for chromosome 1, and both are higher than those for APP mutations but significantly lower than that for late-onset AD. A diagnostic based on presenilin peptides or genes would likely have a market mainly confined to family members at risk, unless in some unexpected way they prove diagnostic for AD more generally. There are enough familial AD families to justify costs of a small niche commercial test, although testing in such families could remain the province of a few academic centers. It would take a dramatic scientific discovery to make the APP gene or chromosome 1 or 14 presenilin genes of broad diagnostic use and thus valuable commercial tests. The main value of discovering the APP gene and presenilin 1 and 2 genes seems likely to be as great scientific advances providing clues to pathogenesis, as well as potential guides for subsequent drug discovery efforts, rather than as diagnostics or therapeutics themselves. Ultimately, a multiple-allele test for multiple different genes on different chromosomes might be developed, involving licenses for these and other genes yet to be discovered.

The situation for APOE testing is substantially different from that for the Mendelian familial Alzheimer genes. The resulting information is about the risk of disease rather than the presence or absence of a gene that directly causes AD. This requires counseling, as does the explanation of genetic risks in familial AD inherited in Mendelian fashion, but it is counseling of a different kind. The APOE test is pertinent to a much larger population, not just to familial clusters with demonstrated risk, so the potential user pool is many times larger. The patent situation is complex, but for different reasons from that of the APP and presenilin genes. To date, only one patent has been issued, "Methods of screening for Alzheimer's disease," to Roses and colleagues, and assigned to Duke University (U.S. Patent #5508167).

The Duke patent has been licensed for the exclusive use of Athena Diagnostics, which offers genotyping as a service. Apolipoprotein had long been studied in cardiovascular disease before its relevance to AD was discovered, so APOE typing itself was not subject to patent. The patent covers APOE typing only for AD. Such a "use patent" is a weaker protection than one claiming all genotyping. A physician can order APOE typing from many clinical laboratories. He or she will not benefit from the other tests and interpretation services available from Athena and is technically infringing the patent if ordering the test to predict or diagnose AD, but it might be difficult for Athena to monitor patent infringement. Even if suspected, infringement could be difficult to prove in court. Since some APOE testing by laboratories other than Athena is legitimate, proof would require showing the infringing party intended genotyping for AD diagnosis and screening, a much harder case than just proving APOE

Table 6.1. Genetic Factors in Alzheimer Disease

Gene and Location	Nature of Inheritance	Faction of AD Population for Which Test Is Relevant	Patent Situation
APP, chromosome 21	Mendelian dominant	Very small (at most 1–3% of cases)	Many patents
Presenilin 1, chromosome 14	Mendelian dominant	No more than 1% of all AD cases	One patent for genetic linkage to chromosome 14, patents on genes presumably pending
Presenilin 2, chromosome 1	Mendelian dominant	Less rare than APP or presenilin 1	
Apolipoprotein E	Risk factor	Common	One-use patent, but no patent for gene or genotyping per se

testing was done at all. And a firm is much more likely to go after an infringing competitor than to single out a few practitioners that constitute their potential market, appearing ham-fisted and greedy.

The difficulty in proving infringement constrains the price Athena can charge, effectively weakening its monopoly and lessening the value of the Duke patent. The need to control the use of the test and limit infringing uses of APOE testing for AD may also be related to Athena's strategy of offering the test only as a direct service, rather than sublicensing to other laboratories. This introduces a substantial "hassle factor" associated with having to draw and send a blood sample to a remote laboratory and wait for the answer, a considerable nonprice constraint on use. The decision to test at a single laboratory is much less likely to lead to widespread testing than a sublicensing strategy to many laboratories, leaving aside cost considerations.

The title of the patent, which refers to screening, suggests that the initial expectation was that APOE testing might be useful for population screening. Other chapters in this volume (chaps. 4 and 5) recount the pros and cons of diagnostic testing and lay out the reasons that such screening is currently deemed premature. The literature from Athena Diagnostics is clear that the test should be ordered only in cases of symptomatic dementia. The test's commercial prospects depend critically on the value of the information the test yields compared with alternative diagnostic tests. This is unsettled. APOE testing is sometimes compared with imaging tests, another expensive item in some dementia diagnostic algorithms. That comparison is spurious, however, in the sense that imaging is much more powerful at ruling out lesions that cause anatomic change, whereas APOE testing to date is a mainly statistical "rule-in" procedure. The ultimate commercial value of APOE testing will depend on price, lowering the nonprice hassle factors, and where it perches in the decision tree—whether it becomes an essential early test, an optional one, or one used only in certain conditions. It will also depend critically on decisions about covering the test under insurance and managed care plans. Given the patient population, most users will be covered by the federal Medicare program, so the decisions of the Health Care Financing Administration and so-called medigap wraparound private insurers will be crucial.

The assumptions about diagnostic testing, including the number of tests and revenue streams, are quite shaky in the near term; they are likely to be catastrophically in error in the long run. Many "wild cards" are likely to overwhelm the short-term projections. Costs will drop, and technology will push hard in the direction of multiple-allele testing. Genetic testing is likely to prove most cost effective with a single disorder but will examine thousands to millions of genetic variants in a single pass at a reasonable cost. In that scenario, AD testing would be just a small part of a much more comprehensive genetic screen, with entirely different market dynamics, technology, cost, and linkage to genetic counseling and other services.

In addition to the technological and cost uncertainties, completely new nonmedical uses of genetic tests could also emerge. Assessing risk factors for AD could dramatically expand the market for tests and, not coincidentally, undermine the possibility of a private market for long-term-care insurance. This is because the risk factor assessment for common diseases is a powerful actuarial tool. Actuarial use of genetic risk factor prediction could approach population screening in size of market, but only if per test costs were pennies or dollars. Broad actuarial testing would depend on a combination of statistical, business, and political factors and would grow dramatically only if it does not provoke a legal response to proscribe or constrain its use.

References

Andrews, L. B., Fullarton, J. E., Holtzman, N. A., and Motulsky, A. G., eds. 1994. *Assessing genetic risks: Implications for health and social policy.* Washington, D.C.: Health and Social Policy, Institute of Medicine, National Academy Press.

Athena Diagnostics. 1996. Alzheimer's Disease Diagnosis Service; and New Athena ADmark Assays for Greater Certainty in AD Diagnosis and Prognosis. Worcester, Mass.

Cockburn, I., and Henderson, R. 1997. Public-private interaction and the productivity of pharmaceutical research. National Bureau of Economic Research Working Paper 6018, Cambridge, Mass.

Cohen, J. 1997. The genomics gamble. *Science* 275:767–72.

Eisenberg, R. 1996. Public research and private development: Patents and technology transfer in government-sponsored research. *Virginia Law Review* 82:1663–1727.

Fox, P. 1989. From senility to Alzheimer's disease: The rise of the Alzheimer's disease movement. *Milbank Quarterly* 67 (1): 58–102.

Gambardella, A. 1995. *Science and innovation: The United States pharmaceutical industry during the 1980s.* New York: Cambridge University Press.

Henderson, R. 1994. The evolution of integrative capacity: Innovation in cardiovascular drug discovery. *Industrial and Corporate Change* 3:607–30.

Henderson, R., and Cockburn, I. 1993. Scale, scope, and spillovers: The determinants of research productivity in the pharmaceutical industry. National Bureau of Economic Research Working Paper 4466, Cambridge, Mass.

Henderson, R., Jaffe, A. B., and Trajtenberg, M. 1997. Universities as a source of commercial technology: A detailed analysis of university patenting, 1965–1988. *Review of Economics and Statistics* (in press).

Katzman, R. 1976. The prevalence and malignancy of Alzheimer's disease: A major killer. *Archives of Neurology* 33:217–18, 304.

Mansfield, E. 1995. Academic research underlying industrial innovations: Sources, characteristics, and financing. *Review of Economics and Statistics* (Feb.): 55–65.

Narin, F., and Olivastro, D. 1992. Status report: Linkage between technology and science. *Research Policy* 21:237–49.

Narin, F., and Rozek, R. P. 1988. Biometric analysis of U.S. pharmaceutical industry research performance. *Research Policy* 17:139–54.

National Academy of Engineering. 1992. *Time horizons and technology investments.* Washington, D.C.: National Academy Press.

Office of Technology Assessment. 1987. *Losing a million minds: Confronting the tragedy of Alzheimer's disease and other dementias.* OTA-BAP-323. Washington, D.C.: Government Printing Office.

———. 1993. *Pharmaceutical R&D: Costs, risks, and rewards.* OTA-BAP-522. Washington, D.C.: Government Printing Office.

———. 1995. *Innovation and commercializing emerging technology.* OTA-BP-ITC-165. Washington, D.C.: Government Printing Office.

PhRMA (Pharmaceutical Research and Manufacturers Association). 1997. PhRMA annual survey 1997. Available from (http://www.phrma.org/facts/data/R&D.html).

Pollen, D. A. 1996. *Hannah's heirs: The quest for the genetic origins of Alzheimer disease.* Rev. ed. New York: Oxford University Press.

President's Commission for the Study of Ethical Problems in Medicine and Biomedical and Behavioral Research. 1983. *Screening and counseling for genetic conditions.* Washington, D.C.: Government Printing Office.

Walkington, R. A. 1997. Financial support for Alzheimer's disease research. Report prepared for the Royalty Fund Advisory Committee, Alzheimer's Association, Washington, D.C.

PART TWO

Ethical Aspects

7

Genetic Testing and Counseling for Early-Onset Autosomal-Dominant Alzheimer Disease

HARRY KARLINSKY, M.D.

The implications of the identification of mutations on chromosomes 1, 14, and 21 associated with the presence of early-onset autosomal-dominant Alzheimer disease (AD) include consideration of their possible use in various clinical circumstances. Specifically, it is now at least technologically feasible to identify mutation carriers in both asymptomatic and symptomatic individuals (i.e., those who are cognitively impaired) from AD families with known mutations. This raises the possibility of predictive and diagnostic testing. Before such testing is undertaken, however, it is important to consider the validity of the proposed genetic tests as well as the complex ethical, legal, and psychological issues that will have an impact on the genetic counseling associated with any proposed AD genetic testing program.

Predictive Testing

One of the difficulties in assessing the utility of apparently disease-causing mutations in the prediction of AD is that definitive data on sensitivity and specificity are not available. These data will eventually emerge from clinicopathological longitudinal studies that include asymptomatic family members whose mutation status is known. In the current absence of such studies, an estimate of specificity requires particular caution in view of the rarity of families with the early-onset mutations identified to date. Although the development of the disease is often cited as virtually certain, there is at least one asymptomatic individual with an APP mutation who is now two standard deviations beyond the family-specific mean age of onset (St. George-Hyslop et al. 1994). Furthermore, it is now becoming increasingly apparent that mutations in the chromosome 1 gene are associated with marked variability in age of onset and possible nonexpression (Bird et al. 1996). Despite the fact that the exact risks are somewhat uncertain, it seems clear that the 50 percent a priori risk of an individual developing AD within these autosomal-dominant families is increased significantly if a known mutation is identified. It therefore seems reasonable that predictive testing be available to such individuals, provided appropriate genetic counseling services are available.

The existing experience in Huntington disease (HD) provides a valuable model of the relevant genetic counseling required for early-onset AD. Like early-onset AD, HD is a progressive incurable neurodegenerative disorder, albeit less genetically heterogeneous than AD. Following the discovery of a linked DNA marker to HD (Gusella et al. 1983), predictive testing programs were established in a number of countries, initially following an "indirect" paradigm but more recently based on "direct" testing following the cloning of the HD gene (Huntington's Disease Collaborative Research Group 1993). Ethical Issues Policy Statements (World Federation of Neurology 1989, 1990) have provided comprehensive recommendations concerning essential genetic counseling aspects of HD predictive testing programs, including the necessity of voluntary participation. Details of essential pretest genetic counseling information have been outlined, including full discussion of the potential personal, familial, and discriminatory socioeconomic consequences of testing. The need for posttest counseling has equally been emphasized.

Following the identification of the APP mutations on chromosome 21, it was proposed that predictive testing for early-onset autosomal-dominant AD could be cautiously offered in research settings, primarily according to the established HD guidelines (Lennox et al. 1994). Indeed, the predictive testing experience for three individuals from a family with an APP mutation has now been reported (Lannfelt et al. 1995). Until additional longitudinal data are available to better define the positive and negative predictive value of the various mutations, test results will need to be cautiously interpreted. Nevertheless, testing still currently provides a significant alteration to the risk of developing AD for asymptomatic members from families with known mutations. A percentage of individuals from other families with early-onset autosomal-dominant disease will likely also request predictive testing, even in the absence of preventive therapies, as more accurate risk status may assist significant life decisions or address the psychological stress of uncertainty in some individuals. Clearly, predictive testing for early-onset AD should not be undertaken without extensive pretest assessment and counseling and full discussion of the potential benefits and burdens of testings. The emotion-laden process of disclosure of test results must be carefully addressed. Finally, long-term follow-up must also be available, regardless of test results, but particularly for psychologically distressed mutation carriers.

As more and more AD-related mutations are being rapidly identified, it may be helpful to outline suggested components of a "generic" predictive testing program that disregards the specific mutation involved. This assumes the important prerequisite that predictive testing is being undertaken only after careful consideration of the positive and negative predictive value of available genetic tests and the potential benefits and harms of testing. If such an analysis concludes that it is reasonable to offer predictive testing to informed voluntary participants, then pretest assessment and counseling, disclosure of test results, and posttest follow-up are essential components of all predictive genetic testing programs for early-onset AD. Details of each of these components follow.

Pretest Assessment and Counseling

In the interests of clarity, pretest assessment and counseling are each discussed under separate headings below. In practice, however, both will quite likely, and appropriately, occur together.

Pretest Assessment

In this discussion, potential participants in predictive genetic testing programs are envisioned to be individuals perceived to be at risk for early-onset autosomal-dominant AD because a family-specific mutation has been identified in other affected family members. Thus, as with traditional genetic counseling, constructing a family tree (pedigree) containing genetic and other relevant information is an essential first step of the pretest assessment. Obtaining and documenting the necessary information can be time consuming. It may, for instance, involve, with appropriate consent, eliciting and evaluating medical, autopsy, and other reports, interviewing various family informants, and examining symptomatic and asymptomatic relatives.

Once an accurate pedigree is constructed, individuals presenting for predictive testing should be assessed to rule out subtle cognitive manifestations of AD, particularly those who are nearing or beyond the mean age of risk within their families. It is notable that some symptomatic individuals have enrolled in predictive testing programs for other disorders as an acceptable means of securing a clinical diagnosis in contrast to the prediction of or prospects of future occurrence of the disease (Meissen et al. 1988). However, individuals with established signs of the disease who are unacknowledged or unsuspected are less likely to be prepared to deal with an unexpected clinical diagnosis and may suffer severe psychological reactions (Bloch et al. 1989). Participants in AD predictive testing programs should therefore be informed as to whether baseline clinical examinations are an integral component of the pretest assessment and provided with the option of not being informed of the examination results. Although not the ideal scenario, even the clinical examination per se should not be compulsory. It will be apparent, however, that examinations that do occur may require a referral to an appropriate specialist, such as a neuropsychologist for detailed cognitive assessment.

Psychological appraisal is also a necessary aspect of the pretest assessment. In practice, this may informally occur throughout the course of the pretest counseling phase. Regardless of the precise timing, it is important to have some sense of the individual's ability to cope with the results of testing, particularly if the mutation is identified. The rationale for a psychological appraisal is clearly evident. For example, 5 percent of at-risk individuals for HD surveyed before predictive testing was available stated that they would choose suicide if given a positive test result (Kessler et al. 1987). Thus, a distinctly cautious approach has been integrated into predictive testing programs for HD, where variables such as psychiatric state, risk of suicide, depression, and level of social support are often formally assessed in interviews and questionnaires (Fox et al. 1989). Although testing should not proceed in acutely suicidal individuals, psychological appraisals will more often lead to deferment of testing than to its absolute exclusion. Psychological appraisals can also be useful in anticipating an individual's response to learning the genetic test results, thereby identifying those individuals requiring the most intensive follow-up support.

Finally, if other criteria for eligibility apply before testing can proceed, they must be considered in the context of the pretest assessment. It might be viewed as obvious, for example, that testing should occur only on a voluntary basis, so requests from third parties—family members or others—should not be considered. It remains unsettled, however, as to whether testing can be imposed as a condition of employability or insurability.

Although an individual could always refuse to be tested in these circumstances, loss of employment or insurability may yet emerge as a valid legal consequence. Also, ideally individuals should be able to participate in predictive testing programs regardless of their financial situation. It is likely, however, that ability to pay will be a criterion for eligibility in some jurisdictions, particularly as long as unfavorable predictive test findings cannot result in beneficial surveillance measures or preventive interventions. Age of majority may also be a legal requirement for testing eligibility in certain jurisdictions, although it would be more appropriate to consider capacity to understand than an arbitrary chronological threshold.

Another issue that may affect eligibility is the possibility that testing of an individual might provide unwanted information to another person. For example, in the initial HD predictive testing programs, an individual at 25 percent risk was considered ineligible for testing if that individual's unaffected at-risk parent did not wish to know his or her own genetic status. The rationale was that should a positive result occur in the tested individual, the at-risk parent would de facto also learn that he or she was a mutation carrier, although such information may have been deliberately unwanted. Similarly, testing of an identical twin would not be done unless or until the co-twin also agreed to undergo testing. Now, however, the consensus appears to be that the right of an adult to know supersedes the rights of other adults not to know: thus, testing in these circumstances is more likely to be viewed as acceptable.

Finally, it is conceivable that in some future circumstances, eligibility for testing might include pretest agreement by a participant to disclose test results to other individuals. For example, the identification of a disease-related gene in a participant might establish a previously unappreciated at-risk status for other family members. If established preventive interventions for AD become available, some predictive testing programs may feel mandatory disclosure of at-risk status to other family members would be a prerequisite for testing the initial participant. The issue of disclosure of test results by the participant, regardless of its voluntary or mandatory nature, should also be discussed in the pretest and follow-up counseling.

Pretest Counseling

Once a preliminary assessment, as described above, has taken place and eligibility for testing has been established, relevant up-to-date information must be conveyed to individuals considering testing to ensure that subsequent participation occurs on the basis of an informed decision. Essential comprehensive information must be provided in four broad subject areas: general information about AD, its genetics in the light of available predictive genetic tests, perceived benefits, and harms of testing, and alternatives to testing. Participants should be encouraged to select one or more partners to join them throughout the process of counseling. It has been suggested in predictive testing programs associated with other disorders that partners should not be genetically related to participants in order to avoid possible vested interests that could bias support. However, it seems preferable that the participant should be able to choose anyone, regardless of the relationship, provided the proposed partner's consent is also obtained (Lennox et al. 1994).

Individuals will be likely to vary widely in the extent and accuracy of their preexisting knowledge about AD. Routinely, therefore, basic aspects of AD should be reviewed, including clinical manifestations, prognosis, and availability of treatment and prevention. It is important that each participant be aware of all risk factors pertaining to his or her situation, and ideally these details should be integrated in an individualized manner into the pretest counseling. If resources are limited, however, some general information about AD can be provided, in the absence of a counselor, in written form, or by means of audiovisual tapes or interactive computer, although the efficacy of these alternative approaches requires rigorous assessment.

Relevant genetic principles should be reviewed, followed by a summary of the genetics of AD. It is likely that many family members will have had limited, if any, prior exposure to the field of genetics, so that conveying the information mentioned can be a significant challenge. Indeed, the potential for misunderstanding is legion. As new AD-related mutations are identified that lend themselves to predictive testing, a growing proportion of potential participants will have been previously unaware of, and therefore less informed about, their family-specific illness. This will be particularly so should predictive testing increasingly encompass those mutations with less than 100 percent penetrance and subject to gene-gene or gene-environmental interactions, or both. Establishing the most effective ways to convey such sophisticated concepts to the lay public remains an ongoing challenge.

Factual information must be provided about the available genetic test (or tests) itself, including how the test is done and how individuals will receive their results. As AD may be associated with nongenetic phenocopies, it must be stressed that the risk of AD from nongenetic causes is not excluded with negative genetic test results. For those AD-related mutations with less than 100 percent penetrance, probability versus certainty of disease occurring must be distinguished. And, finally, it must be stressed that identifying a disease-related gene in an individual does not equate to a diagnosis that the disease is present. Even after genetic counseling, this appears to be a difficult concept for some individuals to grasp. For example, in one study pertaining to HD, a proportion of participants surveyed after counseling still incorrectly equated identification of the gene with diagnosis of the disease (Quaid and Morris 1993).

In some testing circumstances, DNA from other affected and unaffected family members may be requested, which raises its own ethical and legal dilemmas. It is recommended that the participant, rather than members of the predictive testing team, be responsible for approaching other relatives to solicit blood samples for genetic testing, with the understanding that these requests may represent an invasion of privacy.

The participant should then gain a clear understanding of the potential benefits and harms of testing. Even in the current absence of earlier clinical diagnosis or prospects of prevention, predictive testing for early-onset AD will still yield benefits for some individuals, although this can vary widely depending upon the individual's specific circumstances. Benefits may occur, for example, with regard to major life decisions. Marital and reproductive choices, career choices (including the timing of retirement), and advance health care directives could conceivably be influenced by test results, and some participants may view this as helpful. Although details of prenatal testing protocols are beyond the scope of this chapter, the appropriateness of such protocols is an extremely contentious issue, and the availability of prenatal testing will most likely vary depending upon jurisdiction.

For some individuals, simply knowing one's genetic status (i.e., knowledge per se) may be the principal benefit of genetic testing. For these individuals, it is the uncertainty that is hardest to bear. For example, for those who chose to undergo genetic testing for HD, a one-year follow-up program found improved psychological well-being, regardless of the test results, as compared to those who chose to remain uninformed of their risk status (Wiggins et al. 1992). Clearly, for those whose lives are affected by the belief that they have inherited an AD-related gene, the beneficial psychological impact on well-being could be enormous if this belief proves to be erroneous.

Finally, testing may lead to benefits to other family members by providing desired information relevant or necessary to establishing their own risk status. However, individuals must not be coerced into personally unwanted testing by other family members.

Participants must be equally well informed about potential harms of testing. Although test results may facilitate major life decisions, there may be seriously adverse socioeconomic consequences, such as employment, insurance, and financial discrimination. In some jurisdictions, individuals are advised to review and, if necessary, purchase life and health insurance before proceeding with testing.

Rather than benefiting family members, testing may instead prove harmful. Perhaps this occurs most obviously when test results alter genetic risks in other family members who would have preferred to remain uninformed about their own genetic risk status. In some circumstances, altered genetic risk status in one family member may also deleteriously alter family relationships, such as engendering isolation.

Similarly, just as test results may be psychologically helpful, particularly if an AD-related gene is not identified, the detection of a disease-causing mutation may be devastating to vulnerable individuals. It is important, therefore, that participants consider all possible test outcomes, rather than only those expected or desired, and explore the anticipated psychological consequences of each possible test result. Many variables that could influence the psychological impact may need to be reviewed, such as the individual's own experience with AD in other family members, current life circumstances and social supports, personal values, past patterns of behavior and decision making, and life decisions that may be altered by test results. While pretest assessment of expected reactions to test results may not always prove valid, this process helps the participant consider all possible test outcomes.

Finally, it is essential that all participants be aware of their options regarding testing. They must clearly realize that testing can be declined or deferred. In some circumstances, alternatives such as DNA banking and anonymous testing without disclosure to the donor can still benefit other family members, and this option should be presented where appropriate.

Once all relevant information has been conveyed, participants must be given time to fully consider whether they wish to proceed with testing. As "direct" testing can technically proceed without delay, it seems judicious to allow some time to elapse before testing. This is illustrated by a study on decision making in predictive testing in HD, which found that many individuals became more ambivalent about being tested during a relatively lengthy pretest counseling program (Burgess 1994). Although an imposed time delay may be viewed as paternalistic, it seems appropriate to ensure that such an important decision has not been precipitous, particularly when an unpreventable and untreatable disorder such as AD is at issue.

When a participant has difficulty in deciding whether to undergo testing, health care professionals involved in the pretest assessment and counseling may be asked by the participant to make a decision on the participant's behalf. However, most would view the role of health care professionals in these circumstances as facilitative rather than directive and would strongly recommend that the autonomy of the participant be encouraged and respected. Although discussion and exploration should always be supported, including with other significant family members and friends, it is the participant who ultimately must decide.

If the individual reaches a decision to be tested, the clinician will need to collect a blood sample and establish a date for disclosure of test results. Details of posttest follow-up should also be presented at this time. Written consent for testing is recommended and may be a legal requirement in some jurisdictions. Once a decision to be tested has been made, the waiting period before the disclosure session can be one of heightened anxiety during which support may be required (Burgess 1994). The disclosure session should therefore take place as soon as possible.

Disclosure of Test Results

Regardless of whether or not a mutation is identified, the predictive testing experiences in other disorders have established the disclosure of genetic test results as the most emotionally charged interaction of the predictive testing process. For most participants, it will mark the end of a long waiting period filled with uncertainty. It is extremely important, therefore, that participants have a clear prior understanding of what will occur during the disclosure session, including its precise timing and who will be present.

Before scheduling the disclosure session, the participant should be offered alternative times in order to avoid stressful logistical difficulties. In some predictive testing protocols for other disorders, there has been a requirement for the presence of a support person who previously participated in the pretest counseling process. Other protocols, which generally seem preferable, have left this as an option for the participant. If support persons are to be involved, the issue of confidentiality should be discussed before the actual disclosure session. As for which health care professionals should be present, the most important factor is continuity. Ideally, the health care professional most involved in the pretest counseling process should be present, at least in the capacity of support. If this professional is not a geneticist, then, depending on the complexity of the interpretation of the genetic test results, the presence of a geneticist may also be advisable.

Before disclosing results, clinicians should confirm with participants that they still desire this information. Though the pretest counseling process will probably have eliminated those individuals who do not wish to be tested, some participants may withdraw at the last moment, and they should be reminded that they have every right to do so. For this reason, it is also important that those disclosing the test results receive these from the laboratory just before the disclosure session. This not only supports an unbiased stance throughout the pretest assessment and counseling period but also may preserve this lack of bias in future counseling, should relatively last-minute withdrawals by participants occur.

Results should be presented as unambiguously as possible, with careful attention to language. For example, in the scientific community, a positive result implies that a disease-related mutation was identified. However, disclosing results as positive to participants may create confusion and ultimately be viewed as highly insensitive. Instead, it should be stated whether the mutation was identified, followed by an explanation of the effect the test results have on the likelihood of developing the disease.

Immediately upon receiving results, some participants will be likely to experience an intense emotional reaction. At times, it may be helpful to allow some private time to the participant and his or her support person, if present, before continuing with the session. However, if the experience with other disorders is relevant, in many circumstances, the full emotional impact of learning the test results will not occur immediately (Bloch et al. 1992). It is, therefore, extremely important that the details of posttest follow-up again be reviewed. If possible, the health care professionals should explore the intended immediate course of action by the participant. However, given the likely emotional intensity of this session, it is not recommended that much further information be provided, such as details of disease surveillance should the disease-related mutation have been identified. As it is unlikely that further information will be absorbed at this point, such issues should be deferred to the posttest follow-up unless the participant strongly desires additional immediate information.

Posttest Follow-Up

The psychosocial impact of an altered genetic risk status for early-onset AD should not be underestimated, although the impact will obviously depend on the personal characteristics and circumstances of the individual who has undergone testing. As mentioned above, the anticipated intense emotional reactions associated with the conveyance of test results can preclude that forum for meaningful further exploration of the impact of carrier or noncarrier status or the practical steps that become indicated. Further follow-up should therefore be mandatory. Its specific frequency and form will vary, but posttest follow-up should be prompt. For example, the initial guidelines for the molecular genetics predictive test in HD (World Federation of Neurology 1989, 1990) recommended that the counselor have contact with the tested individual within the first week after delivery of the results, regardless of their nature. One immediate consideration is to review the individual's understanding of the test result. As discussed above, predictive tests indicate the likelihood that someone is a carrier of a disease-related mutation but not that the clinical disease per se is now present. Nevertheless, even with intensive counseling, some individuals may still confuse this crucial distinction.

Another immediate consideration is the emotional status of the tested individual. Again, using the illustrative experience of HD, preliminary follow-up research suggests that the period of greatest vulnerability lies in the first month of receiving verification of increased-risk status. Individuals may experience depression or despair over test results, and suicidal ideation needs careful monitoring (Bloch et al. 1992).

Although it is reasonable to assume that the greatest burdens will be endured by those who are shown to carry a disease-related mutation, negative test results may also be accompanied by adverse psychosocial consequences. Again turning to the HD predictive testing experience, some individuals receiving a decreased-risk status for the disease have psychological reactions ranging from denial and disbelief to a complete revamping of a sense of self and outlook on life. Negative ramifications are a greater risk for those individuals who, before testing, had strong preconceived ideas as to the expected test results, had made irreversible lifetime decisions, or had unrealistic and overoptimistic expectations of the benefits of receiving decreased-risk status (Huggins et al. 1992).

Although published data on the short-term psychosocial consequences of predictive testing for other disorders are accumulating, the long-term impact is not known. One significant concern is how individuals at increased genetic risk of developing disease will deal with the onset of symptomatology and clinical diagnosis. It is apparent, for example, that the initial symptomatology of AD (i.e., its subtle intellectual decline) may lead to crippling hypervigilance and mistaken self-diagnosis in family members at empirical risk for this disorder. It is conceivable and a concern that this phenomenon will be accentuated, should individuals be aware that they are carriers of a disease-related mutation. This consideration, among others, indicates the importance of making available long-term support for all participants of predictive testing programs and addressing this protracted time frame in selected research protocols.

It is to be hoped that surveillance and prophylactic interventions for early-onset AD will one day reduce morbidity and mortality in carriers of a disease-related mutation. These future prospects should be conveyed to those individuals in whom the disease-related mutation is detected and a mechanism for follow-up is established.

Diagnostic Testing

Using the known pathogenic mutations, genetic testing of symptomatic individuals with suspected early-onset autosomal-dominant AD from families with known mutations is also now technically feasible. Again, as with predictive testing, genetic test results will need to be cautiously interpreted. Although the identified mutations on chromosomes 1, 14, and 21 appear to be the major genetic determinants of AD in these families, additional as-yet-unknown genetic or environmental factors may modify the penetrance and expressivity of these mutations. An additional issue to consider is that the identification of a pathogenic mutation in a cognitively impaired individual does not necessarily indicate that the mutation is a causal factor in that individual's current symptomatology. Since AD has its recognizable clinical onset in adulthood, the expression of a pathogenic mutation may not occur for decades. Even with the identification of such a mutation in a cognitively impaired individual, other causes of cognitive impairment still need to be considered and excluded (i.e., persons with a mutation may also have other disorders unrelated to this finding, such as depression). It is important to emphasize this point: the detection of a disease-related mutation does not per se establish a diagnosis of AD. The clinical diagnosis of AD is still dependent on the presence of the characteristic cognitive decline and the exclusion of other causes of cognitive impairment or dementia. Finally, an individual without his or her family-specific mutation would still be at risk for AD from other causes, in keeping with age-adjusted general population rates.

Despite the above caveats, testing for mutations may still advantageously enhance clinical diagnostic accuracy, particularly if a specific mutation known to be present in other affected family members of the tested individual is *not* identified (see illustrative case vignette by Karlinsky and colleagues 1994). It is likely that testing cognitively impaired individuals from families with known mutations will be increasingly considered, particularly if it is established that clarifying an affected individual's genotype facilitates the introduction and selection of antidementia drugs.

In addition to the considerations described in the context of predictive testing, testing symptomatic individuals raises additional genetic counseling complexities in the area of consent. As with predictive testing, informed consent must be elicited before testing. However, as symptomatic individuals will have at least some degree of cognitive impairment, a significant percentage may not possess the mental capacity to provide valid informed consent. In these circumstances, a substitute decision maker will need to be identified, a process that will vary according to jurisdiction and of which those providers of genetic counseling should be aware. The competency of affected individuals to consent to testing or assign a substitute decision maker must therefore become routine considerations of pretest genetic counseling. If required, it is important that an acting substitute decision maker receive adequate pretest information so that a genetic test decision in the best interests of the affected individual can be reached.

Other Considerations

The above discussion has focused on asymptomatic and symptomatic individuals from families with known mutations. This circumvents a larger and more difficult question: what is the general role for molecular genetic testing in asymptomatic and symptomatic individuals with suspected early-onset familial AD in whom a family-specific mutation has not been identified? This could occur, for example, if all previously affected family members are deceased. The genetic heterogeneity of AD requires consideration of different test options, but there are problems concerning the sensitivity and specificity of currently available "direct" tests when applied to an unselected population. Furthermore, as not all disease-related genes for AD have yet been identified, it must be stressed that genetic risk may not be entirely excluded with negative results. However, in the event that an individual with a mutation is identified, the potential for predictive testing and diagnostic testing of other interested family members is now facilitated. Those potential benefits for other family members might warrant testing for the AD-related mutations in these circumstances. Benefits will obviously be further enhanced if future therapeutic interventions—both symptomatic and preventive—have selective benefits based on genotype. These issues require further discussion and resolution before widespread introduction of molecular genetic testing of individuals who are either at risk or symptomatic with suspected early-onset familial AD in whom family-specific mutations have not yet been identified.

Conclusion

Three important components to consider must be considered when constructing a predictive testing program for asymptomatic individuals from families with early-onset autosomal-dominant AD: pretest assessment and counseling, disclosure of test results, and posttest follow-up. Although insistence on their inclusion in all predictive testing programs could be criticized as unnecessarily paternalistic and costly, current adherence to such guidelines seems prudent in order to minimize the potential serious consequences associated with predictive testing. Similar recommendations pertain when genetic testing occurs in symptomatic individuals. Although these concepts may seem less than revolutionary in some centers, there is legitimate concern that such factors as the expediencies of commercial testing may lead to unwarranted shortcuts. This, in turn, may be associated with unforseen and unnecessary burdens for the participants.

Acknowledgments

Work on this chapter was supported by the Alzheimer Society of Canada and Riverview Hospital, British Columbia, Canada. The author gratefully acknowledges helpful discussions with Dr. J. Berg, Surrey Place Centre, Toronto and the following members of the Vancouver Collaborative Study of Genetic Testing for Alzheimer's Disease: Dr. M. Bloch, A. Booth, Dr. M. Burgess, Dr. O. Geiger, Dr. B. McKellin, Dr. J. Miller, Dr. D. Sadovnick, A. Smith, Dr. S. Wiggins.

References

Bird, T. D., Levy-Lahad, E., Poorkaj, P., Sharma, V., Lahad, A., Lampe, T. H., and Schellenberg, G. D. 1996. Wide range in age of onset for chromosome 1-related familial Alzheimer's disease. *Annals of Neurology* 40:932–36.

Bloch, M., Adam, S., Wiggins, S., Huggins, M., and Hayden, M. R. 1992. Predictive testing for Huntington disease in Canada: The experience of those receiving an increased risk. *American Journal of Medical Genetics* 42:499–507.

Bloch, M., Fahy, M., Fox, S., and Hayden, M. R. 1989. Predictive testing for Huntington's disease. Part 2, Demographic characteristics, life-style patterns, attitudes, and psychological assessments of the first fifty-one test candidates. *American Journal of Medical Genetics* 32:217–24.

Burgess, M. 1994. Ethical issues in genetic testing for Alzheimer's disease: Lessons from Huntington's disease. *Alzheimer Disease and Associated Disorders* 8:71–78.

Fox, S., Bloch, M., Fahy, M., Hayden, M.R. 1989. Predictive testing for Huntington disease. Part 1, Description of a pilot project in British Columbia. *American Journal of Medical Genetics* 32:211–16.

Gusella, J. F., Wexler, N. S., Conneally, P. M., Naylor, S. L., Anderson, M. A., Tanzi, R. E., Watkins, P. C., Ottina, K., Wallace, M. R., and Sakaguchi, A. Y. 1983. A polymorphic DNA marker genetically linked to Huntington's disease. *Nature* 306:234–38.

Huggins, M., Bloch, M., Wiggins, S., Adam, S., Suchowersky, O., Trew, M., Klimek, M., Greenberg, C. R., Eleff, M., and Thompson, L. P. 1992. Predictive testing for Huntington disease in Canada: Adverse effects and unexpected results in those receiving a decreased risk. *American Journal of Medical Genetics* 41:508–15.

Huntington's Disease Collaborative Research Group. 1993. A novel gene containing a trinucleotide repeat that is expanded and unstable on Huntington's disease chromosomes. *Cell* 72:971–83.

Karlinsky, H., Sadovnick, A. D., Burgess, M. M., Langlois, S., Hayden, M. R., and Berg, J. M. 1994. Issues in molecular genetic testing of individuals with suspected early-onset familial Alzheimer's disease. *Alzheimer Disease and Associated Disorders* 8:116–25.

Kessler, S., Field, T., Worth, L., and Mosbarger, H. 1987. Attitudes of persons at risk for Huntington disease toward predictive testing. *American Journal of Medical Genetics* 26: 259–70.

Lannfelt, L., Axelman, K., Lilius, L., and Basun, H. 1995. Genetic counseling of a Swedish Alzheimer family with amyloid precursor protein mutation. *American Journal of Human Genetics* 56:332–35.

Lennox, A., Karlinsky, H., Meschino, W., Buchanan, J. A., Percy, M. E., and Berg, J. M. 1994. Molecular genetic predictive testing for Alzheimer's disease: Deliberations and preliminary recommendations. *Alzheimer Disease and Associated Disorders* 8:126–47.

Meissen, G. J., Myers, R. H., Mastromauro, C. A., Koroshetz, W. J., Klinger, K. W., Farrer, L. A., Wathins, P. A., Gusella, J. F., Bird, E. D., and Martin, J. B. 1988. Predictive testing for Huntington's disease with use of a linked DNA marker. *New England Journal of Medicine* 318:535–42.

Quaid, K. A., and Morris, M. 1993. Reluctance to undergo predictive testing. *American Journal of Medical Genetics* 45:41–45.

St. George-Hyslop, P. H., MacLachlan, D., Tuda, T., Rogaev, E., Karlinsky, H., Lippa, C. F., and Pollen, D. 1994. Alzheimer's disease and possible gene interaction. *Science* 263:537.

Wexler, N. S. 1992. The Tiresias complex: Huntington's disease as a paradigm of testing for late-onset disorders. *FASEB Journal* 6:2820–25.

Wiggins, S., Whyte, P., Huggins, M., Adam, S., Theilmann, J., Bloch, M., Shelps, S. B., Schechter, M. T., and Hayden, M. R. 1992. The psychological consequences of predictive testing for Huntington's disease. *New England Journal of Medicine* 327:1401–5.

World Federation of Neurology, Research Committee Research Group on Huntington's Chorea. 1989. Ethical issues policy statement on Huntington's disease molecular genetics predictive test. *Journal of Neurological Science* 94:327–32.

———. 1990. Ethical issues policy statement on Huntington's chorea. *Journal of Medical Genetics* 27:34–38.

Implications of Genetic Susceptibility Testing with Apolipoprotein E

KIMBERLY A. QUAID, PH.D.

A major issue for genetic counselors is their comfort level with providing uncertain information to clients. Providing susceptibility data with relatively low sensitivity and specificity is worrisome, because clients may nevertheless make significant life choices based on it. This chapter discusses APOE testing as a paradigm case for genetic susceptibility with a focus on the moral conscience of the counselor and the potential interpretations of data by the client.

A Counselor's Quandary: Risks and Benefits

On April 1, 1996, the front page of the *New York Times* ran a story on genetic testing. Entitled "Breaking Ranks, Lab Offers Test to Assess the Risk of Breast Cancer," the story revealed a developing tension among the genetics community, commercial laboratories, and the public. The essence of the story is this: In the wake of the discovery that as many as 1 percent of Jewish women carry a mutated form of a gene that may predispose them to breast and ovarian cancer, leading scientists and two major commercial testing laboratories agreed informally not to offer the test to the general public. Their reasoning was based on longstanding issues of concern to those in medicine: the risk posed by the gene to the general public was still unclear; it was uncertain what might be done to lessen that risk, once quantified; and, finally, widespread testing might cause more harm than good. Citing women's "right to know," Dr. Joseph D. Schulman, the director of the Genetics and IVF (in vitro fertilization) Institute in Fairfax, Virginia, had just announced his decision to offer the test. This decision, according to a veteran *New York Times* science writer, "enraged" his colleagues (Kolata 1996).

So the battle lines are drawn in a scenario that is likely to be played out many times as the DNA double helix reveals its secrets: How should the dissemination of new genetic tests be handled? On one side are the concerned scientists urging caution and a "Do no harm" approach. On the other side are for-profit laboratories looking at millions of dollars in potential profits and espousing a "Right to know" philosophy. Caught in the middle are those at risk for genetic diseases who are desperately trying to sort out the conflicting information and genetic counselors who are charged with educating consumers and supporting informed decision making.

These issues, with slight variations, have played major roles in genetic testing since 1983, when the gene for Huntington disease (HD) was mapped to a previously unknown location on chromosome 4 using restriction fragment length polymorphisms (Gusella et al. 1983). Huntington disease is a late-onset neuropsychiatric disorder characterized by changes in mood, cognition, and movement. The average age of onset is approximately thirty-nine years. The suicide rate of those affected with HD is seven times the national average. There is no treatment and no cure. Huntington disease is inherited in an autosomal-dominant manner, so each child of an affected parent has approximately a 50 percent chance of inheriting the abnormal gene. Penetrance, the likelihood of developing symptoms if one has inherited the abnormal gene, is virtually 100 percent (Folstein 1989). The discovery of a genetic marker that is linked to the HD gene, and that traveled with the gene during reproduction, made predictive testing for HD possible. The first tests were completed in the summer of 1986, thus heralding the age of predictive medicine based on genetic information.

The potential costs and benefits of predictive testing had been a subject of debate for many years. The potential benefits of testing included the ability to plan for the future, the ability to make informed decisions about childbearing, and a reduction in the anxiety of those at risk (Bates 1981; Craufurd and Harris 1986). The potential negative effects of testing included depression, suicide (Kessler et al. 1987), disruption of family relationships, marital instability (Quaid and Wesson 1995), and discrimination in insurance and employment (Geller et al. 1996). Faced with the realization that the actual consequences of providing this kind information were completely unknown, practitioners initiated predictive testing for HD only through programs with detailed research protocols designed to examine the psychological, social, and economic consequences of testing (Brandt et al. 1989; Fox et al. 1989; Meissen et al. 1988). Offering testing in the context of research protocols had the advantage of providing a wealth of information regarding the consequences of predictive testing for HD. Soon after the initiation of testing, the Huntington's Disease Society of America and the World Federation of Neurology Research Group on Huntington's Chorea published guidelines for testing (HDSA 1989; Went 1990).

The first studies to be published focused on the psychological impact of testing. In 1988, Meissen and colleagues reported that two out of four individuals with an increased risk experienced "severe depression" after testing. Brandt and colleagues reported on twelve persons at high risk and found that two years after testing there were increased scores on the Global Severity Index of the Symptom Checklist (SCL-90) (Derogatis 1983) when compared with baseline. These scores, however, remained within normal limits (Brandt et al. 1989).

Two case studies from the Canadian Collaborative Study of Predictive Testing reported that two of four high-risk cases experienced depression for several months after testing (Bloch et al. 1992) and that 10 percent of those receiving low-risk results experienced some depression after disclosure (Huggins et al. 1992). Another Canadian report on thirty-seven individuals at high risk found no significant differences in average scores on the SCL-90 and the Beck Depression Inventory (Beck et al. 1961) one year after testing when compared with those at low risk. In addition, both of the tested groups were doing better than individuals who had not been tested. These authors concluded that predictive testing for HD had potential benefits for the psychological health of persons who received test results, regardless of whether those results indicated an increased or a decreased risk (Wiggins et al. 1992).

A later study from the Dutch predictive testing program in Leiden reported that the majority of individuals with high-risk results rated their current life situation as "good" or better. The authors attributed this result to denial (Tibben et al. 1993) and cautioned that this manner of coping may lead to increased difficulties in the future.

These various results using objective psychological measures, albeit somewhat mixed, suggested that testing could be done relatively safely in a context of neurological and psychiatric screening, psychological testing, intensive pretest counseling, and follow-up. Based on this information, the number of centers offering testing slowly grew (Quaid 1993).

Low Uptake of Testing

The uptake of testing was less than previously predicted. Before the availability of predictive testing for HD, surveys indicated that between 56 percent (Tyler and Harper 1983) and 77 percent (Stern and Eldridge 1975) would make use of a predictive test that was safe and reliable. Soon after the announcement of the availability of the predictive test, surveys indicated that these numbers remained high (Kessler et al. 1987; Markel, Young, and Penney 1987; Mastromauro, Myers, and Berkman 1987; Meissen and Berchek 1987). However, in actual practice, the number of individuals requesting testing has been fairly low (Craufurd et al. 1989; Quaid, Brandt, and Folstein 1987). Recent estimates suggest that only 5 percent of those at risk for HD have chosen to be tested (World Federation of Neurology 1993). One study examining the reluctance to be tested cited knowledge of increased risk to offspring if the test result was positive, the lack of any effective cure or treatment, and potential loss of health insurance as the major reasons for choosing not to be tested (Quaid and Morris 1993). The use of testing for the prenatal detection of fetuses at risk for HD, believed by some to be the most important use of this technology, was also extremely low (Quaid 1993). Many at-risk or affected parents proceeded with childbearing plans in the hope that a cure would be found in time for their children (Adam et al. 1993).

Several of the more recent studies, my own among them, may offer some clues to this low uptake for testing. Codori and Brandt (1994) reported that, regardless of test outcome, genetic testing resulted in negative as well as positive consequences. They concluded that persons at risk should understand that genetic information will almost certainly result in undesirable as well as desirable consequences. My own investigation into the effects of testing on couples revealed that individuals at increased risk were significantly more distressed during follow- up than individuals who had received a decreased-risk result (Quaid and Wesson 1995). These studies suggest that genetic testing is a serious undertaking that may have profound effects on those tested. They also suggest that experienced investigators should continue to view predictive testing with caution.

New Cautions

With the finding of the HD gene in 1993, direct genetic testing became available (Huntington's Disease Collaborative Group 1993). Direct testing is faster, less expensive, and more readily available. In contrast with testing using linkage, the direct test does not require blood from relatives and usually produces results within two weeks rather than two to three months. As a consequence, individuals requesting testing have less time to consider whether testing is in their best interest. Testing is increasingly available outside of genetics centers and in settings that do not provide pretest or posttest counseling. While these changes have resulted in a demand for HD testing up to four times that for previous testing using linkage, there is some evidence that this new group of testees has fewer social supports than the group that first presented itself for testing (Adam et al. 1995). This new cohort requesting testing may well be more representative of individuals at risk, but this fact may also mean that the previous experimental results based on small self-selected samples may not be generalizable. In other words, this new group of testees may not fare as well. Reports are increasing of children being tested and of people being given test results over the phone or sent results in the mail. As testing is increasingly obtained outside of testing protocols and genetics centers, it is also less likely that any empirical data will be collected to support or refute this prediction of increased negative outcomes.

These changes in testing procedure have led to other changes. Many individuals who call for testing now are unwilling to participate in one session of pretest counseling, let alone several. After ten years of experience offering this testing, first at Johns Hopkins and now at Indiana University, I am still extremely cautious about testing. I remain committed by training and experience to supporting the autonomy of those interested in testing by helping them make the best-informed decision they can. I insist on meeting face to face with every person before testing for at least one in-depth counseling session, which may last several hours. As individuals have become more knowledgeable and testing has become easier, the amount of time devoted to explaining the technical aspects of testing has decreased. However, the psychological ramifications of testing have remained the same and can be severe (Bloch et al. 1996). With the failure of the national health insurance initiative and the growth of managed care, not only have the possible economic ramifications of testing become more urgent, but also it is harder to pay for counseling and testing. The proliferation of knowledge about genetic testing has made the emerging social issues sobering.

New twists continue to surprise. We received a call from a staff member of a local hospital who had a middle-aged individual on the recipient list for a heart transplant. The hospital staff person had just learned that this person was at risk for HD. The staff was insisting on gene testing this individual before they would proceed with the transplant, citing the common practice of using other "outcome" variables to decide who gets donated organs and who does not. Based on his age, this man's risk for developing HD was about 20 percent. His current precarious medical situation was not an opportune time to consider testing, even if he chose that decision freely. The circumstances as they were presented to us suggested that this man would be pressed into testing, although it was not clear that the hospital staff person even considered obtaining his consent. Finally, the point of testing was to make a decision about whether or not to remove him from the list of potential heart recipients. Therefore, testing was clearly not in his best interest. We refused to do the testing, but we are quite aware that with some persistence the hospital might find someone else willing to do the testing with no questions asked. That fact is both depressing and demoralizing.

A Counselor's Worries

As a professional, I find this work draining. Although I had thought that being able to tell some people that they no longer had to worry about HD would balance out having to tell some that they would, it does not work quite that way. I worry about them all. I am not sure that I could say that, on balance, I have done more good than harm. The good, the relief of those who have dodged the genetic bullet, is very good. The bad, informing others that they will one day get a terrible disease about which nothing can be done, is very, very bad. As the studies show, these individuals do cope. They get up in the morning and get dressed and go to work and care for their families. They don't kill themselves, at least not yet. But their sense of loss and grief is profound, and knowing that I have played a part in creating that sense years before the symptoms might start is a burden to me, but one that I, at least, have freely chosen. I have had the additional advantage of having worked with dedicated colleagues in the United States, Canada, and Europe who are committed to providing testing that fulfills the needs of those at risk with the least amount of harm. I have also had the benefit of research that continues to guide and inform my interactions with patients and their families.

The context of genetic testing is changing. The approach taken with HD (initiate testing slowly in the context of research protocols designed to teach us more about the risks and benefits of testing) has become the model in genetics. However, procedures developed for, and information learned about, the relatively rare single-gene disorders are unlikely to be particularly helpful in the face of the prospect of widespread screening for susceptibility to disease. When coupled with the astounding increase in the speed with which discoveries in basic science are translated into marketable products, the possibility of following the HD approach has become a fast-receding luxury. The question of what to replace it with remains.

Alzheimer Disease and APOE

The recent discovery of a gene that heightens susceptibility to the development of AD has once again brought the above question to the forefront of discussions in the genetics community. As illustrated by the breast cancer example, these discussions have been characterized by an unusual degree of emotion. Genetics professionals, attempting to put the brakes on what they see as ill-considered and too-rapid introduction of tests by for-profit companies, find themselves taking stands that might be characterized as at odds with their long-accepted traditions of professional values. In this section, I examine the issue of genetic susceptibility screening with APOE for AD as a paradigmatic case and explore the fundamental tensions that have arisen in the field of genetic counseling as a result of new findings in genetics.

Apolipoprotein E as a Paradigm Case

By the year 2000, an estimated ten million people will have AD (Evans 1990). Characterized by insidious memory loss leading to profound dementia, AD is a devastating disorder, and virtually everyone is at risk. In 1993, the association between the ε4 allele of APOE on chromosome 19 and AD was first reported (Saunders et al. 1993). Since that time, considerable evidence has established the APOE genotype to be the most important genetic determinant of susceptibility to sporadic and late-onset AD (Relkin and National Institute on Aging 1996).

Alzheimer disease is a common late-onset disorder involving the interaction of multiple genes and environmental factors. Environmental factors related to the development of AD include a history of head trauma with loss of consciousness (Mayeux et al. 1993) and low levels of education and socioeconomic status (Mortimer and Graves 1993).

The assessment of genetic risks in multifactorial disorders is complicated (see chap. 1, above). Conveying these risks to individuals is not only hampered by the difficulties in communicating complex genetic information but also colored by the serious psychological, ethical, social, and legal consequences that may result from genetic testing. These facts, when coupled with the large number of people potentially at risk, suggest that APOE genotyping in AD may be considered a paradigm for genetic screening in common late-onset multifactorial diseases.

The Nature of Information

The APOE ε4 allele appears to function in a dose-related manner affecting both susceptibility to disease and age at onset (see chap. 4). However, like other genetic tests based on susceptibility, APOE ε4 is neither sensitive nor specific as a predictor of AD. The parameters of sensitivity, specificity, and predictive value are commonly used to validate clinical tests (Holtzman 1989). Therefore, it might be useful to explore these three concepts in some depth.

Sensitivity is a term that refers to the proportion of people with a particular disease who will be detected (true positives). *Specificity* refers to the proportion of people without the disease who will have a normal test result (true negatives). The *predictive value of a positive result* (PPV) is the proportion of people with positive results who will develop the disease. The PPV increases with increasing disease prevalence. A highly specific test will yield more false positives when the prevalence is low than when the prevalence is high. For this reason, a test used for diagnosis in individuals with symptoms has a higher predictive value than that same test used to screen asymptomatic individuals (Holtzman 1989). In the context of AD, this means that while testing for APOE є4 might be useful as an aid for the diagnosis of individuals presenting with dementia, its utility as a screening test in the general population may be considerably lower.

Apolipoprotein E є4 used as a screening test for AD is neither sensitive nor specific. At least half of patients with AD have no є4 allele; many with this allele never develop the disease (Mayeux and Schupf 1995). One further complication in using APOE є4 as a screening test may be found in the concept of residual risk, the risk that remains after a negative test result. Even if an individual is found through screening to have no copies of є4, he or she is not at zero risk.

This quality of susceptibility testing is problematic from a counselor's perspective. Testing may increase a person's risk assessment if positive, but in no case will testing ever remove it entirely. Many counselors find that individuals have a difficult time understanding even relatively straightforward genetic information. The prospect of educating large numbers of consumers about information as complex as that in susceptibility screening is daunting.

But so what? Why should this matter? Herein lies the peculiar nature of genetic testing. The results of genetic tests pose threats to people's mental health (Kessler et al. 1987), employment, insurance (Geller et al. 1996), and family relationships (Quaid and Wesson 1995). As Charles McKay said, "Predictive testing is, in one sense, a 'treatment' for the uncertainty that is characteristic of the human condition, and not merely for the specific uncertainties of diagnosis or alternative treatment modalities" (McKay 1991a, 249).

I think that it is fair to consider such testing an intervention or treatment. In more traditional, medical-model types of interventions, a treatment (appendectomy, brain surgery, antibiotic therapy) can be successful whether or not a patient comprehends the exact nature of the treatment. But when the intervention itself (in this case, genetic counseling and testing) is the communication of complex information, comprehension is absolutely essential. In contrast to physicians, genetic counselors "cannot be consoled that the treatment worked if the client does not fully understand the information" (McKay 1991a, 248).

Counselors' misgivings are supported by a variety of research findings. Research suggests that the transmitting of information regarding risk, a central component of genetic counseling, is a difficult task and that substantial misunderstanding and misinterpretation may be common (Chase et al. 1986; Wertz, Sorenson, and Heeren 1986). The issue of residual risk, the risk remaining even after a test result is negative, has been considered in the context of screening for cystic fibrosis (CF) because of the large number of mutations in the CF gene and the possibility of unknown mutations. A study on population-based screening for CF found that at least 17 percent of the 427 patients receiving a negative test result incorrectly believed that they were at no risk for having a child with CF (Bekker et al. 1994). This finding is disturbing precisely because concern that individuals would not understand the concept of residual risk led to statements advising against offering CF screening on a population-wide basis (Gilbert 1990; Wilfond and Fost 1990).

These results also suggest that individuals are interpreting risk information as if it provides a yes or no answer. My own experience as well as informal conversations with professionals working with AD patients and their families suggests that healthy individuals who request APOE testing for AD often have a common misperception that this testing will provide an accurate answer with regard to whether or not they will develop AD in the future (Snyder 1994). This tendency to interpret genetic risk factors as deterministic underlies the concern of counselors that individuals will make major life decisions based on information that the counselors believe is not truly relevant.

Justified Paternalism

Is this paternalism? I suppose it is, but I feel that it is justified paternalism. Widespread genetic screening for susceptibility to disease is a new enterprise, and the issue of how to respect individual autonomy while fulfilling one's professional role in helping clients identify what is in their overall best interest still needs to be worked out. To my mind, the benefits of learning one's own genetic makeup are not clear cut. The scientific and clinical significance of much of this information is ambiguous, the medical implications undefined, and the social and psychological consequences unknown. Our society has a long tradition of limiting access to untested medical drugs, devices, and procedures, and medical professionals have long accepted a responsibility not to promote services of unknown benefit and harm (Wilfond and Fost 1990).

Given the fact that, at least for the time being, these tests are being offered in a medical context, the genetics professional retains some responsibility in that individual choice. In the face of all the uncertainties surrounding these genetic tests, the conservative approach is to discourage the use of such tests. While this stance may be viewed as causing damage to an individual's autonomy, at least concrete harms to identifiable individuals will have been avoided (McKay 1991b). This line of thinking has been seen in CF, can be clearly seen in the response of the genetics community to the prospect of widespread susceptibility testing for breast cancer, and has been repeated in their response to apolipoprotein testing in AD.

Consensus

Interest in genetic testing for AD is not new. In 1993, a workshop on genetic predictive testing for familial Alzheimer disease was held in Toronto, Canada, and was attended by participants of diverse professional backgrounds (Lennox et al. 1994). A 1994 issue of *Alzheimer Disease and Associated Disorders* (8:63–147) was devoted to the proceedings of this workshop, which was focused primarily on predictive testing in families with known genetic mutations. The general consensus of that meeting was that testing for autosomal-dominant early-onset AD (at that time limited to direct testing for mutations in the amyloid precursor protein on chromosome 21 and linkage testing for families linked to chromosome 14) could proceed following the model used in HD and the testing guidelines that had been published by the World Federation of Neurology Research Group on HD (Went 1990). This recommendation was not hard to make. Early-onset autosomal-dominant AD is similar to HD in inheritance pattern, age at onset, and severity of symptoms. The assumption was that the psychological and social issues would also be similar, and there existed an enormous fund of research data to inform counselors about how to offer this testing. In other words, this was a familiar scenario, and demand was likely to be low, based on the small numbers of families involved. Testing was able to proceed with little controversy.

The discovery of the AD-APOE association and the potential for population-wide screening was completely different. This finding increased the pressure on the AD community to examine the issue and come to some agreement regarding recommendations for testing. The first group to publish recommendations was the Medical and Scientific Advisory Committee of Alzheimer's Disease International, which met in September 1994 in Edinburgh, Scotland. Under the "Right to Information" section of ethical, scientific, and clinical issues to be considered, this committee explicitly stated the possible conflict between genetics professionals and individuals at risk. It was their view that "a moderately accurate test (e.g., with 80% sensitivity and 80% specificity) would lead to a misclassification of about one in three subjects. Most scientists would reject the clinical use of such a test, given its serious implications. However, perhaps an individual should be able to choose to have the test with the full knowledge that it is only modestly, though significantly, better than chance in predicting outcome" (Brodaty and Medical and Scientific Advisory Committee 1995, 185). The conclusion reached is that the time for presymptomatic predictive testing in general has not yet arrived (ibid.).

A few months later, the joint American College of Medical Genetics (ACMG) and American Society of Human Genetics (ASHG) Test and Technology Transfer Committee developed a ten-member working group. Their consensus statement was published in 1995 and specifically stated: "It would be premature to offer APOE as a genetic test for AD among either members of high-risk families or the general population" (Farrer and American College of Medical Genetics 1995, 1627).

The National Institute on Aging/Alzheimer's Association Working Group held a meeting in October 1995 and published their results in 1996. Citing the lack of accurate estimates regarding genotype-specific AD risk, incomplete knowledge of modifying factors, the current absence of treatment, the uncertainty of disease prediction, the competing risks of mortality from other causes, and the potential for serious psychosocial consequences, this group weighed in against testing. Their final statement was, "The usefulness of APOE genotyping for predicting risk of AD in asymptomatic individuals has not been established in longitudinal population studies and as such is not recommended by this Working Group at this time" (Relkin and National Institute on Aging 1996, 1092).

Thus, other than the statement made by the Alzheimer's Disease International group, no other document mentions what is often considered the role of genetics professionals: to educate, to counsel, and to enable individuals to make their own decisions. The professionals represented in these statements, similar to their colleagues in the breast cancer debate, have taken what one colleague described as a "Just Say No" approach. Not only might this approach be considered paternalistic, it also disregards the fact that concerned individuals continue to seek this information.

Reasons for Testing

Historically, people have sought genetic counseling and testing to obtain information related to family planning. While this may be a consideration for individuals with early-onset autosomal-dominant AD, this reason is unlikely to be a factor relevant to those seeking testing for late-onset AD. With the introduction of predictive testing for late-onset disorders, such as HD, other considerations have come into play. One possibility, not yet realized for AD, is genetic testing as an aid to early diagnosis, treatment, or prevention (Brodaty and Medical and Scientific Advisory Committee 1995). A second possibility is to seek information with which to inform major life decisions regarding schooling, marriage, employment, or insurance (Lennox et al. 1994). The third possibility is just to want to know, with ending uncertainty itself being a motivating factor (Wiggins et al. 1992). The major disadvantages are the significant limitations of the test with regard to sensitivity and specificity and the potential for adverse psychological consequences (Brodaty and Medical and Scientific Advisory Committee 1995). A further point to consider is the fact that, given an estimated market of three million to five million individuals (Helix 1994), providing counseling and testing to even a small portion would overwhelm the providers of genetic services.

One thing to keep in mind is that, in the case of diseases with no treatment or cure (HD and AD), the options for people having a positive test are not medical. While as a counselor I may have a role to play after testing in helping people understand and come to terms with their test results, what they do with that information will depend on their personal strengths and weaknesses as well as their social, financial, and educational resources. For this reason, one might argue that it should be solely the decision of the individual whether or not to be tested. The lack of provisions for education and counseling remain a major drawback to this approach.

Demand for Testing

Estimates of the demand for testing on the part of individuals at risk remain anecdotal. No population-based surveys have been completed that might help us gauge the potential demand for susceptibility testing for AD. One group reported that, while many family members express an interest in testing even if the result were limited to an age-related risk figure, fewer say that they would actually proceed to counseling or testing, should it become available (Brodaty and Medical and Scientific Advisory Committee 1995). While this finding parallels the developments in HD, information gained from experience with other disorders might also be instructive.

In the context of breast cancer, Joseph Schulman stated that "there are fantastic numbers of people who want to know [their status with regard to breast cancer]" (Kolata 1996). One study done in anticipation of the availability of genetic testing for breast and ovarian cancers examined interest in and expectations of the impact of a potential genetic test. Subjects were 121 first-degree relatives of ovarian cancer patients who completed a structured telephone interview of attitudes about cancer and genetic testing and self-report psychological questionnaires to assess overall coping style and mood disturbance. Seventy-five percent of first-degree relatives said that they would definitely want to be tested for BRCA1, and 20 percent said that they probably would. Interest in testing was positively associated with education, perceived likelihood of being a gene carrier, perceived risk of ovarian cancer, ovarian cancer worries, and mood disturbance. These results suggest that the demand for genetic testing for BRCA1 among first-degree relatives of cancer patients may be great and that those who elect to participate may be a psychologically vulnerable population of high-risk women (Lerman et al. 1994).

A more recent study of 484 patients undergoing mammography and 498 patients visiting their obstetrician-gynecologist were asked whether they would take a genetic test to detect a susceptibility to breast cancer. More than 90 percent in both groups said that they would take the test (Chaliki et al. 1995). Predictors of accepting the test were having regular breast examinations by a physician, a belief that mammography effectively detects early breast cancer, and a belief that early breast cancer is curable. Reasons given for accepting the test include "to take extra precautions" if the risk were high (59%) and for reassurance that the risk was low (38%). The authors qualified these results by stating that this is a measure of attitudes and may not predict actual behavior when the test is offered and that these women were not fully educated and counseled regarding the possible significance of test results (e.g., that a negative result per se might not constitute grounds for reassurance). The authors also allude to the complexity of breast cancer genetics and the finding of many different mutations, facts that suggest that an affected relative might be tested first to determine whether or not a known BRCA1 mutation is found. The actual uptake of BRCA1 testing remains to be seen. In contrast to HD or AD, the identification of a higher risk for breast cancer may provide some benefits of early detection or consideration of procedures such as prophylactic mastectomy, factors that might increase the use of this test.

Taken together, these results suggest that individuals like to have the option to be tested but may not actually exercise that option. They also suggest that interest in testing may be high precisely because people may not understand the limitations of the test when applied to populations with no family history, the experimental nature of the testing, and the concept of residual risk. This is surely an argument for offering testing only with the proper education and counseling, exactly the elements that are likely to be lacking as more and more commercial firms offer these tests.

In addition to this problem, three other factors suggest a cause for concern regarding APOE testing as it is currently practiced. The first is a survey of 186 research labs in the Helix network (United States) indicating that 44 percent of laboratories have provided genetic tests directly to consumers (Reilly and Wertz 1995). Second, APOE has long been known to play a role in the transport of cholesterol. As a result, tens of thousands of individuals have already undergone APOE testing in the context of risk assessment for cardiovascular disease. With new information concerning the relationship between APOE type and AD, the possibility exists that these individuals may reinterpret their results without the benefit of education or counseling. Finally, there is the unprecedented entry of biotechnology companies into the arena. These companies have moved into the marketplace in advance of research protocols and the establishment of genetic counseling standards (Brodaty and Medical and Scientific Advisory Committee 1995) and are marketing these tests directly to physicians who may have little or no training in genetics or in the interpretation of complex genetic information.

Several studies suggest that this last factor is cause for concern. Holtzman (1991) examined the ability of physicians to interpret probabilistic information. His results showed a downward trend in the ability of physicians to solve a problem on the predictive value of a test for disease during the course of medical school and house staff training. The inability of physicians to appreciate the magnitude of uncertainty in clinical testing was demonstrated in another study. Specifically, fewer than one-quarter of physicians providing obstetrical care knew the predictive value of a maternal serum alpha-fetoprotein screening test for neural tube defects (Holtzman et al. 1991). Hofman and colleagues found that, while knowledge of genetics and genetic tests is increasing, particularly among more-recent graduates from medical school and physicians who are exposed to genetic problems in their practices, deficiencies remain (Hofman et al. 1993). If the ordering of genetic tests and relaying of results continue to flow out of specialized genetic centers and into the hands of general practitioners, the incidence of serious problems is likely to increase (Giardiello et al. 1997).

Genetic Counseling as a Profession

So who should be offering testing? According to the Code of Ethics of the National Society of Genetic Counselors (NSGC), genetic counselors are health professionals with specialized education, training, and experience in medical genetics and counseling (NSGC 1992). A primary goal of genetic counseling is that the client make a fully informed decision, one that is based on and consistent with his or her own values and full information about the options (Singer 1996). Genetic counseling is a relatively new profession; the first formal program to train master's-level genetic counselors was established at Sarah Lawrence in 1969. The development of this program was in response to a perceived need to provide services to the millions of individuals who had, or were at risk for having children with, inherited diseases and the small number of physicians trained in medical genetics (Marks 1993). As of 1996, twenty programs in genetic counseling graduated approximately 125 genetic counselors per year. Five graduate nursing programs also offer a specialization in genetic counseling. Most training programs combine rigorous course work in statistics and genetics with training in counseling techniques, personality development, and family dynamics. Students entering these programs usually have backgrounds in the biological sciences coupled with a keen interest in working with people.

Since its inception, the field of genetic counseling has placed respect for patient autonomy as its highest value. Historically, adherence to this principle arose in explicit rejection of the eugenics movement of the early twentieth century (Garver and Garver 1991). In fact, according to some writers, the history of eugenics helps explain why genetic counseling exists as a profession at all. Wachbroit and Wasserman (1995) observed that there is no counseling profession associated with other medical tests or procedures of equal complexity or with similar risks to the psychological well-being of individuals. They stated that "the critical difference is that cardiac or oncological testing has had no comparable history of being used against the patient's will and against [his or] her interests" (104).

The principle of respect for patient autonomy is traditionally represented as adherence to a technique of nondirective counseling loosely based on Carl Rogers's notion of client-centered therapy (Fine 1993; Rogers 1951). The stated goal of nondirective counseling is to ensure that the client's rather than the counselor's values determine how genetic information will influence health care decisions (Bartels 1993). Although some controversy exists over what the term *nondirective counseling* actually means, many have interpreted it as requiring the counselor to affect a complete neutrality about the moral issues raised by genetics. Not all agree. This approach has been soundly attacked by at least one critic, who, in the context of prenatal testing, believes that "to leave all decisions to the discretion of parents indicates the low value that our society places upon those with genetic disorders and handicap" (Clarke 1991, 998). A further criticism is that strict adherence to a policy of nondirectiveness may actually work against clients' making decisions that best reflect their own values (Singer 1996). As genetic counseling continues to move from the provision of primarily prenatal services to counseling and testing for late-onset diseases, susceptibilities, traits, and characteristics, the moral complexity of the situations also increases, and the concept of nondirectiveness may not be as useful.

In reality, exceptions to this general rule of respecting a client's autonomy have always been with us. The issue of sex selection is often raised in this context (Wertz and Fletcher 1989). Other possible exceptions include the genetic testing of children for late-onset disorders (Pelias 1991; Quaid 1994; Sharpe 1993), the violation of a client's privacy inherent in informing relatives of their genetic risk (Wertz 1992), and the disclosure of false paternity (Wertz and Fletcher 1989). The personal discomfort of many counselors around these issues has led them to begin to question their duty to grant all client requests and to serious discussions regarding the ability of counselors to set moral limits on the types of service they are willing to provide. These discussions have led some to conclude that client autonomy may be breached in the light of considerations that may include harm to others, the counselor's own moral convictions, or conflict with other recognized principles of biomedical ethics (Walters 1993). If genetics professionals conclude that offering APOE ε4 screening may cause more harm than benefit, they might be considered justified in the decision not to offer testing.

Implications for Genetic Counseling for APOE

Although genetics professionals may prove reluctant to offer the testing, we must be aware that people will continue to seek genetic information. Historically, people have sought genetic counseling because genetic professionals had a specialized body of knowledge regarding base rates and recurrence risks of genetic disorders and other factual information individuals felt they needed to make concrete decisions about current or future pregnancies. Providing this information often required invasive testing procedures, such as chorionic villus sampling or amniocentesis, that could be done only by skilled physicians. In the context of breast cancer, the argument can be made that individuals need an ongoing relationship with a physician to monitor their health and to help them make complex decisions regarding screening regimens and prophylactic surgeries. In cases in which medical professionals can offer no cure or treatment and when the purpose of testing is only to refine risks about which individuals are already aware, then perhaps counselors have less of a role to play than we like to think.

If counselors and other genetics professionals refuse to offer certain tests, it is likely that clients will order tests directly from commercial companies without the benefit of education or counseling. This scenario is unattractive. Clients should make informed decisions whether or not to be tested. The risks of clients ordering their own tests or having them ordered by health professionals who are not well informed are great and include misunderstanding or misinterpreting the meaning of test results, psychological distress, and the possibility that these test results may be used by third parties in ways that consumers might not even begin to imagine.

This is not to say that there are not benefits to be gained from bypassing the medical professionals altogether. These benefits would include lower costs and increased privacy. However, taking this route places the entire burden of testing on patients and their families without guidance as to how to use this information for their own good. It may be that Joseph Schulman, by making genetic tests of uncertain predictive value available to anyone in the general population willing to pay without the benefit of counseling or education, is doing us all a favor by giving us a glimpse of the future. At the very least, he should serve to goad us into action to develop new and better ways to serve our clients in the age of genetics.

References

Adam, S., Wiggins, S., Lawson, K., McKellin, B., and Hayden, M. R. 1995. Predictive testing for Huntington disease (HD): Differences in uptake and characteristics of linked marker and direct test cohorts. *American Journal of Human Genetics* 57 (supp.): A292.

Adam, S., Wiggins, S., Whyte, P., Bloch, M., Shokeir, M. H. K., Soltan, H., Meshino, W., Summers, A., Suchowersky, O., Welch, J. P., Huggins, M., Theilmann, J., and Hayden, M. R. 1993. Five-year study of prenatal testing for Huntington disease: Demand, attitudes, and psychological assessment. *Journal of Medical Genetics* 30:549–56.

Bartels, D. M. 1993. Preface to *Prescribing our future: Ethical challenges in genetic counseling*, ed. D. M. Bartels, B. S. LeRoy, and A. L. Caplan, ix–xiii. New York: Aldine de Gruyter.

Bates, M. 1981. Ethics of provocative test for Huntington's disease. *New England Journal of Medicine* 304:175–76.

Beck, A. T., Ward, C. H., Mendelson, M., Mock, J., and Erbaugh, J. 1961. An inventory for measuring depression. *Archives of General Psychiatry* 4:561–71.

Bekker, H., Denniss, G., Modell, M., Bobrow, M., and Marteau, T. 1994. The impact of population-based screening for carriers of cystic fibrosis. *Journal of Medical Genetics* 31:364–68.

Bloch, M., Adam, S., Hayden, M. R., and the Canadian Collaborative Study of Predictive Testing for HD. 1996. A survey of catastrophic events following predictive testing (PT) for Huntington disease (HD). *American Journal of Human Genetics* 59 (supp.): A333.

Bloch, M., Adam, S., Wiggins, S., Huggins, M., and Hayden, M. R. 1992. Predictive testing for Huntington disease in Canada: The experience of those receiving an increased risk. *American Journal of Human Genetics* 42:499–507.

Brandt, J., Quaid, K. A., Folstein, S. E., Garber, P., Maestri, N. E., Abbott, M. H., Slavney, P. R., Franz, M. L., Kasch, L., and Kazazian, H. H. 1989. Presymptomatic diagnosis of delayed-onset disease with linked DNA markers: The experience in Huntington's disease. *JAMA* 261:3108–14.

Brodaty, H., and the Medical and Scientific Advisory Committee, Alzheimer's Disease International. 1995. Consensus statement on predictive testing for Alzheimer disease. *Alzheimer Disease and Associated Disorders* 9:182–87.

Chaliki, H., Loader, S., Levenkron, J. C., Logan-Young, W., Hall, W. J., and Rowley, P. T. 1995. Women's receptivity to testing for a genetic susceptibility to breast cancer. *American Journal of Public Health* 85:1133–35.

Chase, G. A., Faden, R. R., Holtzman, N. A., Chwalow, A. J., Leonard, C. O., Lopes, C., and Quaid, K. 1986. Assessment of risk by pregnant women: Implications for genetic counseling and education. *Social Biology* 33:57–64.

Clarke, A. 1991. Is nondirective genetic counselling possible? *Lancet* 338:998–1001.

Codori, A.-M., and Brandt, J. 1994. Psychological costs and benefits of predictive testing for Huntington's disease. *American Journal of Medical Genetics* 54:174–84.

Craufurd, D., and Harris, R. 1986. Ethics of predictive testing for Huntington's chorea: The need for more information. *British Medical Journal* 293:249–51.

Craufurd, D., Kerzin-Storrar, L., Dodge, A., and Harris, R. 1989. Uptake of predictive testing for Huntington's disease. *Lancet* 2:603.

Derogatis, L. R. 1983. *SCL-90-R: Administration, scoring, and procedures manual–II for the revised version.* 2d ed. Towson, Md.: Clinical Psychometric Research.

Evans, D. A. 1990. Estimated prevalence of Alzheimer disease in the United States. *Milbank Quarterly* 68:267–89.

Farrer, L. A., and American College of Medical Genetics/American Society of Human Genetics Working Group on APOE and Alzheimer Disease. 1995. Statement on use of apolipoprotein E testing for Alzheimer disease. *JAMA* 274:1627–29.

Fine, B. A. 1993. The evolution of nondirectiveness in genetic counseling and implications of the Human Genome Project. In *Prescribing our future: Ethical challenges in genetic counseling,* ed. D. M. Bartels, B. S. LeRoy, and A. L. Caplan, 101–17. New York: Aldine de Gruyter.

Folstein, S. E. 1989. *Huntington's disease: A disorder of families.* Baltimore: Johns Hopkins University Press.

Fox, S., Bloch, M., Fahy, M., and Hayden, M. R. 1989. Predictive testing for Huntington disease. Part 1, Description of a pilot project in British Columbia. *American Journal of Medical Genetics* 32:211-16.

Garver, K. L., and Garver, B. 1991. Historical perspectives on eugenics: Past, present, and future. *American Journal of Medical Genetics* 49:1109-18.

Geller, L. N., Alper, J. S., Billings, P. R., Barash, C. I., and Beckwith, J. 1996. Individual, family, and societal dimensions of genetic discrimination: A case study analysis. *Science and Engineering Ethics* 2:71-88.

Giardiello, F. M., Brensinger, J. D., Petersen, G. M., Luce, M. C., Hylind, L. M., Bacon, J. A., Booker, S. V., Parker, R. D., and Hamilton, S. R. 1997. The use and interpretation of commercial APC gene testing for familial adenomatous polyposis. *New England Journal of Medicine* 336:823-27.

Gilbert, F. 1990. Is population screening for cystic fibrosis appropriate now? *American Journal of Human Genetics* 46:394-95.

Gusella, J. F., Wexler, N. S., Conneally, P. M., Naylor, S. L., Anderson, M. A., Tanzi, R. E., Watkins, P. C., Ottina, K., Wallace, M. R., Sakaguchi, A. Y., Young, A. B., Shoulson, I., Bonilla, E., and Martin, J. B. 1983. A polymorphic DNA marker genetically linked to Huntington's disease. *Nature* 306:234-38.

HDSA (Huntington's Disease Society of America). 1989. Guidelines for predictive testing for Huntington disease. New York: Huntington's Disease Society of America.

Helix. 1994. Directory of medical genetics laboratories. Seattle, Wash.: Children's Hospital and Medical Center.

Hofman, K. J., Tambor, E. S., Chase, G. A., Geller, G., Faden, R. R., and Holtzman, N. A. 1993. Physicians' knowledge of genetics and genetic testing. *Academic Medicine* 68:625-32.

Holtzman, N. A. 1989. *Proceed with caution: Predicting genetic risks in the recombinant DNA era.* Baltimore: Johns Hopkins University Press.

―――. 1991. The interpretation of laboratory results: The paradoxical effect of medical training. *Journal of Clinical Ethics* 2:241-42.

Holtzman, N. A., Faden, R. R., Leonard, C. O., Chase, G. A., and Ulrich, S. R. 1991. The effect of education on physicians' knowledge of a laboratory test: The case of maternal serum alpha-fetoprotein screening. *Journal of Clinical Ethics* 2:243-47.

Huggins, M., Bloch, M., Wiggins, S., Adam, S., Suchowersky, O., Trew, M., Klimek, M., Greenberg, C., Eleff, M., Thompson, L. P., Knight, J., MacLeod, P., Girard, K., Theilmann, J., Hedrick, A., and Hayden, M. R. 1992. Predictive testing for Huntington disease in Canada: Adverse effects and unexpected results in those receiving decreased risk. *American Journal of Human Genetics* 42:508-15.

Huntington's Disease Collaborative Research Group. 1993. A novel gene containing a trinucleotide repeat that is expanded and unstable on Huntington's disease chromosome. *Cell* 72:971-83.

Kessler, S., Field, T., Worth, L., and Mosbarger, H. 1987. Attitudes of persons at risk for Huntington's disease toward predictive testing. *American Journal of Medical Genetics* 26:259-70.

Kolata, G. 1996. Breaking ranks, lab offers test to assess risk of breast cancer. *New York Times,* April 1.

Lennox, A., Karlinsky, H., Meschino, W., Buchanan, A., Percy, M. E., and Berg, J. M. 1994. Molecular genetic testing for Alzheimer's disease: Deliberations and preliminary recommendations. *Alzheimer Disease and Associated Disorders* 8:126-47.

Lerman, C., Daly, M., Masny, A., and Balshem, A. 1994. Attitudes about genetic testing for breast-ovarian cancer susceptibility. *Journal of Clinical Oncology* 12:843-50.

Markel, D. S., Young, A. B., and Penney, J. B. 1987. At-risk persons' attitudes towards presymptomatic and prenatal testing of Huntington disease in Michigan. *American Journal of Medical Genetics* 26:295-305.

Marks, J. H. 1993. The training of genetic counselors: Origins of psychosocial model. In *Prescribing our future: Ethical challenges in genetic counseling,* ed. D. M. Bartels, B. S. LeRoy, and A. L. Caplan, 15-24. New York: Aldine de Gruyter.

Mastromauro, C., Myers, R. H., and Berkman, B. 1987. Attitudes toward presymptomatic testing in Huntington disease. *American Journal of Medical Genetics* 26:259-82.

Mayeux, R., Ottman, R., Tang, M. X., Noboa-Bauza, L., Marder, K., Gurland, B., and Stern, Y. 1993. Genetic susceptibility and head injury as risk factors for Alzheimer disease among community-dwelling elderly persons and their first-degree relatives. *Annals of Neurology* 33:494-501.

Mayeux, R., and Schupf, N. 1995. Apolipoprotein E and Alzheimer's disease: The implications of progress in molecular medicine. *American Journal of Public Health* 85:1280-84.

McKay, C. R. 1991a. The effects of uncertainty on the physician-patient relationship in predictive genetic testing. *Journal of Clinical Ethics* 2:247-50.

———. 1991b. The physician as fortune teller: A commentary on "The ethical justification for minimal paternalism." *Journal of Clinical Ethics* 2:228-38.

Meissen, G. H., and Berchek, R. L. 1987. Intended use of predictive testing by those at risk for Huntington disease. *American Journal of Medical Genetics* 26:283-93.

Meissen, G. J., Myers, R. H., Mastromauro, C. A., Koroshetz, W. J., Klinger, K. W., Farrer, L. A., Watkins, P. A., Gusella, J. F., Bird, E. D., and Martin, J. B. 1988. Predictive testing for Huntington's disease with use of a linked DNA marker. *New England Journal of Medicine* 318:535-42.

Mortimer, J. A., and Graves, A. B. 1993. Education and other socioeconomic determinants of dementia and Alzheimer disease. *Neurology* 41:1886-92.

NSGC (National Society of Genetic Counselors). 1992. National Society of Genetic Counselors code of ethics. *Journal of Genetic Counseling* 1:41-43.

Pelias, M. Z. 1991. Duty to disclose in medical genetics: A legal perspective. *American Journal of Medical Genetics* 39:347-54.

Quaid, K. A. 1993. Presymptomatic testing for Huntington disease in the United States. *American Journal of Medical Genetics* 53:785-87.

———. 1994. Reply to Sharpe (letter to the editor). *American Journal of Medical Genetics* 49:354.

Quaid, K. A., Brandt, J., and Folstein, S. E. 1987. The decision to be tested for Huntington's disease (letter to the editor). *JAMA* 257:3362.

Quaid, K. A., and Morris, M. 1993. Reluctance to undergo predictive testing: The case of Huntington disease. *American Journal of Medical Genetics* 45:41-45.

Quaid, K. A., and Wesson, M. K. 1995. Exploration of the effects of predictive testing for Huntington disease on intimate relationships. *American Journal of Medical Genetics* 57:46–51.

Relkin, N. R., and National Institute on Aging/Alzheimer's Association Working Group. 1996. Apolipoprotein E genotyping in Alzheimer's disease. *Lancet* 347:1091–95.

Rogers, C. R. 1951. *Client-centered therapy: Its current practice, implications, and theory.* Boston: Houghton-Mifflin.

Saunders, A. M., Strittmatter, W., Schmechel, D., St. George- Hyslop, P. H., Pericak-Vance, M. A., Joo, S. H., Rosi, B. L., Gusella, J. F., Crapper-MacLachlan, D. R., Alberts, M., Hulette, C., Crain, B., Goldgaber, D., and Roses, A. D. 1993. Association of apolipoprotein E allele ε4 with late-onset familial and sporadic Alzheimer's disease. *Neurology* 43:1467–72.

Sharpe, N. F. 1993. Presymptomatic testing for Huntington disease: Is there a duty to test those under the age of eighteen? *American Journal of Medical Genetics* 46:250–53.

Singer, G. G. S. 1996. Clarifying the duties and goals of genetic counselors: Implications for nondirectiveness. In *Morality and New Genetics,* ed. B. Gert, E. M. Berger, G. F. Cahill, K. D. Clousner, C. M. Culver, J. B. Moeschler, and G. H. S. Singer, 125–45. Boston: Jones and Bartlett.

Snyder, L. 1994. Telephone conversation with author, April 7.

Stern, R., and Eldridge, R. 1975. Attitudes of patients and their relatives to Huntington's disease. *Journal of Medical Genetics* 12:217–23.

Tibben, A., Frets, P. G., Van de Kamp, J. J. P., Niermeijer, M. F., Vegtervan der Vlis, M., Roos, R. A. C., Rooymans, H. G. M., Van Ommen, G., and Verhage, F. 1993. On attitudes and appreciation six months after predictive DNA testing for Huntington disease in the Dutch program. *American Journal of Medical Genetics* 46:103–11.

Tyler, A., and Harper, P. S. 1983. Attitudes of subjects at risk and their relatives towards genetic counseling in Huntington's chorea. *Journal of Medical Genetics* 20:179–88.

Wachbroit, R., and Wasserman, D. 1995. Patient autonomy and value-neutrality in nondirective genetic counseling. *Stanford Law and Policy Review* 6:103–11.

Walters, L. 1993. Ethical obligations of genetic counselors. In *Prescribing our future: Ethical challenges in genetic counseling,* ed. D. M. Bartels, B. S. LeRoy, and A. L. Caplan, 131–47. New York: Aldine de Gruyter.

Went, L. 1990. Ethical issues policy statement on Huntington's Disease. *Journal of Medical Genetics* 27:34–38.

Wertz, D. C. 1992. Ethical and legal implications of the new genetics: Issues for discussion. *Social Science and Medicine* 35:495–505.

Wertz, D. C., and Fletcher, J. C. 1989. Fatal knowledge? Prenatal diagnosis and sex selection. *Hastings Center Report* 19:21–27.

Wertz, D. C., and Reilly, P. R. 1995. Laboratory policies and practices on genetic testing of children: A survey of Helix members. *American Journal of Human Genetics* 57 (supp.): A57.

Wertz, D. C., Sorenson, J. R., and Heeren, T. C. 1986. Clients' interpretation of risks provided in genetic counseling. *American Journal of Human Genetics* 39:253–64.

Wiggins, S., Whyte, P., Huggins, M., Adam, S., Theilmann, J., Bloch, M., Sheps, S. B., Schecter, M. T., and Hayden, M. R. 1992. The psychological consequences of predictive testing for Huntington's disease. *New England Journal of Medicine* 327:1402-05.

Wilfond, B. S., and Fost, N. 1990. The cystic fibrosis gene: Medical and social implications for heterozygote detection. *JAMA* 263:2777-83.

World Federation of Neurology Research Group on Huntington's Disease. 1993. Presymptomatic testing for Huntington's disease: A worldwide survey. *Journal of Medical Genetics* 30:1020-22.

Prenatal Genetic Testing for Alzheimer Disease

BONNIE STEINBOCK, PH.D.

This chapter begins with an overview of the ethics debate concerning prenatal genetic testing in the context of increasing genetic information created by human genome research. Throughout, considerable focus is placed on the experience of women. The second half of the chapter considers prenatal genetic testing for late-onset conditions such as AD.

The Purpose of Prenatal Genetic Testing

Prenatal genetic testing is offered to pregnant women or couples to provide them with information that may be relevant to their procreative decision making. In the vast majority of cases, prenatal genetic testing is used to reassure prospective parents that their baby will not have a genetic disorder for which a test is available. As Elias and Annas (1987, 83) note, "since more than 95 percent of all prenatal diagnostic tests are negative, the overwhelming majority of such testing helps lead to the birth of children that might not otherwise have been born." Of course, a negative test is no guarantee that the baby will be born healthy, because the fetus may have an unknown genetic disease or may be affected by environmental causes. In addition, although prenatal genetic testing is highly reliable, there is always the possibility of false positives and false negatives. This is one reason why counseling, which helps people understand the significance of the information they are given, is an important part of prenatal testing.

The most common indication for prenatal diagnosis of a genetic disease is maternal age (thirty-five or more years), which accounts for about 85 percent of the women tested. The relative risk of having a baby with a chromosomal disorder, such as trisomy 21 (Down syndrome), increases exponentially after age thirty. Prenatal genetic testing is also offered when the couple belongs to a racial or ethnic group with a relatively high incidence of a particular genetic disease, such as Tay-Sachs disease for Jews of Eastern European descent or sickle-cell anemia for African Americans. Individuals who have family members with a disease, such as cystic fibrosis, may be advised to have prenatal genetic testing to see if their fetus is affected.

In the relatively few cases where the fetus is determined to have a serious genetic defect, this information can be used by the parents either to prepare themselves for the birth of a handicapped child or, more commonly, to abort and "try again." The decision to terminate a pregnancy is typically based on two kinds of considerations: first, and primarily, the burdens and sacrifices — financial, physical, and psychological — that can be expected to be imposed on the couple or family from the birth of a handicapped child (Kuhse and Singer 1985, 146–53); and second, the view that it is unfair to the child to bring it into the world with a serious disease or handicapping condition. This consideration is most plausible when the child's life is likely to be very brief or extremely limited and either the condition itself or necessary medical interventions inflict prolonged and intractable pain. An example would be the worst-case scenario for spina bifida. The prognosis given to the parents in the famous "Baby Jane Doe" case (see Steinbock 1984) was that their daughter would be completely paralyzed and severely mentally retarded, incapable of learning, responding to people, or recognizing her own parents. In addition, she would be subject to painful and recurrent kidney or bladder infections. Based on this information (which turned out in this case to be unduly pessimistic), the parents felt that life was not a blessing, but rather a burden, to the unfortunate child.

Many genetic conditions have a range of expression. A child with Down syndrome might be only mildly retarded, and capable of living a satisfying life, or severely retarded with associated physical anomalies. A child with spina bifida might be severely retarded and completely paralyzed or might suffer only relatively minor back problems. Prenatal testing can reveal only the presence of disorder, not its severity. Many people believe that the life available to the child in the worst-case scenario is so filled with pain and so devoid of any compensating features that it would be unfair to inflict such a life on anyone. The chance that their afflicted fetus would fall into the worst-case category is an obvious consideration for potential parents.

Some commentators maintain that it is virtually impossible to avoid a birth for the child's sake. From the child's perspective, life and life alone, no matter how limited or painful, might be better than no life at all (Robertson 1974). On this analysis, birth is not a harm or wrong to the child, unless it can be predicted that the child would prefer nonexistence, and this is rarely possible, even in the worst cases. Others maintain that it is unfair to children to bring them into the world if they are deprived of a reasonable chance at life at or above a "decent minimum" (Steinbock and McClamrock 1994, 19). In any event, whether or not being born with serious deformities can be considered a harm to the child, the birth of such a child can impose serious burdens on the parents and other family members. Prospective parents may wish to avoid these burdens even if the child, once born, would not be "better off dead."

Abortion and Prenatal Testing

Despite the fact that prenatal testing can actually facilitate the birth of babies who otherwise would not have been born, most opponents of abortion oppose prenatal genetic testing precisely because it affords prospective parents with an opportunity and a reason to abort. Thus, former surgeon general C. Everett Koop referred to prenatal testing as a search-and-destroy mission. According to abortion opponents, it is as wrong to kill a fetus because it has a genetic handicapping condition as it would be to kill a handicapped newborn.

A different reason for opposing prenatal testing is offered by disability rights advocates, such as Adrienne Asch (1989). Unlike pro-lifers, Asch is not generally opposed to abortion. She agrees with liberals on abortion that fetuses are not children and that women should be able to decide for themselves if they wish to continue a pregnancy. However, the only valid reason for terminating a pregnancy, according to Asch, is to avoid unwanted motherhood. If one has decided to become a mother, then one ought to be willing to accept that child "as is," regardless of disease or defects. Asch questions the parenting ability of those who cannot accept a handicapped child and points out that there is no guarantee that a healthy, normal baby will not develop problems after birth. In addition, she believes that the acceptance of abortion for fetal indications reflects prejudice against disabled persons and the false belief that their lives are not worth living.

Barbara Katz Rothman (1986) objects to prenatal testing on feminist grounds, that is, that such testing does not generally serve the interests of women. Instead, the expectation that one will have genetic testing to avoid the birth of a handicapped child puts women in the awkward position of having "tentative pregnancies." Amniocentesis is typically performed in the fourth month, and results usually take a couple of weeks. By that time, the woman looks and feels pregnant and may have already felt the fetus move. Physically and psychologically the woman may be committed to this pregnancy and this fetus, and yet she may also have to consider abortion. Rothman thinks that women would be better off not being tested, especially since deformed fetuses sometimes spontaneously abort. To those who object that surely the decision to have prenatal testing should be the woman's, Rothman replies that the social pressure to test—and then to abort—may be difficult to resist. Indeed, there may be a tendency to blame a woman who knowingly has a child with a genetic defect. Moreover, few women have the resources to enable them to care properly for a handicapped child, and public resources are seriously inadequate. Thus, the decision to undergo prenatal testing or to abort a fetus with a genetic defect is often not really a choice.

Rothman raises important points. How can we, as a society, lessen the psychological strain on women caused by "tentative pregnancies" and offer them real choices regarding childbirth? The psychological strain can be partly relieved by earlier prenatal testing, such as chorionic villus sampling, which is done in the first trimester, before most women are committed to their pregnancies. However, some women may prefer not to be tested at all, and that choice should be respected. Sufficient resources should be provided to handicapped children with disabilities and their families so that no one willing to care for a child with a disability is forced to abort.

Nevertheless, many women do not want to have a child with a serious disability if they can avoid it. They regard the care of even healthy, normal children as challenging enough. For such women, prenatal testing is a positive good, because it relieves anxiety (in the majority of cases) and enables them to avoid a birth they regard as unfortunate or tragic. For those who accept a woman's right to choose to have an abortion—a position taken by both Asch and Rothman—a fetus is not yet a child, and prospective parents do not have the same obligations to a fetus as they would to a born child. Why, then, should women who choose to undergo prenatal testing be charged with being bad mothers or be made to feel guilty about preferring to have a healthy child? From the fact that parents ought to love and accept their *children,* sick or healthy, disabled or able bodied, it does not follow that prospective parents have the same obligations to *fetuses* or that women are morally obligated to continue a pregnancy when the fetus has a serious disability.

Moreover, the burdens that are likely to accompany the birth and rearing of a child with a disability are at least as severe as other burdens thought to justify abortion. If a woman can justifiably abort because she does not want to interrupt her education or wreck a fledgling career, she can with equal justification abort to avoid the financial, emotional, and physical burdens on herself and her family from having a child with a severe disability. Nor does respecting this choice as morally valid mean that the lives of individuals with disabilities are worthless or that it would be a poor expenditure of resources to enable disabled individuals to lead as rich and full lives as possible (see Buchanan 1996). One can enthusiastically support the rights of existing disabled people without wanting to bring more disabled people into existence. The choices of all women—to be tested or not, to abort or not—should be respected and supported.

Conditions for Morally Acceptable Prenatal Testing

I have suggested above that prenatal testing to avoid the birth of a child with a serious disability is morally permissible. However, the seriousness of the genetic disease or defect is only one factor in determining the appropriateness of prenatal testing. Other factors include the probability of disease and the age at onset (Post, Botkin, and Whitehouse 1992), as well as the possibility of remedial treatment.

To understand how these factors relate to the justification of prenatal testing, consider Tay-Sachs disease, one of the clearest examples of a genetic disease for which prenatal testing is appropriate. First, the impact on health is dire. The child with Tay-Sachs is born apparently healthy. At around nine months of age, signs of psychomotor degeneration appear. By eighteen months, the child is unable to crawl or even lift the head. The disease becomes progressively worse, ending in a vegetative state. Death typically occurs by the age of three to five years. Second, the age of onset is infancy. This differentiates Tay-Sachs from Huntington disease (HD), which is equally severe but does not occur typically until the late forties. Thus, the person with HD can have a healthy, normal life for forty or more years before the disease manifests itself. Third, Tay-Sachs can be diagnosed prenatally with a high degree of certainty, given homozygous status of the fetus. This contrasts with many genetic defects that merely put the child at risk of developing a particular disease. Fourth, there is no cure or even ameliorative therapy for Tay-Sachs. This contrasts with a disease like cystic fibrosis, for which several new genetically engineered drugs and gene therapy are on the horizon.

Even with Tay-Sachs disease, researchers are finding mutations that can result in changes in the age of onset or severity (Kolata 1993). Therefore, the information that can be provided to prospective parents is always a matter of probability and degree of risk. Nevertheless, these four factors—impact on health, age of onset, probability of disease, and potential for therapy—provide a useful framework for discussing the appropriateness of prenatal testing and possible subsequent abortion. As the impact on health, the probability of disease, and the likelihood of therapy diminish, and as the age of likely onset increases, the case for prenatal testing also decreases. For some conditions, like HD, the impact on health is severe, the probability of disease if the fetus carries the implicated gene mutation is high, and there is no cure or therapy, but the age of onset is middle age. This makes the case for prenatal genetic testing much more problematic. Some feel that forty or so "good years" of unaffected existence make up for the horrors of HD; others do not.

Procreative Autonomy and Prenatal Testing

The argument so far suggests that abortion for fetal indications can be morally justified, given certain conditions. The next question is whether prenatal genetic testing should be limited to situations in which these conditions are met, or whether the decision to test should be left entirely up to the pregnant woman or couple. Leaving the decision to the woman or couple runs the risk that some pregnancies may be terminated for relatively benign conditions, such as an easily correctable cleft palate or club foot. On the other hand, disallowing prenatal genetic testing restricts procreative autonomy by preventing people from having information that might incline them to abort. Thus, the fundamental issue is whether people should have the freedom to do what is morally problematic.

Abortion for sex selection provides a dramatic illustration of the problem. In some cultures, the desire for a male child is so strong that women will request prenatal diagnosis for the sole purpose of learning the sex of the fetus, in order to abort if it is a girl. Most people in our culture consider the destruction of a healthy fetus just because of its sex to be immoral, either because of the sexist attitude it expresses or because such abortions reflect insufficient respect for potential human life or both. Many physicians will refuse to screen a fetus for sex if they believe that the parents will use the information to abort a fetus of the "wrong" sex.

Are such refusals justifiable? The first point to note is that it is relatively easy to get around such refusals. All a couple need do is pretend to have a health-related concern. For example, although screening for Down syndrome is not recommended until after age thirty-five, many younger women request amniocentesis, a not unreasonable request, since most babies with Down syndrome are born to women in their twenties (Elias and Annas 1987, 84). There would be no way for a physician to know that the couple's real concern was the sex of the fetus, rather than its health status. Suppose, however, that the couple are truthful about their reason for wanting prenatal diagnosis: they intend to abort a female fetus. On the one hand, we can sympathize with the physician's reluctance to participate, even indirectly, in an abortion that she or he finds repugnant. On the other hand, physicians are not authorized to quiz women on the validity of their reasons for terminating a pregnancy. If physicians have neither the right nor the responsibility to monitor a woman's reasons for abortion in general, it is hard to see why an exception should be made in the case of abortion for sex selection.

In any event, is sex selection always or necessarily wrong? Imagine a woman in her late forties who has already borne five sons and finds to her amazement that she is again pregnant. If she were to decide to abort, few people would regard her decision as unjustified or her reason — that she has completed her family and is through with childbearing and child rearing — as trivial. But now suppose that the woman has always wanted a girl. She could face a sixth child, she thinks, if it were the longed-for daughter. In such a case, it is far from clear that using prenatal testing to determine the sex of the fetus would be morally wrong.

In some countries, the desire for a son is so strong that women undergo numerous pregnancies to have a male child. We may regard such a preference as sexist and unenlightened, but it exists and has implications for the lives of women living in these cultures. Repeated pregnancies take a serious toll on their health and force them to bear more children than they can adequately feed and clothe. The lives of the girls who are born in the attempt to get a son are often substandard, as they typically receive less food and medical attention than their brothers. Preventing the births of girls who will be neglected or allowed to starve seems a morally preferable option. The automatic and absolute rejection of sex selection fails to take into consideration the social realities in which it may occur.

The lesson to be derived from the example of sex selection is this. From a "pro-choice" perspective, the decision to abort belongs to the pregnant woman. Procreative freedom for women means that women have the right to choose to abort, even if they choose for reasons that most people consider trivial or frivolous. No physician should be coerced or pressured into performing abortions, but physicians who do perform abortions do not have the liberty to decide when a termination is justified. Physicians can offer their patients advice and counsel, but ultimately they should respect the woman's right to make this decision and her related right to have information that she deems relevant to the decision. To withhold such information on the ground that it would lead to an abortion of which the doctor disapproves is paternalistic and violates the woman's procreative rights.

Therefore, if a test for a genetic condition is available, it should not be withheld because, in the physician's judgment, abortion would not be justified. A quite separate question is whether a particular test should be made generally available. This is a question of social policy. An important consideration in deciding whether a genetic test should be made available is its reliability, raising the question of how good a predictor it must be. A test that does not give reasonably accurate information is not medically warranted. Another consideration is the potential for social stigmatization and discrimination. For example, carriers of sickle-cell anemia were harshly discriminated against in the 1970s after the military, schools, and employers adopted screening tests, despite the fact that carriers remain unaffected by the disease (Reilly 1977). Discrimination can also result from prenatal genetic screening. For example, insurance companies might refuse to give health insurance to children born with genetic diseases detected prenatally on the grounds that such diseases are preexisting conditions. The social impact of genetic testing must be considered along with its medical appropriateness before a test is put on the market and made available to consumers.

Application to Late-Onset Diseases like Alzheimer Disease

It may be thought bizarre that anyone would even consider prenatal genetic testing for AD. For AD typically develops at the very end of life, in the seventies, eighties, or even nineties. Abortion cannot be contemplated to avoid burdens to the parents, because they will probably be dead before the onset of the disease. Nor do considerations of the interests of offspring seem persuasive in this case, because the disease typically does not affect the person until after a life of normal length and health. It is unfortunate to undergo dementia at the end of life, and something to be avoided if possible. However, we all have to die of something, sometime. The prospect of eventual illness and deterioration is not a reason against getting born.

It may be argued that AD is a particularly terrible disease and that it would be better never to have been born than to manifest the dementia characteristic of AD, even though this typically occurs quite late in life. This view is most persuasive when we think of AD patients who scream continually or fight their caretakers or smear themselves with their own feces. They seem to be miserably unhappy. Others argue that the lives of AD patients are not necessarily terrible. They may be "pleasantly senile." Although they cannot enjoy the pursuits they enjoyed when they were not demented, they can enjoy their limited lives. However, many people consider the loss of personality, autonomy, and dignity in a demented existence to be a tragic end to life, regardless of whether the patient suffers. The thought here is, "I do not want to live like that," where the "I" is the person I am now, with my convictions, talents, and personality traits. This thought is often combined with the idea that the competent individual has the right to make medical decisions, including the forgoing of treatment, for a future, noncompetent self.

Some commentators argue that competent individuals should not be allowed to make medical decisions for their future incompetent selves because the incompetent individual is likely to have very different interests. Someone who enjoys a pleasant demented existence should not be killed or allowed to die just because "someone else" (i.e., the prior competent self) is repelled by dementia (Dresser and Robertson 1989). Others argue that it is wrong to view the incompetent person as a different self. They maintain that human beings retain their identity over time and have a legitimate interest in who they were and who they become. Moreover, it is perfectly reasonable to allow the self-while-competent to make choices about medical treatment, because noncompetent individuals cannot make such choices (Rhoden 1989).

Whether the desires of the "then" self should take precedence over the desires of the "now" self (Post 1995, 307–21) in the context of treatment decisions remains controversial. However, this debate has little relevance in the context of prenatal diagnosis, because the decision—to abort or not abort—is being made neither by the "then" self nor the "now" self but by others, namely, the prospective parents. The decision to abort is not based on their own interests, since late-onset diseases are unlikely to cause burdens of care. The question then is whether abortion is morally justified on the basis of the interests of the child who would be born. Surely the case cannot be made. Admittedly, some people would prefer to die before they develop dementia; at least one of Dr. Jack Kevorkian's assisted-suicide patients was in the early stages of AD. Perhaps there are even people who would prefer nonexistence to a life that ends in dementia. However, this is surely an unusual view. Most people, if they were able to make the choice, would not choose nonexistence over a life that ended in AD after a normal, healthy life. Therefore, a "proxy chooser" (Feinberg 1987) making the choice for an as yet unborn child could not rationally assume that the child would prefer nonexistence to life with AD at age eighty or even that the child would view his or her life as being below a decent minimum.

Early-onset AD presents a different situation. The disease begins to manifest itself between the ages of thirty and sixty, and some individuals have shown signs of dementia as early as twenty-five. Early-onset AD thus looks more like HD in terms of impact on health, age of onset, and the present absence of treatment or cure. However, there is an important difference between early-onset AD (an estimated 1–2% of all AD cases) or HD and the common late-onset AD, and that difference is the ability to predict the development of the disease. Experts concur that, at this time, no genetic test for late-onset AD can identify who will develop the disease. The APOE genotype has been discovered to be the single most important genetic determinant of susceptibility to AD, but some individuals with that genotype do not develop AD and some who have a different genotype do. The consensus is that while APOE genetic testing may prove useful in diagnosing individuals with cognitive impairment, it is not appropriate to use as a predictive test in asymptomatic patients at this time (National Institute on Aging/Alzheimer's Association Working Group 1996, 7). Furthermore, AD is a multifactorial disease. It is affected by environmental as well as genetic factors, making it unlikely that there will ever be a reliable genetic test to determine who will and who will not develop the disease.

Parental Autonomy and Professional Responsibility

Some individuals may respond that even if a prenatal test can reveal only that the fetus is at increased risk of AD, they would want to know that. It is possible that a woman or couple would choose abortion even if they cannot be told if the fetus will develop AD but only that it has an increased risk of doing so. This position might be based on two factors: (1) a belief that AD is sufficiently awful that it should be avoided even though it is possible to have years of healthy life before it manifests itself, and (2) severe aversion to risk. Even if late-onset AD cannot be reliably predicted by means of a genetic test, some people may prefer to abort rather than take a risk of having a child who will someday develop AD. Faced with such a person, what should a physician or genetic counselor do?

In thinking about this question, we need to balance respect for procreative and parental autonomy with professional responsibility. Physicians and genetic counselors have responsibilities that go beyond merely giving clients what they want. It is entirely proper for professional organizations to assess genetic testing for reliability and predictive value and make recommendations for appropriate use. At this stage, it would be inappropriate to offer to test for APOE when performing amniocentesis.

But what if someone with a strong family history of AD specifically requests such testing? What should the response of a physician or genetic counselor be? Most would be likely to find the request idiosyncratic, even bizarre, based as it is on an extreme aversion to a late-onset disease combined with extreme risk-aversiveness in general. However, respect for patient autonomy requires that the physician or counselor not substitute his or her own values for those of the patient. Professional responsibility requires the professional first of all to provide as accurate scientific information as possible, stressing that no genetic test can identify a fetus as one that will or will not develop AD. It would also be appropriate for a counselor to point out that if the woman aborts this pregnancy because the fetus has a gene associated with heightened risk of AD, she may get pregnant again only to find that the next fetus is definitely afflicted with a worse genetic disease, such as trisomy 13 or 18. It is important to remember that we cannot control everything in our lives, and the obsessive attempt to avoid even small risks of bad outcomes may lead to worse outcomes. A discussion of this sort is entirely consistent with, indeed required by, professional responsibility (Lancaster, Wiseman, and Berchuck 1996). Ultimately, however, the decision rests with the patient or client, assuming the desired test is available and the client is willing to pay for it.

It is unlikely that very many patients will both know about the possibility of prenatal diagnosis for an increased risk of AD and insist on being tested, contrary to the recommendation of their physician or genetic counselor. The more important questions are when, if ever, a genetic test should be recommended by a provider and if it should be covered by insurance. The purposes of such testing are primarily to avoid excessive burdens on the prospective parents and family and secondarily to avoid a lifetime of disability for the child. Because neither purpose is achieved with prenatal diagnosis for AD, offering or covering such a test would be bad, indeed absurd, social policy.

References

Asch, A. 1989. Reproductive technology and disability. In *Reproductive laws for the 1990s*, ed. S. Cohen and N. Taub, 69–124. Clifton, N.J.: Humana Press.

Buchanan, A. 1996. Choosing who will be disabled: Genetic intervention and the morality of inclusion. *Social Philosophy and Policy* 18:18–46.

Dresser, R. and Robertson, J. A. 1989. Quality of life and nontreatment decisions for incompetent patients: A critique of the orthodox approach. *Law, Medicine, and Health Care* 17:234–44.

Elias, S. and Annas, G. J. 1987. *Reproductive genetics and the law.* Chicago: Year Book Medical Publishers.

Feinberg, J. 1987. Wrongful life and the counterfactual element in harming. *Social Philosophy and Policy* 4:145-78.

Kolata, G. 1993. Cystic fibrosis surprise: Genetic screening falters. *New York Times,* Nov. 16, 1993.

Kuhse, H., and Singer, P. 1985. *Should the baby live? The problem of handicapped infants.* New York: Oxford University Press.

Lancaster, J., Wiseman, R., and Berchuck, A. 1996. An inevitable dilemma: Prenatal testing for mutations in the BRCA1 breast-ovarian cancer susceptibility gene. *Obstetrics and Gynecology* 87:306-9.

National Institute on Aging/Alzheimer's Association Working Group. 1996. Apolipoprotein E genotyping in Alzheimer's disease. *Lancet* 347:1091-95.

Post, S. G. 1995. Alzheimer disease and the "then" self. *Kennedy Institute of Ethics Journal* 5:307-21.

Post, S. G., Botkin, J. R., and Whitehouse, P. 1992. Selective abortion for familial Alzheimer disease? *Obstetrics and Gynecology* 79:794-98.

Reilly, P. 1977. *Genetics, law, and social policy.* Cambridge: Harvard University Press.

Rhoden, N. K. 1989. Litigating life and death. *Harvard Law Review* 102:375-446.

Robertson, J. A. 1974. Involuntary euthanasia of defective newborns: A legal analysis. *Stanford Law Review* 27:213-52.

Rothman, B. K. 1986. *The tentative pregnancy.* New York: Viking.

Steinbock, B. 1984. "Baby Jane Doe in the courts." *Hastings Center Report* 14:13-19.

Steinbock, B., and McClamrock, R. 1994. When is birth unfair to the child? *Hastings Center Report* 24:15-21.

PART THREE

Social Issues

Genetics and Long-Term-Care Insurance

Ethical and Policy Issues

ROBERT H. BINSTOCK, PH.D., AND

THOMAS H. MURRAY, PH.D.

As indicated in chapter 4, an estimated three million to four million Americans have Alzheimer disease (AD). From the time that someone experiences symptoms of AD, he or she can live for many years, in some cases for several decades. Whatever the remaining years of life, for much of that period a person with AD requires full-time, round-the-clock, long-term-care services.

A wide range of medical, nursing, social, legal, financial, and other long-term-care services that can be of value to persons with AD, to lessen their suffering and to optimize their functioning, have been identified through program development and research (table 10.1). Some of these services are also of value to family members and others who provide care for AD patients because they can reduce the physical, emotional, and financial burdens of caregiving.

Such long-term-care services, of course, are not only important to persons with AD. The service needs of AD patients and their families are inextricably linked with the overlapping and parallel needs encountered by any of us—regardless of illness, disability, family situation, or age—who are faced with issues of long-term care (see Office of Technology Assessment 1990). Altogether, nearly thirteen million persons in the United States need long-term care; about 19 percent of them reside in nursing homes and other institutions, and 81 percent reside at home or in other community settings where the bulk of care is provided on an unpaid basis by families and others (General Accounting Office 1994).

Nonetheless, AD patients comprise from one-quarter to one-third of Americans who need long-term care. According to the Alzheimer's Association (1996), at least one-half of people with AD are in nursing homes; the balance reside at home or in other community-based settings.

The provision of services to AD patients is becoming increasingly prob-

Table 10.1. Possible Services Needed for People with Alzheimer Disease and Their Families

Diagnosis	Supervision
Acute medical care	Home health aide
Ongoing medical supervision	Homemaker
Treatment of coexisting medical conditions	Personal care
Medication and elimination of drugs that cause excess disability	Paid companion or sitter
	Shopping
Multidimensional assessment	Home-delivered meals
Skilled nursing	Chore services
Physical therapy	Telephone reassurance
Occupational therapy	Personal emergency response system
Speech therapy	Recreation and exercise
Adult day care	Transportation
Respite care[a]	Escort service
Family or caregiver education and training	Special equipment (ramps, hospital beds, etc.)
Family or caregiver counseling	
Family support groups	Vision care
Patient counseling	Audiology
Legal services	Dental care
Financial and benefits counseling	Nutrition counseling
Mental health services	Hospice
Protective services	Autopsy

Source: Based on Office of Technology Assessment 1990, 16.

Note: These services may be needed by and can be provided for persons who are living at home, in a nursing home, or in another care setting, such as assisted living housing, a continuing care retirement community, a board-and-care facility, or an adult foster home.

[a] Respite care includes any service intended to provide temporary relief for the primary caregiver. When used for that purpose, homemaker, paid companion or sitter, adult day care, temporary nursing home care, and other services included on the list in the table are regarded as respite care.

lematic, however, whether they are formal, paid services or provided on an informal, unpaid basis by family members and other caregivers. Out-of-pocket payments for care are becoming larger and unaffordable for many. The safety net that government programs provide by financing long-term care is seriously threatened by federal and state budgetary politics as the twentieth century comes to a close. And broad societal trends suggest that informal care will become less feasible for family members in the future.

In this context it seems likely that the demand for private sector long-term-care insurance will grow substantially. At present long-term-care insurance polices are held by fewer than 5 percent of older Americans. But various studies suggest that the percentage of policyholders may grow substantially in the years ahead as market and public policy changes take place (Crown, Capitman, and Leutz 1992; Friedland 1990; Rivlin and Wiener 1988; Wiener, Illston, and Hanley 1994). Indeed, for many AD patients and their families, long-term-care insurance may become the principal means through which they can access formal, paid care for services.

As long-term-care insurance becomes a more important phenomenon in American society the advent of genetic testing that can identify the risk of developing AD raises some significant social issues. Should genetic testing be used by long-term-care insurance providers as a screening device to deny coverage or charge much higher than standard rates to healthy applicants who are discovered to be in a higher-than-average risk pool for contracting AD?

This chapter addresses this question in terms of the serious ethical and public policy issues that it raises. First, it portrays the present situation and trends in the financing of long-term care for AD patients and others, with attention to the likelihood that consumer demand for long-term-care insurance will increase substantially in the future. Then it addresses issues of fairness that bear on the use of genetic information in underwriting long-term-care insurance and considers circumstances and principles that might justify public policy proscribing such underwriting practices.

Overview of Expenditures for Long-Term Care

Aggregate expenditures for long-term care are sizable and very likely to increase in the decades immediately ahead. The total bill in 1993 was $75.5 billion; of this amount, 72 percent was spent on nursing home care and 28 percent on home and community-based care (Wiener, Illston, and Hanley 1994). Out-of-pocket payments by individuals and their families account for 44 percent of the total (51% of nursing costs and 27% of home- and community-based services are financed in this fashion). Only 1 percent is paid for with private insurance benefits. The remaining 55 percent is financed by federal, state, and local governments.

Paying the costs of long-term care out-of-pocket can be a catastrophic financial experience for patients and their families. The average annual cost of a year's care in a nursing home was $46,000 in 1995 (Levit et al. 1996), and in some homes the cost was more than $100,000. While the use of a limited number of services in a home or other community-based setting is less expensive, noninstitutional care for patients who would otherwise be appropriately placed in a nursing home is not cheaper (Weissert 1990).

The costs of care will undoubtedly grow in the future. Price increases in nursing home and home- and community-based care have consistently exceeded the general rate of inflation. Trends in long-term-care labor and overhead costs indicate that this pattern will continue.

Dozens of governmental programs are sources of funding for long-term-care services, including Medicaid, the Veterans Administration, Social Security's Title XX for social services, and the Older Americans Act (General Accounting Office 1995). Yet, each source regulates the availability of funds with rules as to eligibility and breadth of service coverage and changes its rule frequently. Consequently, persons with AD and their caregivers often find themselves ineligible for financial help from these programs and unable to pay out-of-pocket for needed services. In one study, about 75 percent of the informal, unpaid caregivers of AD patients reported that they did not use formal, paid services because they were unable to afford them (Eckert and Smyth 1988).

The Prominent Role of Medicaid in Financing Care

Medicaid, the federal-state program for health care of the poor, is the major source of the 55 percent of long-term care that is financed by government programs. Medicare, by comparison, pays for short-term subacute nursing care in nursing homes and at home, but it does not provide reimbursement for long-term care.

Medicaid finances the care—at least in part—of about three-fifths of nursing home patients (Wiener and Illston 1996) and 28 percent of home and community-based services (American Association of Retired Persons 1994). The program does not pay for the full range of home care services that are needed for most clients who are functionally dependent (Binstock, Cluff, and von Mering 1996). Most state Medicaid programs provide reimbursement only for the most "medicalized" services that are necessary to maintain a long-term-care patient in a home environment; rarely reimbursed are supports such as chore services, assistance with food shopping and meal preparation, transportation, companionship, periodic monitoring, and respite programs for family and other unpaid caregivers.

Medicaid does include a special waiver program that allows states to offer a wider range of nonmedical home care services, if limited to those patients whose services will be no more costly than Medicaid-financed nursing home care. But the volume of services in these waiver programs—which in some states combine Medicaid with funds from the Older Americans Act, the Social Services Block Grant program, and other state and local government sources—is small in relation to the overall demand (Miller 1992).

Although many patients are poor enough to qualify for Medicaid when they enter a nursing home, a substantial number become poor only after they are institutionalized (Adams, Meiners, and Burwell 1993). Persons in this latter group deplete their assets in order to meet their bills and eventually "spend down" and become poor enough to qualify for Medicaid.

Still others become eligible for Medicaid by sheltering their assets—illegally or legally with the assistance of attorneys who specialize in so-called Medicaid estate planning. Because sheltered assets are not counted in Medicaid eligibility determinations, such persons are able to take advantage of a program for the poor without actually being poor.

Asset sheltering has become a source of considerable concern to the federal and state governments as Medicaid expenditures on nursing homes are increasing rapidly—projected to triple from 1990 to 2000 (Burner, Waldo, and McKusick 1992). An analysis in Virginia estimated that the aggregate value of assets sheltered through the use of legal loopholes in 1991 was equal to more than 10 percent of what the state spent on nursing home care through Medicaid in that year (Burwell 1993). A study drawing on interviews with state government staff who determine Medicaid eligibility in four states—California, Florida, Massachusetts, and New York—found a strong relationship between a high level of financial wealth in a geographic area and a high level of Medicaid estate planning activity. Most of these workers estimated that the range of asset sheltering among single applicants for Medicaid was between 5 percent and 10 percent and for married applicants between 20 and 25 percent (Burwell and Crown 1995).

The prevalence of asset sheltering will probably decline in the years ahead. Federal and state laws are continually closing the loopholes that make this practice feasible. Indeed, in 1996 Congress passed legislation that makes it a federal crime to shelter assets and then apply for Medicaid.

A More Limited Role for Medicaid in the Future

From the mid-1980s until the mid-1990s a number of national policy makers were sympathetic to the inability of individuals and their families to pay for services and the anxieties of becoming impoverished through spending down and becoming dependent on the Medicaid program. Since then, however, the main concern in Washington, as well as in the states, has been to limit Medicaid expenditures. In this new context, the most likely prospect is that public resources for long-term care will be even less available, in relation to the need, than they have been to date.

In the early 1990s advocates for the elderly, as well as younger disabled persons, were optimistic that the federal government would establish a new program for public long-term-care insurance that would not be means-tested, as is Medicaid. A number of bills introduced from 1989 to 1994 included some version of such a program, including President Bill Clinton's failed proposal for health care reform (see Binstock 1994). None of these proposals became law. The major reason was that the various proposals for a new federal long-term-care policy would cost tens of billions of dollars each year just at the outset and far more as the baby boom generation reaches old age.

By 1995, however, legislative focus had shifted from creating a new program to curbing the costs of public expenditures for long-term care. Medicaid's outlays for long-term care had been growing at an annualized rate of 13.2 percent since 1989 (General Accounting Office 1995). Congress proposed in 1995 to cap the rate of growth in Medicaid expenditures in order to achieve savings of $182 billion by 2002, to eliminate federal requirements for determining individual eligibility for Medicaid (as an entitlement), and to turn over control of the program to state governments through capped block grants. President Clinton's veto of the budget bill killed this proposal, but it resurfaced in 1996 with proposed reductions totaling $72 billion (Congressional Budget Office 1996).

This approach for changing Medicaid remains on the policy agenda. If it becomes law, state governments would have to face a number of critical allocation issues. The resolution of these issues would vary, of course, from state to state. But it seems likely that generally throughout the states Medicaid spending would be much less than is projected at present, and the program's function as a financial safety net for persons with AD and their families would be substantially weakened.

Some analysts have predicted that considerable reductions in current state Medicaid spending will almost certainly occur unless federal law requires states to increase their funding for the program (e.g., General Accounting Office 1995) and that nascent home- and community-based services will be decimated in at least half of the states (e.g., Kassner 1995). Whether or not these specific predictions come true, if provisions to cap and block-grant Medicaid do become law, they will almost certainly engender conflict within states regarding the distribution of limited resources between persons with AD and other constituencies.

The Possibility That Informal Care Will Decline

In addition to cash expenditures, long-term care is substantially financed by the in-kind, informal caregiving services of families and friends. A number of research efforts have documented that about 80 percent of the long-term care provided to older persons outside of nursing homes is presently provided on an in-kind basis by family members—spouses, siblings, adult children, and broader kin networks. About 74 percent of dependent community-based older persons receive all their care from family members or other unpaid sources: about 21 percent receive both formal and informal services; and only about 5 percent use just formal services (Liu, Manton, and Liu 1985). The vast majority of family caregivers are women (see Brody 1990; Stone, Cafferata, and Sangl 1987). The family also plays an important role in obtaining and managing services from paid service providers. But it is possible that families may do substantially less of this work during the next few decades.

The family, as a fundamental unit of social organization, has been undergoing profound transformations that will become more fully manifest over the next few decades as baby boomers reach old age. The striking growth of single-parent households, the growing participation of women in the labor force, and the high incidence of divorce and remarriage (differentially higher for men) all entail complicated changes in the structure of household and kinship roles and relationships. There will be an increasing number of "blended families," reflecting multiple lines of descent through multiple marriages and the birth of children outside of wedlock through other partners. This growth in the incidence of step- and half-relatives will make for a dramatic new turn in family structure in the coming decades. Already, such blended families constitute about half of all households with children (National Academy on Aging 1994).

As such changes begin to coincide with the growth of three- and even four-generation families, what emerges is a very complex picture that has hardly even begun to be analyzed and understood with respect to its potential ramifications. One clear implication, however, is that while kinship networks in the near future will become much more extensive than in the past, they will also become more complex, attenuated, and diffuse (Bengtson, Rosenthal, and Burton 1990).

There is much room for speculation and debate about the implications of these trends for the functioning of the family as a source of unpaid care for persons with AD. However, early research evidence of a weakened sense of filial obligation in blended families (National Academy on Aging 1994) does give cause for concern. If these changes in the intensity of kinship relations continue and significantly erode the capacity and sense of obligation to provide informal care for persons with AD, then a greater portion of such care will need to come from paid service providers.

The Role of Private Insurance

For reasons discussed above, financing of long-term care for persons with AD through out-of-pocket payments or through government programs is likely to become more and more difficult in the years ahead. The extent of unpaid care could also diminish. Hence, the use of private insurance care for persons with AD and others who need long-term care may grow considerably.

Private insurance to cover the costs of long-term care is a relatively new product. According to the Health Insurance Association of America, the number of policies ever sold increased from 815,000 in 1987 to 2.9 million in 1992; but the number of active policies at any given time is lower (Wiener, Illston, and Hanley 1994).

A good policy can largely defray the expensive costs of care. Consider the example of an individual (as opposed to a group) insurance policy offered by the Teachers Insurance and Annuity Association (TIAA), which receives the highest quality ratings from independent insurance-rating agencies. Nursing home benefit rates are $100 a day, which virtually covers the national average cost of a nursing home. Coverage for home health care or adult day health care (at a center outside the home) is $50 a day. Average daily rates, however, vary considerably among specific communities and particular homes. In Ohio, for instance, nursing home rates range from $90 to $150 a day. In New York City the average daily rate is $220, but in the Riverdale section of the city the rate is as high as $300.

The benefits are limited, however, with respect to when they first become available and how long they will be paid. From the time that eligibility for benefits is determined there is a ninety-day waiting period before benefits are paid; in effect, this is a deductible amounting to $9,000 for nursing home care and $4,500 for home and adult day health care. The maximum amount of benefits that will be paid under the TIAA policy range from $110,000 to $225,000, depending upon the amount of the premium paid for the policy. There is also the problem of price inflation in long-term-care services over time. Teacher's Insurance and Annuity Association offers a 5 percent inflation option on its benefits, but this may not be enough to cover the full rate of inflation in long-term-care costs. Nonetheless, the policy can defray a high percentage of expenses for from three to eight years.

As indicated above, at present only 1 percent of long-term-care expenditures are financed by private insurance. Among people sixty-five and older, fewer than 5 percent hold policies.

Why do so few persons own long-term-care policies? Part of the problem seems to be that the product is presently unknown to most potential customers. In addition, the current level of pricing may be too high for many of them. At age sixty-five, for instance, the annual premium for TIAA's lowest maximum in benefits is $833, and for the highest it is $1,028. At age seventy-five, these premiums climb to $1,846 and $2,229, respectively. For a high percentage of older people these prices seem unaffordable. Among persons aged sixty-five and older, 39.6 percent have a pretax income of less than 200 percent of the poverty threshold—$14,618 for an individual and less than $18,440 for a married couple where the man is aged sixty-five (Department of Commerce 1996). Among individuals aged seventy-five and older, 54 percent are below the poverty threshold.

Yet, there is considerable room for increase in the number of people holding long-term-care policies. Although premiums are unaffordable for a large proportion of the older population, there remains a huge segment of the potential market that can afford premiums—perhaps as many as fifteen million people. Marketing of the product, and, thus, potential customer familiarity with it, is growing each year. As it does, people are also becoming more sophisticated about the optimum age for purchasing coverage—the trade-offs between lower premiums at younger ages and the risks of needing long-term care at older ages.

Moreover, insurance companies initially set artificially high prices for premiums because they had little experience regarding how much they would have to actually pay out in benefits. Rates are now gradually becoming much lower as the companies become more experienced with the financial risks to which their policies expose them. As recently as 1991, the best quality policies—providing substantial benefits over a reasonable period of time—charged premiums much higher than the TIAA policy, averaging $2,525 for persons aged sixty-five and $7,675 for those aged seventy-nine (Wiener and Illston 1996). Some studies conducted prior to these contemporary changes in insurance—as well as the cost-control political environment of the Medicaid program—projected that early in the twenty-first century the percentage of the older population that might be covered by long-term-care insurance would increase significantly as new marketing techniques are developed and public policies are enacted to induce the purchase of policies (see Crown, Capitman, and Leutz 1992; Friedland 1990; Rivlin and Wiener 1988; Wiener, Illston, and Hanley 1994). Although other studies suggest a potential for an even higher percentage of customers, they assume relatively limited packages of benefit coverage (see, e.g., Cohen et al. 1987).

A variation on the private insurance policy approach to financing long-term care is continuing care retirement communities (CCRCs), which promise comprehensive health care services—including long-term care—to all members (Chellis and Grayson 1990). Customers of CCRCs tend to be middle- and upper-income persons who are relatively healthy when they become residents and pay a substantial entrance charge and monthly fee in return for a promise of "care for life." It has been estimated that about 10 percent of older people could afford to join such communities (Cohen 1988). Most of the one thousand CCRCs in the United States, however, do not provide complete benefit coverage in their contracts, and those that do have faced financial difficulties (Williams and Temkin-Greener 1996). Because most older people prefer to remain in their own homes rather than join age-segregated communities, an alternative product termed "life care at home" (LCAH) was developed in the late 1980s and marketed to middle-income customers with lower entry and monthly fees than those of CCRCs (Tell, Cohen, and Wallack 1987). There are, however, only about five hundred LCAH policies currently in effect (Williams and Temkin-Greener 1996).

Genetics, Ethics, and Insurance

In the decades immediately ahead, private insurance is very likely to become a major resource through which many persons with AD and other diseases can finance their long-term care. In this context insurance companies will seek, of course, to insure favorable risk pools—that is, clienteles who are less likely, on average, to be eligible for benefit payments. As they do, the advent of genetic testing for AD will generate significant ethical and public policy issues.

Ever since attention was first focused on the ethical, legal and social implications of the Human Genome Project, the possibility that insurers might want to use genetic information in deciding whom to insure, for what risks, and at what rates has been seen as important. The first task force established by the Ethical, Legal, and Social Issues (ELSI) Working Group for the U.S. Human Genome Project was created to deal with the subject of genetics and insurance.

The task force's report, *Genetic Information and Health Insurance* (NIH/

DOE 1993), considered the likelihood that health insurers might actually use potentially predictive genetic information, examined critically the ethical basis for such use (in the practice insurers call "underwriting"), and offered recommendations about what limitations ought to be placed on the use of genetic information in health insurance. These same issues are directly relevant to long-term-care insurance and the availability of genetic information related to AD.

Narrow and Broad-Based Concepts of Genetic Information

One can take a narrow or a broad view of what constitutes genetic information, and the decision on which conception to adopt was the initial challenge faced by the task force. The narrow view—a view adopted in most of the recent laws directed against genetic discrimination or for the protection of genetic privacy—limits attention to the results of direct-DNA tests. These are tests that look at the DNA itself for mutations or polymorphisms that might predict the likelihood of future disease. With this narrow view, other kinds of tests are ruled out. These would include, for example, tests of the protein products made by genes or the metabolites of those proteins, as well as other kinds of genetic information, including family histories.

The broad view of genetic information, in contrast, does include these latter types of tests and information. It emphasizes that genetic information about the likelihood of disease is important in itself, regardless of the precise form in which it is derived. At present, the most common, and probably the most useful, genetic information is in the form of family health histories rather than direct-DNA tests. Even in the future, the most clinically significant genetic information may be about what happens "downstream" from the gene—in the enzymes, structural proteins, neurotransmitters, and assorted molecules coded for by genes.

The task force, which included representatives from the insurance industry and groups with genetic diseases along with several experts, rejected the narrow concept of genetic information. It noted that the typical medical record contained a health history, including information about diseases affecting other family members, and that this information is, on any fair reading, genetic information. It also noted that well-established biochemical tests for known genetic diseases such as sickle-cell anemia or the sweat chloride test for cystic fibrosis are not direct-DNA tests. The task force therefore adopted the broad view of genetic information because it would encompass the full range of clinically, and actuarially, relevant information about genetic differences among individuals.

Insurers and Genetic Information

At present there is little evidence that insurers are making systematic use of the new direct-DNA testing technologies. As long as these tests are relatively expensive and the usefulness of the tests for underwriting purposes is not confirmed, insurers are unlikely to engage in widespread direct-DNA testing. Insurers do, however, insist on their right to know if an applicant has had genetic tests of any kind. To do otherwise, they argue, would result in asymmetrical information and would place them at a disadvantage by putting them at risk of what they term "adverse selection" in their pools of insurees.

The task force acknowledged that there is little likelihood that insurers will affirmatively require applicants to undergo direct-DNA tests until such tests could be justified on a cost-benefit basis, that is, until the money saved (by the insurer) through requiring the tests significantly exceeded the incremental costs of testing. No one can say with certainty just when that would happen for any particular test. But experts involved in developing genetic testing technology are confident that the cost of such tests will decline rapidly and significantly.

In any event, it does not take widespread direct-DNA testing for reports of genetic discrimination to appear. Some published studies have identified possible incidents of genetic discrimination, including discrimination by insurers (Billings et al. 1992; Lapham, Kozma, and Weiss 1996), although there are no reliable estimates of incidence or prevalence. However, when the unsettling reports of genetic discrimination are added to the prospect of attractive cost-benefit ratios in the near future and mixed with the concept of "actuarial fairness" — a principle of distributive justice favored by insurers — the result is worrisome.

Insurers and Actuarial Fairness

In the insurance industry, actuarial fairness is the claim that fair treatment of persons requires classifying them according to their risks and making underwriting decisions — whether to offer a policy, with what terms, at what cost — in accordance with those risks. Under actuarial fairness, insurers claim they would be acting unjustly if they offered essentially the same terms and rates to persons with different risks. The individual with lower risks would have been treated unfairly (Clifford and Iuculano 1987). Actuarial fairness seems to reflect a reasonable moral view about fairness for some insurance products, for example, insurance against damage to property or goods for a business. Why should company A pay for company B's carelessness or willingness to take much greater risks? But actuarial fairness seems much less able to account for widespread convictions about fairness in other spheres—health insurance in particular.

Norman Daniels offers a critical examination of what he calls "the Argument from Actuarial Fairness," the "moral judgment that fair underwriting practices must reflect the division of people according to the actuarially accurate determination of their risks" (Daniels 1996, 179–80). If we think of insurance as the prudent sharing of risk, then the practice of tying premiums to the likelihood of claims seems sensible. As Daniels points out, however, this is not a morally neutral presumption. It may be valid for certain insurance products, business loss and liability policies, for example. But its application to health insurance, the target of Daniels' analysis, is dubious. He argues that actuarial fairness is equivalent to fairness per se only if "individuals are entitled to benefit from any of their individual differences, especially their different risks for disease and disability" (Daniels 1996, 181). The plausibility of this claim depends upon deeper disagreements about justice, illness, and access to health care. Daniels claims that people have no such entitlements; some other philosophers, especially those of a libertarian bent, argue otherwise.

An alternative approach to the problem of distributive justice in health insurance involves an effort to understand the shared meaning of the social good that is health care and of the principle of distribution appropriate to that social good. Walzer (1983) argues that health care in the contemporary United States is part of the sphere of security and welfare, a sphere in which the proper distributive principle is need. This analysis has been extended to the use of genetic information in health insurance (Murray 1992). Indeed, public opinion appears to support the claim of a fairly widespread social understanding that health care, and the insurance that helps pay for it, ought to be available according to need and not mere ability to pay or other possible distributional principles.

Fairness and Long-Term-Care Insurance

What happens when these perspectives on fairness in health insurance are applied to long-term-care insurance? Is it likely that insurers will want to use genetic information in writing long-term-care insurance policies? Would that be unfair—not in actuarial terms, but according to our shared conception of justice?

Insurers can be expected to be concerned about any asymmetry of information—any situations in which potential customers know things relevant to risks that the insurer does not also know. They are likely to insist that they have access to relevant genetic information, including the results of genetic tests for predisposition to or risk of Alzheimer dementia. Even though risk factors may have dubious clinical relevance for individual patients, insurers find them of great interest. Insurers deal with populations, and a factor that can predict substantial differences in underwriting costs for certain populations might be considered very useful by an insurer, even if a physician would be reluctant to give clinical advice to an individual based on the same information. The APOE allele system might be such a factor.

In cases of dominant mutations, where the inheritance is 50 percent, insurers will want to know the family health history as well as the results of any genetic test. For polymorphisms with lower predictive value, such as the APOE alleles, again insurers will want to know any health-related information the applicant has that is actuarially relevant. Whether a double dose of APOE ε4 is sufficiently predictive to warrant the attention of actuaries is not a question we are qualified to answer conclusively.

It is important to note that insurers can acquire and use genetic information without specifically requiring applicants to take genetic tests. For one thing, medical records frequently contain genetic information, at least in the form of family health histories. Applications for health insurance (and presumably for long-term-care insurance), unless they are under large group policies, may be underwritten—that is, evaluated for their risk of a claim. The application typically includes an authorization for the insurer to obtain medical information about the applicant from physicians and others. The insurer may request a statement from the applicant's physician, who in turn is likely to delegate the task of responding to office staff. It appears that most of time the response is simply to copy and send the medical record, rather than to answer the specific questions posed by the insurer (Stone 1996). Applicants, it might be said, have the option of refusing to give permission for the insurer to obtain the applicant's medical records. But insurers have the right to refuse to consider the application, and they surely exercise that right.

In addition to obtaining genetic information from medical records, insurers have available another strategy for using genetic information. Where it is permitted by law, an insurer could offer preferred policies to those people who voluntarily come forward with genetic information that indicates they do not have any elevated risk for something like dementia. It could work like this: Company A offers a standard policy, at a relatively high rate, for people with no genetic information about their risk for dementia. It also offers a "preferred" policy for applicants who can show that they do not have any of the dominant mutations associated with AD, nor do they have any APOE ε4 alleles. Company A is not forcing anyone to get genetic information, but it is encouraging a division in the market for long-term-care insurance between those with and those without known genetic risks.

Would using genetic information about the risk of AD be unfair in the context of long-term-care insurance? Insurers are likely to regard such use as fair, if actuarial statistics support its predictive power. But would it be deemed fair by the public? by those who, because they have a genetic predisposition to AD, will find long-term-care insurance unaffordable or completely unattainable? by those whose rates may be increased if insurers are not allowed to take into account genetic predispositions for dementia?

The likelihood of a rate increase for long-term-care insurance depends on several factors: the actuarial predictiveness of genetic mutations and polymorphisms linked to AD; the magnitude of the "adverse selection" effect — how much the decision to purchase a long-term-care policy will be a function of knowledge on the customer's part that she or he is at increased genetic risk of dementia and the financial impact of such selectivity in applications on the insurer; and whether long-term-care insurance remains a purely voluntary market. If insurers are prohibited by law from using any genetic information, including information about the future likelihood of dementia, then people will have the right to purchase such policies, but their price might rise substantially.

The insurance industry vigorously defends its desire to have access to the same genetic information that applicants have concerning their risks. The industry also wants to be able to use that information in underwriting for individual applicants. A recent article by a physician associated with the insurance industry states the implications of actuarial fairness bluntly: "Harsh as it may sound to the ears of a society that subscribes to egalitarian principles, solidarity ends with a negative genetic test" (Pokorski 1997).

One way to try to answer the question of fairness here is to ask whether long-term-care insurance in this context is more like traditional health insurance — a form of insurance intended to meet needs for health care that can occasionally incur catastrophic costs — or a means to protect assets for one's heirs that might otherwise be consumed in payments for long-term care. We can expect difficulties either way we choose, assuming that genetic predispositions for dementia have actuarial significance. If we ban the use of genetic information by insurers, and if substantial adverse selection occurs, long-term-care insurance is likely to become less available and affordable. If we permit the use of genetic information, then people who through no fault of their own have genetic predispositions to dementia are likely to have great difficulty getting affordable long-term-care insurance and, unless they shelter their assets, are likely to see them diminished or exhausted by the cost of their care.

Fairness and Public Policy

Is there need for public policy concerning issues that involve the availability to insurers of genetic information, as broadly conceived, about an individual's risk for AD? Whatever policies we might adopt should reflect our deepest societal convictions regarding justice and fairness on these issues.

There are two major reasons why individuals purchase long-term-care insurance, and they are strongly intertwined. One reason is to make sure that they have a way to pay for long-term care that they may need. The other is to protect their assets, to avoid spending them down to pay for long-term care.

During the early 1990s the merits of using public policy to protect assets from being spent down on long-term care were debated. At that time it seemed like a major federal long-term-care benefit program (in addition to Medicaid) would be established, funded at a level of tens of billions of dollars in its first year (see Binstock 1994).

The major concern of advocates for such a program, led by the national Alzheimer's Association, was and is that middle-class persons would become poor through spending down to pay for long-term care and then become dependent on a welfare program, Medicaid, to pay nursing home and home care bills. (This concern does not, of course, extend to very wealthy persons.) There is a distinct and understandable middle-class fear—both economic and psychological in nature—of having to use savings and sell a home to finance one's own long-term care.

One element in this anxiety is the desire to maintain one's feelings of self-esteem and independence. In American culture such feelings tend to be inextricably bound up with material worth, particularly in older years when a paid-off mortgage and the accumulation of some savings provide a symbol of one's independence and responsibility.

Another element is the loss of a capacity to provide some measure of security for one's children and grandchildren. The desire to leave a modest inheritance to help assure security and opportunity for one's family is understandable and even laudable. Giving our offspring a decent start in life and making to them a modest gift upon our death seems a reasonable goal. Indeed, for many Americans who care deeply about their families, perhaps the worst scenario for their dying would be one in which their families were physically, emotionally, and financially exhausted by their dying. Indeed, the impulse to care for our survivors is a good one and something we ought to encourage. Additionally, the peace of mind in knowing that something can be left to those we loved in life can offer comfort to people nearing the end of life.

Yet the prospect that an expensive government program might be used to protect assets from being spent down on long-term care generated a number of issues of fairness, explicit and implicit. Why shouldn't people spend their income and assets on long-term care? Why should tax dollars foot the bill? Why should it be government's responsibility to preserve inheritances? Should government take a more active role than it already does in preserving inequalities in economic status from generation to generation? On what basis should some persons be taxed to preserve the inheritances of others? Should the taxing power of government be used to preserve the psychological sense of self-esteem that for so many persons is bound up in their lifetime accumulation of assets—their material worth?

These questions had barely permeated into the arena of public discussion when they became moot. With the failure of President Clinton's proposal for comprehensive health care reform in 1994 and the emergence in 1995 of an entirely new political milieu regarding federal policy initiatives, the prospects for a major new federal long-term-care program faded and remain dim (see Binstock 1997).

The issues for debate change somewhat when one focuses on private long-term-care insurance and the prospect of public policies that might regulate the use of genetic information by insurers. Concerns about using the taxes paid by some to preserve the assets and inheritances of others become irrelevant. Other aspects of fairness come to the fore.

At the threshold it is worth reiterating that long-term-care insurance is largely of benefit to the middle-class and of little benefit to the very rich and prosperous. The TIAA policy described earlier in this chapter, for example, offers maximum lifetime benefits ranging from $110,000 to $225,000, depending on the size of premiums. Some policies offer larger maximum benefits. But none of the mainstream insurance products provide benefits that will protect much more than a relatively modest life-time accumulation of assets—say, a paid-off home and $100,000 to $200,000 in savings—from being exhausted on long-term care for persons with AD.

In this context the central question is this: Should government take steps to protect middle-class persons from underwriting practices that draw on genetic information? There is a precedent for government intervention, targeted to the middle class, in matters of financing long-term care.

In the early 1990s the Robert Wood Johnson Foundation financed an experimental program in four states, the prime goal of which is to reduce Medicaid spending by providing an asset-protection incentive for people to purchase long-term-care insurance. It is designed to enable middle-class persons to avoid spending down and yet have Medicaid pay for some of their long-term care. At the same time it has the purpose of reducing the period that Medicaid will pay for long-term-care services that will be needed by an individual.

Through this Partnership for Long-Term Care Program, state governments agree to exempt individuals who apply for Medicaid eligibility from having to spend down assets in order to qualify for the program, if they have previously had some long-term care paid for by a state-certified private insurance policy. In California, Connecticut, and Indiana, the Medicaid agencies will allow a dollar of asset protection for each dollar that has been paid by insurance. In New York the experimental program protects the assets of wealthy as well as middle-class people; after three years of private insurance coverage for nursing home services or six months of home health care, protection is granted for all assets in determining a person's Medicaid eligibility, although the individual's income must be devoted to the cost of care along with Medicaid payments. The outcomes of these experiments have yet to be evaluated (see Meiners 1996).

The goal of a public policy prohibiting insurers from using AD-related genetic information in underwriting long-term-care insurance would be different from that of the Robert Wood Johnson policy experiments. The goal would be to protect middle-class people who have a genetically based risk of contracting AD — protect them from being excluded from obtaining such insurance or having to pay an exorbitantly high price for it.

What form might such a public policy take? In principle, state governments could regulate the sale of long-term-care insurance policies that provide a modest amount of maximum lifetime benefit payments. They could prohibit insurers from using genetic information (broadly conceived) that pertains to an individual's risk of developing AD when underwriting such policies.

Could such a policy, essentially targeted to help the middle class, be justified by societal convictions about fairness? The shared understandings about justice supporting such a policy are less than fully formed. The argument could be this: The ability to purchase reasonably affordable long-term-care insurance can provide both peace of mind for purchasers and a modicum of security for their survivors. Because it is socially desirable to encourage people to care for their families and because a decent measure of financial security is seen by many Americans as a thing we legitimately want to leave to our descendants, there is likely to be a widely shared belief that people ought not to be barred from doing so due to a genetic predisposition utterly beyond their control. If this analysis is correct, then denying access to long-term-care insurance may be a form of injustice.

If the issue of fairness is framed in terms of ensuring access to long-term care for persons with AD, then the case for public policy intervention becomes even stronger. In this framework one can turn again to Walzer's analysis, in which health care (including long-term care) is part of a sphere of justice where the proper distributive principle is simply the need for care.

For American society to share this view of justice, however, an evolution in cultural perceptions of long-term care will need to take place. For most of this century long-term care — and especially the care of persons with AD — has been a comparatively neglected backwater in the overall American health care scene. Until recently, except for occasional nursing home scandals and fires — and subsequent ad hoc activities in response to these events — long-term care has received little attention from the medical profession and society at large. It has been eclipsed by the glamour and prestige of hospital-based medical care that is inherently dramatic because it deals with acute episodes of illnesses and trauma and their relatively high-tech and "quick fix" dimensions of diagnosis and intervention.

In effect, long-term care has not been perceived as part of health care. Long-term care has not even been covered through traditional health insurance mechanisms such as employee benefit plans. When concerns are expressed about the fact that forty million Americans are not covered by health insurance, coverage for long-term care is not part of the discussion.

The structure of the health care delivery system and the financing that underpins it have also engendered a functional reality, as well as a perception, that separates long-term care from other forms of health care. Few health care provider organizations integrate acute and long-term care in an effective fashion. Separate sources of financing for acute and long-term care tend to engender this fragmentation, even when acute and long-term care services are part of the same organization (see Meiners 1996).

Yet, there are good reasons to believe that long-term care will come to function and be perceived more widely as part of the continuum of health care that is needed by all of us (see Binstock, Cluff, and von Mering 1996). The federal government has been sponsoring a number of demonstration projects that integrate acute and long-term care through various financing mechanisms. The proliferation of Medicare health management organizations (HMOs) is beginning to encourage contractual arrangements between them and long-term-care providers.

As the baby boom cohort begins to approach the ranks of old age, the importance of long-term care—the formidable volume of need for it, the difficulties of financing it, and the challenges of delivering it effectively—is likely to become increasingly accepted throughout American society. Such acceptance will bring with it a widespread understanding that long-term care is not simply social care but health care by another name. This perception may enfold long-term care into the shared understanding of justice in health care that dictates that it should be distributed according to need. In turn, this would provide a moral foundation for public policy that would bar the use of genetic information in underwriting long-term-care insurance.

References

Adams, E. K., Meiners, M. R., and Burwell, B. O. 1993. Asset spend-down in nursing homes: Methods and insights. *Medical Care* 31:1–23.

Alzheimer's Association. 1996. *1996 Advocate's guide.* Washington, D.C.: Public Policy Division, Alzheimer's Association.

American Association of Retired Persons, Public Policy Institute. 1994. *The costs of long-term care.* Washington, D.C.: American Association of Retired Persons.

Bengtson, V. L., Rosenthal, C., and Burton, L. 1990. Families and aging: Diversity and heterogeneity. In *Handbook of aging and the social sciences,* ed. R. H. Binstock and L. K. George, 263–87. 4th ed. San Diego: Academic Press.

Billings, P. R., Kohn, M. A., de Cuevas, M., Beckwith, J., Alper, J. S., and Natowicz, M. R. 1992. Discrimination as a consequence of genetic testing. *American Journal of Human Genetics* 50:476–82.

Binstock, R. H. 1994. Older Americans and health care reform in the 1990s. In *Health care reform in the nineties,* ed. P. V. Rosenau, 213–35. Thousand Oaks, Calif.: Sage Publications.

———. 1997. The old-age lobby in a new political era. In *The future of age-based public policy,* ed. R. B. Hudson. Baltimore: Johns Hopkins University Press.

Binstock, R. H., Cluff, L. E., and von Mering, O., eds. 1996. *The future of long-term care: Social and policy issues.* Baltimore: Johns Hopkins University Press.

Brody, E. M. 1990. *Women in the middle: Their parent-care years.* New York: Springer Publishing.

Burner, S. T., Waldo, D. R., and McKusick, D. R. 1992. National health expenditures projections through 2030. *Health Care Financing Review* 14 (1): 1–29.

Burwell, B. 1993. *State responses to Medicaid estate planning.* Cambridge, Mass.: SysteMetrics.

Burwell, B., and Crown, W. H. 1995. *Medicaid estate planning in the aftermath of OBRA '93.* Cambridge, Mass.: MEDSTAT Group.

Chellis, R. D., and Grayson, P. J. 1990. *Life care: A long-term solution?* Lexington, Mass.: Lexington Books.

Clifford, K. A., and Iuculano, R. P. 1987. AIDS and insurance: The rationale for AIDS-related testing. *Harvard Law Review* 100:1806-25.

Cohen, M. A. 1988. Life care: New options for financing and delivering long-term care. *Health Care Financing Review* (ann. supp.): 139-43.

Cohen, M. A., Tell, E., Greenberg, J., and Wallack, S. S. 1987. The financial capacity of the elderly to insure for long-term care. *Gerontologist* 27:494-502.

Congressional Budget Office. 1996. *The economic and budget outlook: An update.* Washington, D.C.: Government Printing Office.

Crown, W. H., Capitman, J., and Leutz, W. N. 1992. Economic rationality, the affordability of private long-term care insurance, and the role for public policy. *Gerontologist* 32:478-85.

Daniels, N. 1996. The Human Genome Project and the distribution of scarce medical resources. In *The Human Genome Project and the future of health care,* ed. T. H. Murray, M. A. Rothstein, and R. F. Murray Jr., 173-95. Bloomington: Indiana University Press.

Department of Commerce, Bureau of the Census, Economics and Statistics Administration. 1996. *Poverty in the United States, 1995.* Current Population Reports, Consumer Income, no. P60-194. Washington, D.C.: Government Printing Office.

Eckert, S. K., and Smyth, K. 1988. *A case study of methods of locating and arranging health and long-term care for persons with dementia.* Washington, D.C.: U.S. Congress, Office of Technology Assessment.

Friedland, R. 1990. *Facing the costs of long-term care: An EBRI-ERF policy study.* Washington, D.C.: Employee Benefits Research Institute.

General Accounting Office. 1994. *Long-term care: Diverse, growing population includes millions of Americans of all ages.* GAO/HEHS-95-62. Washington, D.C.: Government Printing Office.

―――. 1995. *Long-term care: Current issues and future directions.* Washington, D.C.: Government Printing Office.

Kassner, E. 1995. *Long-term care: Measuring the impact of a Medicaid cap.* Washington, D.C.: Public Policy Institute, American Association of Retired Persons.

Lapham, E. V., Kozma, C., and Weiss, J. O. 1996. Genetic discrimination: Perspectives of consumers. *Science* 274:621-24.

Levit, K. R., Lazenby, H. C., Braden, B. R., Cowan, C. A., McDonnell, P. A., Sivarajan, L., Stiller, J. M., Won, D. K., Donham, C. S., Long, A. M., and Stewart, M. W. 1996. National health expenditures, 1995. *Health Care Financing Review* 18 (1): 175-214.

Liu, K., Manton, K. M., and Liu, B. M. 1985. Home care expenses for the disabled elderly. *Health Care Financing Review* 7 (2): 51-58.

Meiners, M. R. 1996. The financing and organization of long-term care. In *The future of long-term care: Social and policy issues,* ed. R. H. Binstock, L. E. Cluff, and O. von Mering, 191-214. Baltimore: Johns Hopkins University Press.

Miller, N. A. 1992. Medicaid 2176 home and community-based care waivers: The first ten years. *Health Affairs* 11:162-71.

Murray, T. H. 1992. Genetics and the moral mission of health insurance. *Hastings Center Report* 22:12-17.

National Academy on Aging. 1994. *Old age in the twenty-first century.* Washington, D.C.: National Academy on Aging.

NIH/DOE (National Institutes of Health/Department of Energy) Joint Task Force on Genetic Information and Insurance. 1993. *Genetic information and health insurance.* Bethesda, Md.: National Institutes of Health.

Office of Technology Assessment. 1990. *Confused minds, burdened families: Finding help for people with Alzheimer's and other dementias.* Washington, D.C.: Government Printing Office.

Pokorski, R. J. 1997. Insurance underwriting in the genetic era. *American Journal of Human Genetics* 60:205-16.

Rivlin, A. M., and Wiener, J. M. 1988. *Caring for the disabled elderly: Who will pay?* Washington, D.C.: Brookings Institution.

Stone, D. A. 1996. The implications of the Human Genome Project for access to health insurance. In *The Human Genome Project and the future of health care,* ed. T. H. Murray, M. A. Rothstein, and R. F. Murray Jr., 133-57. Bloomington: Indiana University Press.

Stone, R., Cafferata, G. L., and Sangl, J. 1987. Caregivers of the frail elderly: A national profile. *Gerontologist* 27:616-26.

Tell, E. J., Cohen, M. A., and Wallack, S. S. 1987. New directions in lifecare: An industry in transition. *Milbank Quarterly* 65:551-74.

Walzer, M. 1983. *Spheres of justice: A defense of pluralism and equality.* New York: Basic Books.

Weissert, W. G. 1990. Strategies for reducing home care expenditures. *Generations* 14 (2): 42-44.

Wiener, J. M., and Illston, L. H. 1996. Health care financing and organization for the elderly. In *Handbook of aging and the social sciences,* ed. R. H. Binstock and L. K. George, 427-45. 4th ed. San Diego, Calif.: Academic Press.

Wiener, J. M., Illston, L. H., and Hanley, R. J. 1994. *Sharing the burden: Strategies for public and private long-term care insurance.* Washington, D.C.: Brookings Institution.

Williams, T. F., and Temkin-Greener, H. 1996. Older people, dependency, and trends in supportive care. In *The future of long-term care: Social and policy issues,* ed. R. H. Binstock, L. E. Cluff, and O. von Mering, 51-74. Baltimore: Johns Hopkins University Press.

ERIC T. JUENGST, PH.D.

The Ethical Implications of Alzheimer Disease Risk Testing for Other Clinical Uses of APOE Genotyping

One of the unusual features of using apolipoprotein E (APOE) genotyping to assess the risks of developing Alzheimer disease (AD) is that it would involve a genetic test that can be performed for other clinical purposes as well. Apolipoprotein E genotyping is already used by cardiologists to help determine the risks of hyperlipidemia and its clinical sequelae, atherosclerosis and myocardial infarction. In fact, the same allele of the APOE gene, the $\epsilon 4$ allele, seems to convey the highest risk for both coronary artery disease (CAD) and AD (Assman et al. 1984; Cumming and Robertson 1984; Davignon, Gregg, and Sing 1988; Kosunen et al. 1995; Menzel, Kladetzky, and Assman 1983; Utermann, Hardewig, and Zimmer 1984). This versatility has gone almost entirely unremarked in the burgeoning literature on genetic testing for AD risk (except by Wachbroit 1996), but it is one of the aspects of AD genetic testing that is most likely to set a precedent, as other genetic tests are increasingly shown to be clinically versatile as well.

Moreover, the precedents that APOE genotyping may have to set for managing versatility in genetic testing are startling. To be consistent with our most relevant current policies and practices, it appears that, short of major societal change, all uses of a versatile genetic test will have to be governed by the protocols required by its most problematic use. Indeed, to live up to our current commitments, in the many practice situations in which it is impossible to meet the clinical requirements for AD risk testing, APOE genotyping should already be abandoned as a clinical tool. Or so I argue below.

Background

"Beanbag genetics" is the epithet that the evolutionary biologist Ernst Mayr employed to criticize his predecessors' simple-minded interpretation of the Mendelian principle that genes (and traits) assort themselves independently between generations. Unlike colored beans in a bag, Mayr argues, genes rarely have only one phenotypic effect and are never entirely disconnected from one another (Mayr 1963, 263). Since then, the phenomena to which he referred— pleiotropy, heterogeneity, and linkage—have become foundational for much of modern genetics, undergirding both the gene hunting of the Human Genome Project and the functional analysis of genes to which so much of basic biomedical research has turned.

Despite the best efforts of science, however, beanbag genetics has shown stubborn persistence in medicine. "Genetic diseases" are still usually identified by self-contained causal associations between a particular allele of a specific gene and a single (though not necessarily simple) clinical syndrome, complicated at most by the magic of mysterious environmental factors. The medical advantage of thinking this way about genetic risk factors is clear: it allows one to apply the doctrine of specific causation to these health problems (Baird 1990). If deleterious alleles can be considered the specific (e.g., necessary and sufficient) pathogens for these diseases, their presence in the body becomes a powerful diagnostic and predictive sign and a justification for initiating preventive or palliative interventions. Thus, where medical geneticists are able to tell a convincing causal story of this sort, they like to name not just specific alleles but the genes themselves after the particular disease that their mutant variants can cause (viz., the Huntington gene, CFTR, or BRCA1), as if the genes were pathognomonic signs of the disease itself. Where medical researchers cannot yet tell a clear story, as in the genetics of schizophrenia, the search goes on, motivated by the hope that one or two major loci might account for the problem (for AD, see Breitner 1994).

As genomic research extends Mayr's arguments into human biology, of course, this simple "beanbag" model for medical genetics is breaking down. Almost all the DNA-based descriptions of new disease genes have underscored the fact that multiple alleles at a given locus can produce the same clinical phenotype, and in most cases multiple loci are implicated as well. The effect of this heterogeneity is to mute the predictive power of any particular genetic approach to risk assessment for these conditions, and the expressions of caution that dominate most current genetic testing policy statements are a reflection of this uncertainty (Holtzman 1989).

Now, with the association of the APOE genotypes with differential risks for acquiring AD, the other side of Mayr's challenge to beanbag thinking—the problem of pleiotropy—asserts itself. It should not, of course, be surprising that mutations at the genomic level should ramify through the body's systems in more than one direction and end up causing widely different types of health problems. As medicine relearns human physiology from the genome up, the multipotency of the APOE alleles is likely to become the norm rather than the exception: every genotypic change probably has multiple phenotypic effects, just as any particular effect is likely to have multiple genotypic causes.

But this molecular biological truism has thorny implications for the management of clinical testing. Imagine the day in which APOE allele testing has become a standard tool in cardiology alongside cholesterol serum testing. Cardiologists promoting preventive care for heart disease may feel inadequately prepared to discuss genetic and geriatric issues with their young, healthy patients. Can these physicians appropriately perform APOE genotyping on their patients for their own purposes without special reference to the implications for AD risk and the protocols for education, counseling, and consent recommended for AD testing? If so, what should be done with test results that suggest that some patients, should they successfully avoid heart disease, face an increased genetic risk to suffer AD in their later adulthood? Today, the same questions face research cardiologists, who have already performed APOE genotyping on thousands of their patients for research purposes and who, presumably, would like to continue to do more.

There are at least three directions to explore in seeking guidance on these questions, each of which holds some claim to providing precedence: (1) existing recommendations policies regarding predictive risk assessments for AD; (2) the literature in general medical ethics regarding the provision of unsolicited medical advice; and (3) clinical geneticists' traditional practices regarding the disclosure of unanticipated information subsequent to genetic testing. Unfortunately, as the next three sections show, the guidance that these sources provide holds out little hope, short of major societal reform, for any use of APOE testing outside the context of AD testing.

Genetic Testing for AD Risk

Clinicians interested in the potential utility of APOE testing for cardiology can be forgiven for not greeting the association between APOE alleles and AD risk as great news. Presumably, the ethicolegal requirements of informed consent would now require them to disclose to their patients that information on

AD risk would be contained in the results of any APOE genotyping (Wachbroit 1996). Moreover, on the face of it, the clinicians' commitment to candor and the patient's right to know would also seem to require that they divulge the AD risk results when patients ask for that information after testing has been conducted. If the concept of "look-back liability" becomes established in the courts, there may even be a legal cost to pay in not recontacting old patients to disclose this new information (Pelias 1991). And, of course, the clinicians' commitment to competence means that all of those disclosures should be performed according to the professional standards of care established for that task. Unfortunately, if those standards follow the recommendations emerging from the current discussion of APOE genotyping for AD risk, it will almost never be possible for other clinicians to offer APOE testing in the setting of their medical services.

Most current professional practice recommendations on APOE genotyping for AD risk assessment take as their model the protocols developed in medical genetics to govern the clinical introduction of presymptomatic testing for Huntington disease (HD) (Lennox et al. 1994; and Medical and Scientific Advisory Committee 1995). Ironically, the genetics of HD and the dynamics of HD testing are about as close as one can get to the ideal of beanbag medical genetics. With HD, a highly penetrant set of mutations makes genetic testing a powerfully predictive tool: it is so deterministic that even linkage analysis is commonly called "presymptomatic" testing, as if carrying the markers were diagnostic of the disease itself. Using this kind of testing as a paradigm sets the ethical standards for APOE genotyping for AD risk quite a bit higher than they have been to date in cardiological contexts, because the model's focus is on protecting the patient from risks of the testing procedure itself rather than on preventing the harms it predicts. Toward this same goal, the current position statements on AD risk testing all emphasize three points: (1) the relative uncertainty of AD testing, (2) the psychosocial burden of generating information on AD risk, and (3) the consequent necessity for fully educated and voluntary consent on the part of those tested.

Predictive Uncertainty

The major caution sounded by all the recent statements regarding the possible use of APOE genotyping for AD risk assessment concerns the remaining uncertainties about the predictive power of the association. Even the strongest advocates of the genetic association argue that at this point, APOE genotyping is best reserved for use in clarifying a differential diagnosis of AD rather than as a predictive risk assessment tool (Roses 1995). Far from serving as a pathognomonic sign, "it is clear already, that carrying the ϵ4 allele is neither a necessary nor a sufficient condition to acquire AD pathology" (Lovestone 1995, 2). As a result, until the scientific meaning of the association can be better understood, there is a widespread consensus that "the use of APOE genotyping to predict future risk of AD in asymptomatic individuals is not recommended at this time" (Relkin and National Institute on Aging 1996, 347).

Clinicians in other fields may see this negative recommendation as good news. If APOE genotyping is not yet a useful tool in assessing AD risk, then it generates no AD risk information worth disclosing to their patients, and clinicians can continue performing the test according to their own protocols. On this interpretation, only if and when APOE genotyping becomes sanctioned as an AD risk assessment tool would other clinicians need to become concerned about disclosing the implications about AD risk to their patients. Moreover, this interpretation would work, if not for another major point of consensus about APOE genotyping for AD risk.

The Social Risks of Genetic Risk Information

One of the important common themes across the several sets of recent recommendations on APOE genotyping for AD risk is that generating information about genetic risk for AD carries its own burden of possible harms. Beyond the risk of the disease itself, studies of other forms of genetic testing have documented the reality and severity of the social risks of stigmatization and discrimination based on the overinterpretation of genetic risk information by other people and institutions (Billings et al. 1992).

In sum, these studies warn that, because of the causal power they are often (mistakenly) given, genetic risk factors also tend to play a disproportionate role in the social identification of those who carry them, reducing their identities to their carrier status. Genetic information can identify health risks we inherit from and share with our families and explain those risks at what seems to be a very basic biologic level. Together, the familial and constitutional connotations of genetic information make it easy to interpret genetic health risks as a reflection on the recipients' identify and label them accordingly. To the extent that genotypic labels are interpreted as indicative of hidden weaknesses within individuals, this reductionistic understanding of genetic test results simply exacerbates any stigmatization that the target disease (like AD) may already carry. Thus, there is widespread acknowledgment in the discussions of APOE genotyping for AD risk that gathering the information can have negative consequences for patients in any social context in which latent health problems are viewed as a liability, from employment and insurance to personal relations.

Moreover, and more important, this social risk does not depend on either the patient's knowing the information or the actual scientific validity of the information. If parties outside the therapeutic relationship, including patients' families and institutions privy to medical records like the patients' insurers, labor under the belief that APOE genotyping will predict AD risk, their reactions can still harm the patient. This is why it actually makes some prudential sense to model the AD risk-testing protocol against the more deterministic example of HD: our experience with other genetic tests suggests that the most predictable social risks of AD testing will be those that follow from people interpreting the test results in the beanbag manner, as if they were equivalent to an HD test.

In essence, setting the social risk protection standards high even when our scientific confidence is low is simply a way of establishing "universal precautions" against the iatrogenic risks of this medical genetic intervention. Thus, the most recent recommendations regarding APOE genotyping urge that "in deciding whether or not to carry out APOE genotyping for any purpose, physicians and patients should bear in mind that genotype disclosure can have adverse effects on insurability, employability, and the psychosocial status of patients and family members" (Relkin and National Institute on Aging 1996, 1091). Presumably, the scope of "any purpose" should also include the purposes of the cardiologists, and the implication of "patients bear[ing] in mind" is that the metarisks of the AD association are also material risks that their patients should consider before consenting to APOE genotyping.

Education, Counseling, and Fully Informed Consent

The protections that are being recommended in the face of the predictive uncertainties and the metarisks of APOE genotyping for AD risk all take the form of making sure the patients being tested appreciate what they are undertaking before they undergo the test. All the current statements stress the need for testing to be voluntary on the part of patients and for it to be performed within the context of a formal education and counseling protocol. Thus, there appears to be widespread consensus now that:

- The complex nature of AD and the competing risks of death and dementia from other causes affect both the interpretation of the APOE genotype test results and the ensuing counseling. Future clinical applications of genotyping should be offered only when pretest and posttest counseling, education, and support are available.

- Provision for posttest interpretation, counseling, and support services must be made, and this includes referral for psychiatric care, support groups, and pastoral care (Relkin and National Institute on Aging 1996, 1093). Moreover, as this recommendation suggests, the adequacy of the support services in this context is usually closely linked to the involvement of appropriate professional expertise in the process. For example, the Medical and Scientific Advisory Committee of Alzheimer's Disease International is not unusual in insisting that "counseling requires access to a skilled competent professional, usually within a specialized genetics unit, who is knowledgeable about the tests and their meaning" (Medical and Scientific Advisory Committee 1995, 186).

It is interesting to note that the NIA-sponsored Relkin statement even recommends that the pretest consent and counseling process include "disclosure of risks associated with other disorders related to APOE, such as mortality from myocardial infarction" (Relkin and National Institute on Aging 1996, 1093). By the same token, to the extent that the metarisks associated with AD testing are real, then other clinicians would seem to be under a similar obligation to reveal the risks associated with AD testing. But if they are to do so correctly, they should also be following the pretest education and posttest counseling protocols now recommended. Of course, given the lack of appropriate professional expertise, resources, and time, these are also just the requirements that will often be impossible to fulfill outside the context of AD testing.

Providing Unsolicited Medical Advice

At this point, the cardiologists might interrupt to argue that the whole analysis has gotten off on the wrong foot. Perhaps it begs the question to attempt to assess their obligations by reference to recommendations for AD risk assessment, since they are putting the tool of APOE genotyping to an entirely different use. In becoming preoccupied with the (still hypothetical, after all) psychosocial risks of APOE genotyping for AD testing, we risk ignoring, and losing, the very real benefits that the testing can provide for other problems.

The first professional obligations of the cardiologists, they might argue, must lie with using the best tools at their disposal to address the problems with which their patients present them. The fact that their best tool—be it a scalpel, sedative, or DNA test—can be misused in other clinical settings to the detriment of patients does not constitute an argument for them to forgo its appropriate use. If thalidomide proves to be a useful tool in the treatment of HIV disease, we would not expect internists to forgo its use because, in obstetrical contexts, it carries severe iatrogenic risks. Even more to the point, we would not expect a psychiatrist assessing a patient's depression to avoid eliciting a drinking history, simply on the grounds that the information, once in the record, could be misused to stigmatize the patient as an alcoholic.

From that perspective, it may not seem clear whether cardiologists should even raise the specter of the social risks of AD risk testing with their patients. One of the most powerful ways in which physicians respect the autonomy of patients is to let them set the agenda of a therapeutic encounter. Out of respect for their patient's privacy and dignity, physicians do not turn every visit into a comprehensive physical examination: in fact, the invitation to search for unanticipated health problems is itself a very special kind of doctor's appointment. Instead, physicians are expected to attend to the complaints on which the patient has solicited their advice. Of course, their assessment of those complaints may lead to unanticipated diagnoses. But, outside of primary care check-ups, we would not ordinarily expect a physician to initiate a discussion of potential health problems entirely unrelated to the patient's complaint and outside the physician's specialty. Thus, patients would not expect an orthopedic surgeon to comment on a (potentially stigmatizing) dermatological condition in the course of assessing a broken bone and might even feel that their privacy had been invaded if that were done. Medical discretion, after all, involves both seeing and selective not-seeing in almost every medical encounter.

Would disclosing the fact that, in performing APOE genotyping to assess their cardiological problems, the cardiologist will also learn something about their (potentially stigmatizing) AD risk breach the dictates of medical discretion? Fortunately, there is a relatively clear ethic in medicine governing the circumstances in which it becomes required to impose one's knowledge on unsuspecting patients. This ethic is framed in several ways in the literature, but in essence the criteria are similar to those that govern the limits of the physician's "duty to warn" in legal contexts (Pelias 1991). In short, the duty to provide unsolicited medical advice increases proportionately with the following:

1. the seriousness of the health problem that has been uncovered (Moseley 1985; Ratzan 1985; Reilly 1980)
2. the certainty with which the physician can predict or diagnose the health problem, including the physician's competence to make that clinical judgment (Moseley 1985; Ratzan 1985; Reilly 1980)
3. the danger involved in continued neglect of the problem (Moseley 1985)
4. the efficacy of available measures to prevent or treat the problem (Moseley 1985)
5. the extent to which the problem is likely to be unrecognized by the patient before the onset of clinical symptoms (Ratzan 1985).

Unfortunately for the cardiologists, attempting to apply these standards to the problem of disclosing unsolicited information about AD risk simply returns us to the problem of the social risk that has been created by the public association of APOE genotypes with AD risk. In terms of what APOE genotyping can actually reveal about the risks of AD, one might make a case for nondisclosure: the risks of AD are not certain enough to warrant a warning by professionals untrained to do so. However, it does not take specialty training to be able to recognize and assess the social risks involved in APOE genotyping: one merely has to know the ways in which information about health risks can work against the interests of patients in our current health care coverage system. Moreover, these are risks that could easily lie unrecognized by patients until the onset of their problems, and risks that can be avoided (if only by forgoing the testing). To the extent that the extrapolations of social risk from other forms of genetic testing are well founded, and to the extent that the cardiologist's patients are living within our current U.S. health care system, these criteria would suggest that the social risks of APOE testing, even though they flow from other clinical uses of the testing, do warrant unsolicited disclosure and, therefore, forewarning.

Disclosing Unanticipated Findings in Reproductive Medicine

Even when health professionals accept responsibility for communicating unanticipated findings, they sometimes wrestle with the best ways to accomplish such disclosure. Here, cardiologists might look to gynecology for guidance. For example, in the context of medical evaluations of amenorrhea, gynecologists have long had to be prepared for the fact that their patient's problem may be due to a genetic condition called "testicular feminization," or "XY female syndrome." In these cases, a genetic error early in development leads chromosomally male fetuses to develop the secondary sexual characteristics of a female. Externally, these individuals grow up as normal women, but they lack ovaries and a uterus. Moreover, they have the remains of testes in their body cavities, which should be removed to prevent the moderate risk of cancer that they pose. A simple karyotype of the patient's chromosomes can confirm this diagnosis (President's Commission 1983).

In cases like these, the impulse to invoke the "therapeutic privilege" is strong: the physician seems caught between the obligation to inform the patient's decision making and the obligation to prevent psychosocial harm to the patient. Some have argued that in this circumstance, the bare fact that the young woman carries a Y instead of an X chromosome is irrelevant both to the clinical problem about which she is seeking help (her amenorrhea) and the most important clinical implications of her condition: her sterility and cancer risks. Although the gynecologist learns something from the karyotyping that carries high psychosocial risks for the patient, it is not something relevant to the patient's care, and it can, therefore, be properly ignored. One authoritative group has made the following recommendation: How the information is presented depends, of course, on the patient's level of education and her knowledge of human biology, but basically the person needs to be told that she did not develop a uterus and ovaries (and hence cannot bear children) and has nonfunctional reproductive tissue that must be surgically removed in order to avoid a risk of cancer (President's Commission 1983, 63).

Cardiologists might argue similarly that, while they can anticipate learning a patient's AD risk through APOE genotyping, they can best protect the patient's interests by avoiding the disclosure of that information. If the patients are unaware of their AD risk status, they cannot be traumatized by the information or penalized by others for knowing it. At most, the cardiologist should warn their patients that APOE test results might be used in insurance underwriting, since its use in CAD risk assessment alone makes that true. But extensive counseling about AD in that context, cardiologists might argue, would be just as inappropriate as the crude explanation by a gynecologist that a patient's amenorrhea is due to the fact that she is really a man.

Unfortunately, invoking the principle of nonmaleficence to justify nondisclosure in these contexts is an incomplete and ultimately unsatisfactory response. In the gynecological context, for example, the President's Commission approach is silent about why the patient did not develop female reproductive organs or what exactly that "nonfunctional reproductive tissue" was. This creates the risk that the patient will discover or be told the complete story eventually, without having been prepared to interpret it correctly or to cope with its psychosocial impact. By avoiding the issue in seeking to protect the patient from unnecessary harm, the physician actually does the patient a disservice.

For the same reasons, applying this approach to APOE genotyping in cardiology is also ultimately self-defeating. To the extent that the public's interest in AD encourages publicity about the genetic association between the APOE ε4 allele and AD, the likelihood that the patients themselves or their relatives will make the relevant connections increases. If they have not been prepared to interpret that association correctly, they are likely to assume the psychosocial burden of an overly deterministic reading and end up worse off than they would have been after disclosure and counseling in the clinical setting.

Again, in the case of testicular feminization, the more comprehensive approach is to disclose all the information yielded by the karyotype test of the patient's chromosomes but to frame the explanation in a way that minimizes its psychosocial impact and equips the patient to respond to the reactions of others. That is, after starting with the partial explanation recommended by the President's Commission, as stated above, one could explain that the patient has no uterus because she never had the genes to code for one, due to a genetic defect in one of her sex chromosomes. This frames her female development as correct and the inheritance of her Y chromosome as the mistake rather than the other way around. (Taken literally, it also suggests that the Y chromosome is pathological; something that, for her, is undoubtedly true.)

This comprehensive strategy would allow the cardiologists to better prepare their patients for what they may eventually learn anyway. Unfortunately, again, it does not provide a shortcut around the patient education, testing, and counseling protocols recommended for using APOE genotyping to assess AD risk. In this case, those protocols are, presumably, the best comprehensive guides to preparing patients to understand and cope with their risk status in a helpful way.

Conclusion: The Problem of "Spoiler Associations"

In sum, it seems that the genetic association of the APOE genotypes with AD risk, however uncertain, should be a scientific claim with large practical repercussions within some parts of medicine. To the extent that patients perceived by others to be at risk of AD are thereby at risk for stigmatization and discrimination, those social risks of APOE genotyping must be disclosed to all candidates for the test, regardless of why the test is indicated. Where such disclosures cannot be conducted against the standards of care being recommended by the most expert community—the AD medical community—the testing should probably be forgone until such time as the social risks of testing are reduced by public education and public policy reform.

The ironic, and frustrating, final point is that the social risks of using APOE genotyping for AD risk assessment will end up having a far greater impact on practice in other medical specialties than in AD risk assessment itself. For the moment, at any rate, relatively little APOE genotyping seems justified in the context of AD risk assessment: at best, it will be relevant in the differential diagnosis of affected patients, for whom the social risks of predictive testing are superseded by the social risks of diagnosis. Since predictive testing for AD risk is not recommended, the only contexts in which the disclosure of its social risks will become necessary, and the only patients to whom the AD medical community's recommendations regarding pretest and posttest education and counseling will apply for the foreseeable future, will be those of the cardiologists and their colleagues.

The challenge posed by APOE genotyping is probably not going to be unique in genetic testing. It suggests an ominous lesson for professional policy: that wherever a "spoiler association" comes along that conveys high levels of psychosocial risks to the results of a genetic test, the protocols involved in the use of any genetic test will escalate to the level required by the most volatile use, and the test's versatility will be compromised accordingly. On the other hand, spoiler associations do offer one benefit: they bring the social policy problems that underlie the social risks of the most volatile use in to the ken of a wider group of clinicians in a forceful way. As beanbag medical genetics give way to medical genomics, it will be increasingly and painfully obvious that the institutions and systems that put a social price on learning about our genetic risk factors are everyone's concern.

References

Assman, G., Schmitz, G., Menzel, H.-J., and Schulte, H. 1984. Apolipoprotein E polymorphism and hyperlipidemia. *Clinical Chemistry* 30:310–13.
Baird, P. 1990. Genetics and health care: A paradigm shift. *Perspectives in Biology and Medicine* 33:203–13.
Billings, P., Kohn, M., De Cuevas, M., Beckwith J., Alper, J. S., and Natowicz, M. R. 1992. Discrimination as a consequence of genetic screening. *American Journal of Human Genetics* 50:476–82.
Breitner, J. C. 1994. Genetic factors. In *Dementia,* ed. A. Burns and R. Levy, 281–92. London: Chapman and Hall.
Cumming, A. M., and Robertson, F. 1984. Polymorphism at the apoE locus in relation to risk of coronary disease. *Clinical Genetics* 25:310–13.
Davignon, J., Gregg, R. E., and Sing, C. F. 1988. Apolipoprotein E polymorphism and atherosclerosis. *Arteriosclerosis* 8:1–21.
Holtzman, N. 1989. *Proceed with caution: Predicting genetic risks in the recombinant DNA era.* Baltimore: Johns Hopkins University Press.
Kosunen, O., Talasniemi, S., Lehtovirta, M., Heinonen, O., Helisalmi, S., Mannermaa, A., Paljarvi, L., Ryynanen, M., Riekkinenen, P., and Soininen, H. 1995. Relation of coronary atherosclerosis and apolipoprotein E genotypes in Alzheimer patients. *Stroke* 26:743–48.
Lennox, A., Karlinsky, H., Meschino, W., Buchanan, J., Percy, M. E., and Berg, J. M. 1994. Molecular genetic predictive testing for Alzheimer's disease: Deliberations and preliminary recommendations. *Alzheimer Disease and Associated Disorders* 8:126–47.
Lovestone, S. 1995. The genetics of Alzheimer's disease: New opportunities and new challenges. *International Journal of Geriatric Psychiatry* 10:1–7.
Mayr, E. 1963. *Animal species and evolution.* Cambridge: Harvard University Press.

Medical and Scientific Advisory Committee, Alzheimer's Disease International. 1995. Consensus statement on predictive testing for Alzheimer disease. *Alzheimer Disease and Associated Disorders* 9:182-87.

Menzel, H.-J., Kladetzky, R.-G., and Assman, G. 1983. Apolipoprotein E polymorphism and coronary artery diseases. *Arteriosclerosis* 3:310-15.

Moseley, R. 1985. Excuse me, but you have a melanoma on your neck! Unsolicited medical opinions. *Journal of Medicine and Philosophy* 10:163-70.

Pelias, M. 1991. The duty to disclose in medical genetics: A legal perspective. *American Journal of Medical Genetics* 39:347-54.

President's Commission for the Study of Ethical Problems in Medicine and Biomedical and Behavioral Research. 1983. *Screening and counseling for genetic conditions.* Washington, D.C.: Government Printing Office.

Ratzan, R. 1985. Unsolicited medical opinion. *Journal of Medicine and Philosophy* 10:147-62.

Reilly, P. 1980. When should an investigator share raw data with the subjects? *IRB: A Journal of Human Subjects Research* 24:5, 12.

Relkin, N. R., and National Institute on Aging/Alzheimer's Association Working Group. 1996. Apolipoprotein E genotyping in Alzheimer's disease. *Lancet* 347:1091-95.

Roses, A. 1995. Apolipoprotein E genotyping in the differential diagnosis, not prediction, of Alzheimer's disease. *Annals of Neurology* 38:6-14.

Utermann, G., Hardewig, A., and Zimmer, F. 1984. Apolipoprotein E phenotypes in patients with myocardial infarctions. *Human Genetics* 65:237-41.

Wachbroit, R. 1996. Disowning knowledge: Issues in genetic testing. *Philosophy and Public Policy Report* 16:14-19.

12

Justice, Rights, and Alzheimer Disease Genetics

LEONARD FLECK, PH.D.

The fundamental problem of health care justice in our society may be framed this way: What does it mean to be a just and caring society when we have only limited resources to meet virtually unlimited health care needs? A more specific formulation of this question relative to our topic would be this: Is a just and caring society morally obligated to include funded access to genetic testing for Alzheimer disease (AD) in the Medicare program? in the Medicaid program? in the core benefit package of some future form of national health insurance, perhaps something like the Clinton proposal for managed competition? Or is it the case that access to such testing is fairly and justifiably left to individual ability to pay? That is, would it be morally correct to say that the poor, the working poor, the uninsured, the poor elderly, and so on would not be treated unjustly if, as a practical economic matter, they were denied access to such testing?

Let us sharpen up just a bit more the precise question we intend to address. At least three known genetic mutations associated with chromosomes 1, 14, and 21 are autosomally dominant and result in an early-onset version of AD (onset in the early forties to mid-fifties). Predictive testing is currently available for these mutations in research settings. In addition, there is testing available for APOE on chromosome 19, one allele of which is associated with an increased susceptibility for AD with varying ages of onset (see chaps. 2–4, above). For genetic testing for AD of any of the varieties alluded to above, genetic counseling is strongly recommended. The minimum cost of such testing is about $300. Is an individual treated unjustly if he or she wants one of these tests but is denied it because he or she is unable to afford the cost of the test? My primary goal in this chapter is to provide a rationally defensible answer to this moral problem. To accomplish that goal, however, I need to address the much larger question of what, if any, genetic tests a just and caring society is morally obligated to provide to all its citizens, given all the other health care needs that exist in our society, including currently unmet health care needs as well as rapidly emerging, foreseeable health care needs.

This last is a much larger and more complicated question than may be evident at first. If the number of genetic tests available were relatively small in number, and if the demand for the tests were very modest, then this would not be so challenging a moral problem. However, we are beginning to see the rapid proliferation of a broad range of genetic tests. As the task of mapping and sequencing the entire human genome is brought to a conclusion by the year 2003, it is likely that anywhere from several hundred to more than a thousand genetic tests will be available. Some of these tests can be used predictively to establish that an individual will be afflicted with a particular genetically based disorder over the course of his or her life; other tests establish susceptibility over the course of a lifetime; others can be used diagnostically to confirm or reject a suspected diagnosis. Some of these tests might be used premaritally for purposes of determining whether specific individuals contemplating marriage to each other might be at elevated risk of having a child who would be afflicted with a specific serious genetic disorder that would adversely affect the length or quality of life. These tests could also be used to test eight-cell embryos before implantation (when, for example, a couple knew they were at elevated risk of having a child with a serious genetic disorder) or else to test fetuses in the late stages of the first trimester for purposes of determining whether or not that pregnancy would be completed.

In addition to these varying contexts in which genetic testing is an option, we need to remember that there is an enormous range of genetically related medical and behavioral disorders that we might test for. For example, we could test for Tay-Sachs or hemophilia or cystic fibrosis or Huntington disease (HD) or manic depression or various obsessive-compulsive disorders or breast cancer (BRCA1/BRCA2) or colon cancer or multiple sclerosis or muscular dystrophy or juvenile diabetes or familial Alzheimer disease (FAD) or AD associated with various alleles of APOE on chromosome 19. This is a very short list, hardly representative of the genetic tests we can do today, much less what will be possible in the near future. The question we need to come back to is this: Are all of these tests in the various testing contexts mentioned above on the same moral plane as far as fair access to needed health care is concerned? Or do some of these tests in some of these contexts make stronger moral claims than others to limited societal resources for health care? If so, where on this priority scale would various tests in various contexts for AD fit?

Would they be high-priority genetic tests or low-priority genetic tests? And are there in fact objective morally relevant criteria for assigning priorities for various genetic tests?

Let me give several concrete examples to illustrate the questions above.

1. If we have two thirty-year-old individuals, one of whom has three close relatives who died of breast cancer and the other of whom has two grandparents who were diagnosed with Alzheimer disease in their early eighties, would they have equally strong moral claims to genetic testing for themselves? That is, would a just and caring society be equally obligated to assure funded access to such tests for both individuals?

2. If we have two thirty-year-old pregnant women, one of whom is concerned about having a child with cystic fibrosis because of family history and the other of whom is concerned about having a child at future risk for AD because two grandparents were diagnosed with the disease in their early eighties, would they have equally strong moral claims to prenatal genetic testing at twelve weeks?

3. If three couples wished to have children of their own but they knew they were respectively at risk for having a child with cystic fibrosis, a child that would inherit the breast cancer gene (BRCA1), and a child that would inherit a double dose of the ε4 allele of APOE (and thus a significantly heightened susceptibility to AD), and if all three couples wished to employ in vitro fertilization and embryonic genetic analysis so that they could choose embryos for implantation that were free of the feared genetic disorders, then would all three have equally strong moral claims to embryonic genetic analysis (at a cost of about $30,000 per successful pregnancy)? That is, could any of these couples persuasively claim that they were treated unjustly if there were public funding at some level for one of these genetic analyses but not for another?

The larger contextual question is, again: Among all the health care needs that exist in our society, how high a priority ought to be assigned to these various genetic tests in various contexts?

Framing the Problem of Health Care Justice

In the first part of this chapter I want to lay out a number of working assumptions that constitute a framework for thinking through as a problem of health care justice the issue of access to genetic testing for AD. I believe these assumptions are well supported in the relevant literature I cite, but many of them are controversial matters for philosopher-medical ethicists as well as for thoughtful members of our society at large.

1. *There are presumptively problems of justice in health care.* Health care is not correctly thought of as being simply another consumer good in our society that is properly distributed on the basis of ability to pay. That is, there is some package of health care services that a just society is morally obligated to guarantee to all its citizens, whether or not they individually have the ability to pay for those services. Libertarians, such as H. Tristram Engelhardt (1996, 375–410), will deny this assumption. However, the two considerations that speak most in favor of this assumption are that huge public investments in medical education and research (such as the Human Genome Project) have generated the medical miracles from which any of us might benefit and that access to needed health care is as closely linked to protecting fair equality of opportunity in our society as is education, which we guarantee a large measure of to all our citizens (Daniels 1985, 19–85; Fleck 1989a).

2. *There is no generic, unlimited right to health care.* Individuals do have moral rights to specific health care services, but these rights will be derived from a specific conception of health care justice (Churchill 1987; Daniels 1985, 1–17; Fleck 1989b). If we did believe there was an unlimited right to health care, virtually the entire economy could be hijacked to meet health care needs at the expense of all other social needs. An outcome like that appears to be neither rational nor morally defensible.

3. *Health care needs, as opposed to health care desires, make presumptively just claims to health care resources. But because health care needs are virtually unlimited and health resources limited, only some health care needs will generate actual obligations of justice.* As Daniel Callahan writes, "Medical need is not a fixed concept but a function of technological possibility and regnant social expectations" (1987, 134). Any survey of contemporary medicine over the last ten years will yield a long list of advances in virtually every field of medicine, whether it is heart disease or cancer or stroke or AIDS or rehabilitation medicine or diagnostics or genetics or home health care, and virtually all these advances have represented net additions to the total cost of health care. To give one illustration of the "endless needs" problem, about twenty-five hundred heart transplants were performed in the United States in 1995, at a cost of about $150,000 per transplant. We did only that limited number because we had only that many transplantable hearts. However, it is estimated that up to 350,000 individuals could have benefited, with up to five extra years of life expectancy, on average, if they had had access to one of these heart transplants. (This is out of 730,000 individuals who died of heart disease in 1995 in the United States.) It is unfortunate, but not unjust, that those 347,500 individuals died who could have lived if they had had access to a heart transplant.

It is expected that by the year 2000 we will have a working model of a totally implantable artificial heart (TIAH). There will be no natural limit to the number of these devices that we can produce, though obviously economic issues will have to be faced. The cost of transplantation for these devices will be roughly the same as that of natural heart transplants, which would mean there is a potential for $52 billion per year in additional health costs that would be attached to this one device alone. About 70 percent of these individuals would be over age sixty-five (i.e., eligible for Medicare), which would mean a potential annual addition to Medicare costs of $35 billion (in constant 1995 dollars). This one device alone potentially would generate a much-expanded pool of health care needs—expensive needs. Intuitively, it seems clear we are talking about needs. This device could mean the difference between life and death for some 347,500 individuals. Furthermore, if all, or some fraction, of these 347,500 individuals were to die because, say, the federal government chose not to make this a Medicare-covered benefit, then it would take some compelling moral argument to generate the conclusion that such deaths were merely unfortunate rather than morally criticizable.

One further observation must be made regarding the "endless needs" problem. It has to do with what Callahan (1990, 45–47) refers to as the "ragged edge" (63–65) that is often associated with emerging medical technologies. There is no bright line that separates morally compelling from morally optional uses of (or needs for) the technology. If it is clear that an individual will die in two years from a terminal cancer but will die in two months from heart failure without a heart transplant, then can a just and caring society deny that individual an artificial heart because we know he or she has no chance of surviving five years? In practice, for instance, with respect to access to kidney dialysis, we have proved neither able nor willing to make such limiting choices, the result being an even more rapidly expanding domain of health needs and health costs. This leads to the fourth working assumption.

4. *The need for health care rationing is inescapable.* We must distinguish between health care needs that a just and caring society is morally obligated to meet and those that are beyond justice, either in the domain of social beneficence or in the domain of markets and ability to pay. We need to have a morally defensible approach to prioritizing health care needs. The "inescapability" of rationing means that no feasible efforts to weed out inefficiencies, fraud, excess profits, or abuse in the health care system will generate sufficient resources to meet all health care needs. David Eddy (1994) probably offers the most concise defense of this claim: rationing means that identified individuals will be denied access to health care that will prove to be only marginally beneficial to them

and not cost-worthy from some social point of view. Some (Brody 1988) see health care rationing as being morally abominable because identified individuals are denied access to health care that they themselves see as being needed in a strong sense, such as the individual who will die in two weeks without an artificial heart transplant but who will die no matter what in two years as a result of his terminal cancer. But I have argued (Fleck 1994a) that just approaches to health care rationing are possible, that the serious moral wrongs associated with rationing have nothing to do with identified individuals (Fleck 1994b) but have, rather, to do with approaches to rationing that are arbitrary, capricious, discriminatory, and hidden from public scrutiny.

Oregon has provided us with some important lessons in this regard in its health care priority-setting process. The most important of these include the following: (1) piecemeal, uncoordinated rationing decisions are likely to be unjust; (2) rationing decisions made publicly are open to critical assessment and correction; (3) those directly affected by rationing decisions should have a fair opportunity to participate in the making of those decisions (i.e., establishing priorities, making reasonable trade-offs); (4) firm budgets are needed to give structure and coherence to a priority-setting process, so that what is being given up is clear to all; (5) stable, rationally and justly determined health priorities, explicitly agreed to by all, will be immune to special pleading, which always represents a threat to just agreements; and (6) those who are least well off in terms of health should have presumptively stronger just claims to health resources as long as they can benefit sufficiently from access to those resources (Fleck 1994a, 374–77).

5. *No single conception of health care justice can yield a morally defensible set of rationing protocols and health care priorities.* Instead, we need a more complex, pluralistic conception of health care justice to achieve that goal. The extreme heterogeneity of health needs, the large range of effectiveness, cost, and uncertainty associated with interventions in various clinical circumstances, the complexity of individual clinical circumstances (especially young individuals with numerous costly medical problems only partially and marginally responsive to medical interventions), the social burden of the aggregated costs of common medical needs, the strong social desire for medical innovation and the concomitant costs and uncertainties associated with clinical experimentation, and the large range of costs associated with various degrees of individual irresponsibility for health maintenance — all of these features of our health care system conspire against the likelihood that any single theory of health care justice can yield an approach to health care rationing and priority setting that will be fair enough.

Thus, if we are tempted by a utilitarian approach to health care justice because we wish to maximize needs met at the lowest possible cost (certainly a reasonable goal), then there is great moral risk that the elderly, disabled, or seriously chronically ill persons (all those who are least well off in terms of health) will suffer needlessly and die prematurely as a result of unmet health needs. On the other hand, if we are committed to a strong egalitarian conception of health care justice, then there is a moral risk that those with the greatest health needs that are only marginally responsive to costly interventions will squander limited resources that ought to be used to meet a much broader range of health needs. Or, alternatively, if we are committed to a strong libertarian conception of health care justice, then it is likely that poor or uninsured persons will suffer needlessly and die prematurely for lack of access to costly needed health care.

The conclusion I draw from this is that an adequate conception of health care justice for purposes of rationing and priority setting will have to be pluralistic and contractarian. That is, the conceptions of health care justice alluded to above (along with Norman Daniels' fair-equality-of-opportunity account [1985]) should be thought of as single strands in a more comprehensive conception of health care justice whose task would be to determine the contextual relevance and moral "pull" of a particular strand relative to other strands and to the particular problem of health care justice that needed to be addressed. Such a conception would be pluralistic because no one strand would be morally hegemonic over the other strands in all the problem areas of health care justice. This conception would be contractarian in the Rawlsian sense, in that the detailed weighings and balancings among the various strands would be a product of free rational agreements, fair terms of cooperation mutually agreed to by all who could be affected by the rationing protocols and health care priorities that would emerge from this conception of health care justice (Rawls 1993, 3–47).

6. *No philosophically articulated conception of health care justice can be finely enough elaborated to yield uniquely morally correct judgments of health care justice for all the real-world problems of health care rationing and priority setting that will need to be resolved.* Thus, when the resources of a conception of health care justice have been exhausted in a particular problem setting, we ought to turn to rational democratic deliberation as the fairest approach to resolving the rest of the problem. The world of health care is empirically too complex and too subject to rapid changes induced by technological, political, economic, organizational, and cultural factors that are constantly reshaping and recreating problems of health care justice and health care rationing. No conception of health care justice will have the conceptual and methodological resources

needed to yield uniquely and optimally just resolutions to the complexly detailed rationing and priority-setting problems that will be precipitated by such a milieu.

Instead, it will often be the case that some number of alternative rationing protocols and health care priority settings might be chosen that could all be described as being "fair enough" or "just enough." It would not be morally desirable to allow power relations, or some other nonrational mechanism, to be the basis of such a decision if we can identify a morally preferable, rational alternative. If our overarching moral objective is to preserve fair terms of cooperation mutually agreed to for our overall scheme of health care rationing and priority setting, then rational democratic deliberation (as I have described elsewhere [Fleck 1994a]) is such a morally preferable alternative. Its greatest moral virtue is that it is a public process that, when done well, yields autonomously imposed (and, therefore, presumptively morally legitimate) rationing protocols.

To give one quick illustration of what rational democratic deliberation means in practice, imagine that all of us (you, my readers) belong to the same managed care plan. It has 100,000 members. We all want high-quality care, but we want a care package overall that is both fair (meets high-priority health needs) and affordable. We know that there are two types of contrast agents used for CAT scans: high-osmolality contrast agents (HOCAs) and low-osmolality contrast agents (LOCAs). High-osmolality contrast agents cost $10 each, while LOCAs cost $120 each. The virtue of LOCAs is that they reduce by a factor of ten the risk of anaphylactic shock when that agent is introduced into the system of someone who is highly sensitive to the dye. Anaphylactic shock is dangerous and scary, but there are always trained emergency personnel around to respond to and reverse the shock.

But there is a risk of failure with HOCAs. That is, there might be one chance in 100,000 that the shock is not reversed in a timely way and that person dies. This is where our suggested rationing protocol comes in. We could, if we wished in our managed care plan, avert that death by giving everyone LOCAs. But the cost of averting that death would be $11 million per 100,000 CAT scans. Is a just and caring managed care plan morally obligated to spend those resources in that way? I cannot conceive a morally compelling argument that would yield an affirmative answer to that question. Hence, we can collectively judge through rational democratic deliberation whether we would adopt for our future selves a rationing protocol that would restrict all of us to HOCAs. Given the cost, it is easy to imagine that we would collectively agree that other higher-priority health needs were more deserving of those resources. But if we were a highly risk-averse group, we might decide to give up some other set of health benefits. Many decision analysts might regard such a choice as marginally rational at best, but it would still be a morally and democratically legitimate social choice.

Just Prioritization of Genetic Services: Some Key Principles

With the above moral framework in mind, we can now turn to the question of how high a priority various genetic tests and genetic interventions in a variety of clinical contexts ought to have relative to all the other health needs that are out there competing for limited health resources. Again, for the purposes of this chapter I would remind the reader that the most we can hope to accomplish is to lay out a rough framework and principles that will define a direction for further analysis. In this area, morally defensible conclusions will be highly sensitive to shifting and emerging empirical details related to genetics.

I begin with a moral claim that may not resonate well with most Americans, but that I have argued elsewhere (Fleck 1994c) is morally defensible. It will rarely be unjust to fail to develop some life-saving or life-prolonging medical technology. We have come to expect a constant stream of medical innovations, but, from a moral point of view, these are matters of social beneficence, not social justice. That is, no one could justifiably claim that he or she was treated unjustly, or that any basic moral rights were violated, if as a society we decided we would not complete, for instance, the development of the artificial heart. If we consider this scenario from the perspective of our various strands of health care justice, it seems that none would be likely to condemn such a social decision. The life-years that would be saved through the artificial heart would be very expensive life-years and late-in-life years for the most part. Utilitarians could easily believe that other less expensive life-years ought to be saved first; and egalitarians would easily imagine less expensive health needs of less fortunate individuals in our society that would make stronger just claims to those resources. And, from the point of view of fair equality of opportunity, many younger life-years would make a stronger just claim to those resources.

Second, at least some possible and emerging genetic tests and interventions that represent high-priority health care needs would make strong just claims on limited health care resources. I believe our investment in the Human Genome Project represents social beneficence, as does our investment in the artificial heart. However, issues of social justice are still there and need to be addressed. For the future, it will most likely be the case that we will have to scale back our investments in medical innovations. The choices we make there will not be "beyond justice." That is, considerations of health care justice ought to shape our social investment decisions regarding medical innovation (outside of private capital investment).

Imagine, for example, that we have the capacity to perfect germ-line genetic engineering. What I have in mind is the capacity to identify serious genetic deficiencies in eight-celled embryos that would have been conceived in vitro, then deleting those defective genes and replacing them with good copies of the gene that would normally be there. My question is this: If we have limited resources for investing in medical innovation, then should investment in perfecting the artificial heart be a higher or lower priority than perfecting germ-line genetic engineering? That is, which choice should a just and caring society make? My intuitive judgment is that the germ-line engineering would make the stronger moral claim.

For the sake of concreteness I will impute a cost of $100,000 per engineered embryo resulting in a live birth. It is hard to imagine that all births in the United States could be engineered in this way (given aggregate costs), so we will imagine instead that the technology would be aimed at preventing the birth of children with serious genetic defects that would seriously adversely affect the quality and length of their lives. Future children at risk for cystic fibrosis or juvenile diabetes or fragile X syndrome would be the sort of cases I have in mind. A broad-based program of premarital or postmarital genetic screening would likely tell us where our engineering efforts ought to be applied. This sort of engineering certainly seems more morally compelling than developing and disseminating artificial hearts from the point of view of a fair-equality-of-opportunity account of health care justice. The artificial heart, after all, would mostly go to older individuals who had had the opportunity to live a long and full life. The germ-line engineering would be aimed at dramatically improving life prospects for these embryonic future children from the very beginning. As nearly as I can tell, both utilitarian and egalitarian conceptions of health care justice would endorse this priority, at least as long as it was the case that there was no invidious discrimination along racial or economic lines among embryos. Likewise, I cannot conceive a libertarian objection to this ordering.

It may be the case that some readers find this example too futuristic. It is easy enough to conjure up a current example, namely, preimplantation genetic diagnosis. Less dramatic results can be accomplished here, but they are still of substantial moral significance. Here we are restricted to genetically analyzing some number of embryos for a single genetic defect, then implanting those who are free of that defect. The costs are not small, about $30,000 per achieved birth. Still, when we compare outcomes from the point of view of health care justice for the beneficiaries of the artificial heart and preimplantation genetic diagnosis, it seems the same considerations outlined above would speak in favor of awarding higher priority to the preimplantation genetic diagnosis, *at least as long as genetic deficiencies we sought to eliminate adversely affected the length and quality of life of these future children.* I emphasize this last point because, as I argue later, this moral argument would not succeed if we wanted to screen embryos for the ε4 allele of APOE, which would mean that these embryos were significantly more susceptible to being afflicted with AD in their later years.

Third, for many real or potential genetic interventions (i.e., various types of genetic testing or future gene therapy), analogues in contemporary medicine can give us a good fix on the moral priority that such interventions ought to have with regard to making just claims on limited health care resources. Norman Daniels articulated a critical principle of health care justice in his fair-equality-of-opportunity account (1985), especially with regard to making many kinds of health care rationing decisions. In essence, his argument is that in many contexts access to needed health care is as strongly connected to protecting equal opportunity as is education in our society. What we are morally obligated to do as a just society is to assure all who have the capacity access to a normal range of opportunities in our society. This permits a just differential range of responses to a variety of health needs in different health contexts. Thus, from this point of view we have no obligations of justice to sustain the lives of individuals in a persistent vegetative state, no matter what their age, nor do we have any obligations of justice to sustain the lives of anencephalic infants. In both cases there is literally no opportunity range that these individuals are capable of accessing.

Using Daniels' account, we can also argue that if we have a very healthy eighty-year-old individual with a failing heart whose only hope for survival is a heart transplant, it would be neither unjust nor uncaring for a society to deny that individual a heart transplant because, in part, he would already have had a full opportunity to access a normal range of opportunities in that society. In addition, giving that individual a heart transplant would necessarily mean denying it to a younger individual who would have had less opportunity to access that normal opportunity range.

Some children are born with a medical condition known as necrotic small bowel syndrome. The only thing that can save their lives is total parenteral nutrition (TPN). Total parenteral nutrition is very expensive, costing more than $300,000 per year. In addition, TPN has the unfortunate side effect of destroying the livers of these children, which means they will usually die by the age of four unless they get a liver transplant, which may extend their lives an extra two years. At best, they will be able to access only a small part of a normal opportunity range, given their medical circumstances. I want to suggest that a just and caring society could give very low priority to sustaining the lives of these children, given the high costs and marginal benefits to them, especially if there are substantial unmet health needs for other children which, if met, would result in their being able to access more of, and more securely, the normal opportunity range of our society.

I turn now to the issue of what kind of priority a just and caring society ought to assign to various types of gene therapy relative to other therapies intended to address other health needs. All current efforts at gene therapy are highly experimental. But there is considerable therapeutic promise. In many cases the hope may be that very precisely targeted genetic therapies will have longer-lasting or permanent therapeutic effects without the problematic side effects of current, relatively crude pharmacologic therapies we rely upon now.

One such early therapy was aimed at severe combined immune deficiency (SCID), or what is colloquially referred to as the "bubble boy" syndrome because these children are without a functioning immune system and, hence, must be completely isolated from the normal environment. Positive effects have been very modest and costs very high. From the point of view of health care justice, we can say that this case is comparable to that of children afflicted with necrotic small bowel syndrome. This implies that so long as there is reasonable scientific justification for believing these experimental efforts may bear substantial fruit for these unfortunate children, we ought (justly) to fund modest experimental efforts. These are children who have no other options. But, if we hit a costly scientific dead end, meaning that we were able to keep these children alive for perhaps four years for a million dollars, after which they were doomed to die shortly, then sustaining the lives of these children would be justly relegated to a low priority as far as health care justice was concerned.

There are also some significant efforts in gene therapy aimed at cystic fibrosis, mostly in older children and young adults. Again, success has been modest. It seems that repeated therapeutic efforts are needed to introduce properly functioning genes into the lungs of affected individuals. If this were to become a more or less permanent plateau for this sort of therapeutic intervention, then it would be morally akin to kidney dialysis. If costs were in the vicinity of $25,000 per year, that would be an additional reason for assigning it roughly the same sort of priority regarding just claims to limited resources as dialysis. There is some legitimate cause for moral concern because this would be another halfway technology, the sort of technology that transforms fatal problems into very expensive chronic problems that have the potential to skew unjustly societal health priorities. But, again, to get our moral bearings, from the point of view of protecting fair equality of opportunity, gene therapy for cystic fibrosis would deserve higher priority than funding for artificial hearts, or at least those artificial hearts that would go to a substantially older population.

A number of efforts involving gene therapy are aimed at fetuses. The likelihood of success here may prove much greater than gene-therapeutic efforts aimed at children or adults. There might be large gains in cost effectiveness, especially if there were minimal or no need for postnatal booster therapeutic efforts. Still, it would be reasonable to assume that these efforts would be costly at the level of individual treated fetuses, perhaps $30,000 each, to force the realization that not all genetic disorders should be thought of as having equal priority for fetal genetic therapy. A reasonable general rule for establishing just health priorities for fetal therapy might be this: First priority ought to be given to fetal gene therapies aimed at disorders that to a high degree adversely affect length of life or quality of life for children. Only after resources permitted the effective treatment of those disorders would resources be allocated for treating in utero genetic disorders that would otherwise manifest themselves in young adulthood or in midlife. Examples in this latter category would be breast cancer (BRCA1 or BRCA2), HD, or FAD. What should quite likely be a low-priority option for fetal genetic therapy would be late-in-life genetic disorders, especially those that involve susceptibilities to disease, such as AD associated with ε4 alleles of APOE. Before concluding this section, I need to make a few observations regarding the problem of background justice with regard to emerging genetic technologies. These genetic technologies ought to radically reorder our societal health care priorities, if we would hope to be a just and caring society. In the past we have taken our genetic endowment as a fixed given as far as judging what sort of opportunity range an individual could lay just claim to with the help of therapeutic resources. That is, many individuals were doomed to live short lives of greatly diminished quality because of their genetic endowment. This was merely unfortunate, not unjust. Genetic advances directly challenge that assumption and will often require us to see problems of health care justice in that genetic endowment. This suggests the possibility that there ought to be a large reordering of health priorities in the direction of assuring that all future children, regardless of the economic class of their parents, ought to be assured as healthy an initial genetic endowment as technological capacity and societal resources would permit.

At present the therapeutic potential of gene therapy is just that—potential, and highly speculative. However, embryonic genetic analysis combined with selective implantation seems to be quite effective for addressing some range of genetic disorders. While it is presently regarded as experimental therapy, it is easy to imagine that it might become soon enough an acceptable therapeutic option. The likely moral problem that would emerge is that the middle class would agitate for insurance coverage for the procedure. This would add to total insurance premiums. As things are now, the federal and state governments exclude insurance premiums paid by employers from taxable income. This tax expenditure amounted to more than $80 billion in 1995. Potential tax revenues, then, are diminished as employers pay for increasing health insurance premiums for the middle class. But the middle class today also resists more strongly cost shifting in health care that was previously used to subsidize costs for health care for uninsured persons. They also resist increased taxes aimed at paying for the health needs of poor people under the Medicaid program. Morally speaking, the net result of these technological advances in health care is that the middle class and their children benefit while those who are less well off in terms of health (and in terms of opportunity) become even less well off in relative terms. General medical advances in the past have only marginally widened this gap, but genetic advances have the potential for widening that gap greatly.

Genetic Priorities and Alzheimer Disease: A Moral Assessment

In this concluding section I return to the central issue that precipitated this inquiry: If we wish to be a just and caring society, and if we have only limited resources for meeting virtually unlimited health care needs, then how high a priority ought we to assign various genetic tests and various genetic interventions in a range of clinical contexts that are aimed at AD? I outlined three clinical scenarios to which we now return.

In the first of those scenarios I imagined two thirty-year- old women who wanted genetic testing for themselves. One wanted to be tested for the breast cancer gene (BRCA1) because three close relatives had died of breast cancer. The other wanted APOE testing to establish her risk for AD because two of her grandparents were diagnosed with AD in their early eighties. Would a just and caring society with limited resources to meet virtually unlimited health needs be equally obligated to provide genetic testing to both these women? I would give a negative answer to this question.

The following considerations would seem to justify making the moral distinction I endorse in this case. First, there are therapeutic options available for dealing with breast cancer, whereas there are no therapeutic options for

AD. The woman at risk for breast cancer has a morally compelling need to know because she can avail herself of more frequent mammograms, be more diligent in breast self-exams, consider prophylactic mastectomy, and so on. But nothing can now be done preventively with respect to AD (although this may change). No dietary changes or exercise routines or additional medical vigilance will alter any outcomes. Second, if a reasonable moral touchstone for priority setting in health care is protecting fair equality of opportunity, then clearly the woman at risk for breast cancer has more to lose in terms of access to life opportunities. Consequently, society would have a stronger moral obligation to meet her needs. As a society we already invest disproportionate resources in meeting the health care needs of elderly people. To be sure, there are still significant unmet health needs that elderly persons have and to which our society ought to be more attentive. But APOE testing for AD is not likely to be among those needs.

Third, the woman at risk for AD may claim that she too has a "need to know," that there is no other way to alleviate her anxieties in this matter. But then there is a brute empirical fact that must be recognized, namely, that APOE represents a gene that confers a certain susceptibility to AD, which will vary depending upon the specific allele one may have. The logical implication of this is that although the individual may have a "need to know," the APOE test will not yield the knowledge that she seeks. Her anxious feelings ought not to be ignored; they deserve a compassionate response. But that compassionate response cannot include giving her access to that to which she has no just claim. She is free to use her own resources to purchase the test; but if she lacks those resources, then denial of access is not unjust.

My second scenario pertained to prenatal testing. We again have two thirty-year-old women, both pregnant. One is concerned about having a child with cystic fibrosis because of family history; the other is concerned about AD because two grandparents were diagnosed with AD in their early eighties. Is a just and caring society with only limited resources to meet virtually unlimited health care needs equally obligated to provide prenatal genetic testing for both women? Again, I would answer this question in the negative. Similar moral considerations as above warrant this response. Someone could argue that neither condition is curable and that both women might wish to choose abortion as a response to what they learn from the prenatal test. This is true. But in one case the test might give the woman the opportunity to assess the availability of familial, medical, and social support services available for children with cystic fibrosis in her community. There is no comparable investigation that the other woman could engage in, since the medical problem that concerns her would emerge late in life. In short, the woman concerned about AD has the moral right to spend her own resources for prenatal testing, but there is no basis for a just claim to limited social resources.

In my third scenario we have three couples who are all interested in preimplantation genetic diagnosis. They are respectively concerned about cystic fibrosis, breast cancer, and AD, all because of pertinent family history. Is a just and caring society with only limited resources for meeting virtually unlimited health care needs morally obligated to provide equal support for all three of these couples for in vitro fertilization and preimplantation genetic diagnosis? Again, I defend a negative answer to this question. Here, we are clearly talking about a very expensive intervention, at $30,000 per successful pregnancy. From a pure cost-effectiveness perspective (which has implications for health care justice), a $30,000 investment that will prevent the birth of a child with cystic fibrosis or eliminate an 80 percent risk that a woman will be afflicted with breast cancer is a rational decision. (There is the alternative of artificial insemination by donor at only 10 percent of the cost of this intervention, but this raises some other complicated issues we need to pass over.) There are potential savings associated with the AD embryo, but they would be far into the future and speculative at best.

As far as protecting fair equality of opportunity is concerned, we would accomplish the most in choosing an embryo free of cystic fibrosis, and the second most in choosing an embryo free of the BRCA1 gene. There are strong moral claims here because there is a large potential for loss in both cases. But this would not be true with respect to the embryo at risk for AD, even if that embryo were to have a double dose of the ϵ4 allele of APOE. Again, a free society should most likely permit the couple concerned about an embryo at risk late in life for AD to purchase preimplantation genetic diagnosis at their own expense, so long as no one else is denied access to this technology who has a stronger just claim to it. Again, the positive thrust of the argument here is that a just and caring society will have strong obligations to fund fair access for all to preimplantation genetic diagnosis when future children are at risk for genetic disorders that will adversely affect either their length of life or their quality of life and, hence, their capacity to access the normal opportunity range of that society.

Before concluding, I need to consider two other scenarios related to AD and health care priorities. This first is an imaginative scenario, but it has significant analytic power from a moral point of view. Many AD researchers believe that the neurofibrillary tangles and plaques associated with AD appear in the brain over a period of many years, much like atherosclerotic heart disease.

Imagine that a drug were invented that could forestall the formation of those plaques and tangles for about ten years if an individual started to take that drug in his or her mid-forties. We will assign a relatively modest cost to the drug of $500 per year. Would a just and caring society with limited resources to meet virtually unlimited health care needs be morally obligated to underwrite the costs of that drug at social expense? Would a just and caring society also be morally obligated to underwrite the costs of APOE genotyping? Again, negative answers are warranted for both these questions.

The basic facts with respect to APOE genotyping are these. According to Roses (1995), about 17 percent of individuals with AD have the $\epsilon 4/\epsilon 4$ haplotype of APOE, and they are faced with a mean age of onset of sixty-eight. About 43 percent of individuals with AD have the $\epsilon 3/\epsilon 4$ haplotype of APOE, with a mean age of onset of seventy-five. About 33 percent of individuals with AD have the $\epsilon 3/\epsilon 3$ haplotype of APOE, with a mean age of onset of eighty-four. Again, the reader is reminded that this is a susceptibility gene and that only varying fractions of these groups of individuals will in fact be afflicted with AD. The $\epsilon 4/\epsilon 4$ group has the highest lifetime risk for individuals who survive to age eighty. It might seem that they have some presumptive just claim to the drug that would forestall AD by ten years.

However, to accomplish that, everyone would have to undergo APOE genotyping around age forty-five. That in itself would be a substantial social cost. But even then it would be practically impossible to restrict funded access to this drug to the $\epsilon 4/\epsilon 4$ group. If they gained a ten-year reprieve from AD, then they would be better off on average than the $\epsilon 3/\epsilon 4$ group, who would then contend that fairness required they had access to the funded drug as well, which would trigger exactly the same demands from the $\epsilon 3/\epsilon 3$ group. This is a perfect example of the "ragged edge" problem I identified earlier. Now you have literally tens of millions of individuals demanding access to this drug and adding $20 billion to $30 billion per year to the cost of health care for elderly people in our society, unless very substantial offsets were found in reduced nursing home costs. An outcome like this badly skews allocations of resources away from unmet health needs that make much stronger just claims to limited resources. This conflict of unmet health needs would obtain both among elderly people and between elderly and nonelderly persons in our society. For these reasons, predictive APOE genotyping in such a scenario at social cost would be unjustified. (The argument in support of this conclusion is presented more fully in Fleck 1996.)

One last scenario: Allen Roses speculates that APOE genotyping might be warranted in a diagnostic situation where there is substantial clinical evidence that a patient has AD (see chap. 4, above). As things are now, these patients routinely undergo an MRI scan at a cost of about $1,200. But Roses argues that if a patient is either the ϵ4/ϵ4 or ϵ3/ϵ4 haplotype of APOE (test costs estimated at $300), then the diagnosis of AD is 99 percent certain without the MRI. That is, there is less than a 1 percent chance that the presenting signs of dementia are attributable to something other than AD, such as a brain tumor. This would represent a savings of $900 to a managed care plan or Medicare. Could a patient claim that he or she was treated unjustly if access to an MRI in these circumstances were denied? This is one of those questions to which no conception of health care justice can give a clear, unequivocal moral answer. This is a question that, as suggested earlier, is best addressed through a process of rational democratic deliberation. There are at best marginal benefits involved. If the beneficiaries of Medicare, or the members of a managed care plan, believe that those savings can be better used to meet what they judge for themselves are higher-priority health care needs, then their collective agreement gives moral legitimacy to that MRI rationing protocol.

In conclusion, genetic testing for AD associated with APOE and other genetic interventions aimed at AD associated with APOE have only the lowest priority as far as just claims to limited health care resources are concerned.

References

Brody, B. 1988. The macro-allocation of health care resources. In *Health care systems: Moral conflicts in European and American public policy,* ed. H. Martin-Sass and R. Massey, 213–16. Dordrecht: Kluwer Academic Publisher.

Callahan, D. 1987. *Setting limits: Medical goals in an aging society.* New York: Simon and Schuster.

———. 1990. *What kind of life: The limits of medical progress.* New York: Simon and Schuster.

Churchill, L. R. 1987. *Rationing health care in America: Perceptions and principles of justice.* Notre Dame, Ind.: University of Notre Dame Press.

Daniels, N. 1985. *Just health care.* Cambridge: Cambridge University Press.

Eddy, D. 1994. Health system reform: Will controlling costs require rationing services? *JAMA* 272:324–28.

Engelhardt, H. T. 1996. *The foundations of bioethics.* 2d ed. New York: Oxford University Press.

Fleck, L. M. 1989a. Just health care. Part 1, Is beneficence enough? *Theoretical Medicine* 10:167–82.

———. 1989b. Just health care. Part 2, Is equality too much? *Theoretical Medicine* 10:301–10.

———. 1994a. Just caring: Oregon, health care rationing, and informed democratic deliberation. *Journal of Medicine and Philosophy* 19:367–88.

———. 1994b. Justice, age rationing, and the problem of identifiable lives. In *Health care for an aged population,* ed. C. Hackler, 93–105. Albany: State University of New York Press.

———. 1994c. Just genetics: A problem agenda. In *Justice and the Human Genome Project,* ed. T. Murphy and M. Lappe, 133–52. Berkeley: University of California Press.

———. 1996. Just caring: The moral and economic costs of APOE genotyping for Alzheimer's disease. *Annals of the New York Academy of Science* 802:128–38.

Rawls, J. 1993. *Political liberalism.* New York: Columbia University Press.

Roses, A. 1995. Apolipoprotein genotyping in the differential diagnosis, not prediction, of Alzheimer's disease. *Annals of Neurology* 38:6–14.

Managed Care Issues in Genetic Testing for Alzheimer Disease

STEVEN MILES, M.D.

Managed health care differs from fee-for-service medicine in that the functions of insurance (spreading health risk by enrolling and collecting premiums from many people of whom only some will use health care) and the clinical care of those enrolled are combined within one framework. A managed health care plan is best defined as one that holds a group of clinicians collectively accountable for providing a comprehensive set of health care services to a defined population for a specified budget. This definition of a managed health plan encompasses staff-model health maintenance organizations (HMOs) that collect insurance premiums and employ clinicians as well as "preferred provider" networks, in which insurers contract with independent groups of clinicians who share financial risk for the cost of treating member-patients.

Little is known about how managed care systems differ from or resemble conventional indemnity health insurance in enrolling or managing persons with dementing disorders. First, the incidence of dementia before age sixty-five is very low, and managed care insures a relatively small percentage of persons who are on Medicare (Welch 1996). Second, the ability to measure the prevalence of dementia, especially early dementia, in managed care programs is limited. Third, it is essential and yet nearly impossible to separate trends in genetic insurance discrimination by managed care plans from comparable trends in traditional employer-based insurance and the increasing use by employers of inadequate and unregulated insurance products (the Employee Retirement Income Security Act self-insurance). Finally, the few studies of genetic insurance discrimination (referenced below) do not distinguish managed health care plans from traditional indemnity insurance.

Dementia can occur before or after retirement. Persons with dementia would be high-cost users of some kinds of health care services. Dementia is disabling. It is also relevant to applicants for long-term-care insurance, in that persons with dementia would be more likely to need more-costly nursing home care. Thus, Alzheimer disease (AD) testing is relevant to health, disability, and long-term-care insurance and the services paid for by this insurance, as well as for any managed care system that insures and services persons at risk of AD.

Managed care systems compete as insurers and as health care providers. As insurers, they try to minimize the treatment obligations that they assume (Light 1992). If a system enrolls individuals or populations with a greater-than-average proportion of costly medical needs, such as those resulting from dementia, then premiums must increase for all other plan members to provide resources for the needs of other persons with chronic disease and routine or catastrophic needs as well as satisfy corporate needs for capital. Insurers have an incentive to charge high-risk persons more than their actuarially increased health care costs in order to discourage their enrollment rather than simply to recoup the costs of caring for them (Alper, Geller, and Barash 1994). This raises the issues of enrollment practices, genetic screening, how to inform persons of the insurance consequences of being tested, and how to protect persons from insurance discrimination.

As health care providers, systems try to maximize their reputation for high-quality care and attractive resource allocations to build market share. Some services are offered because the plan is required to do so by law (such as covering maternity inpatient care for at least two days), others because they are necessary to meet the standard of care (e.g., a plan must offer cardiac catheterization for persons with heart attacks). Still other services (e.g., birthing rooms) are offered, at the discretion of the plan, to attract members. The issue of whether and how a plan allocates health care resources to heroic, innovative, chronic, primary, hospital, or palliative care or services, like genetic testing for dementias, that do not offer any immediate therapeutic benefit raises questions about the ethics of resource allocation.

Issuing Insurance

The ultimate goal of policies addressing the use of genetic tests by insurers is to prevent insurers from acting unfairly toward, or harming, individuals (Reilly 1995). This section considers how these goals apply to (1) insurance pricing or issuing that is adjusted on the basis of genetic data, (2) genetic screening, and (3) safeguarding consent for testing.

Genetic Testing and Discriminatory Insurance Pricing or Issuing

Ethically, genetic tests to confirm the diagnosis or prognostication for dementia do not differ from genetic tests that diagnose or prognosticate other diseases. Recently enacted laws, however, significantly differ in how they proscribe insurance discrimination that is specifically based on genetic information. Some bar insurers from using genetic tests as the basis for declining to issue insurance or adjusting premiums because of higher or lower risks of disease. Others define genetic discrimination as an insurance barrier that relies on any genetic test, clinical data, or family history that reveals a heritable disease (Rothenberg 1995). The broader definition would include diseases, for example, sickle-cell anemia, that are diagnosed by gene products rather than DNA analysis. It would also include recognizable clinical syndromes for which genetic markers or tests are not developed but which are recognized as having a genetic basis.

Though federal law gives employers virtually unlimited flexibility with regard to the scope, design, and provision of pension benefits including health, disability, and long-term-care insurance, several federal laws are relevant to genetic discrimination by insurers. For example:

- A model Genetic Privacy Act would proscribe discrimination in issuing or pricing insurance policies based on the broadest definition of "genetic information," one that encompasses gene tests and other clinical or biochemical evidence, including family history, of a heritable disorder (Annas, Glantz, and Roche 1995). This would clearly prohibit health insurance discrimination based on the identification of a heritable form of dementia.

- The 1996 federal Health Insurance Portability and Accountability Act is designed to protect insured workers with preexisting conditions or risk factors for preexisting conditions who are at risk of losing insurance as they change jobs and thereby change to new employer-purchased policies. It bars health insurance discrimination based on genetic testing. Although diagnosed and clinically present genetic disorders are not addressed in the language pertaining to the ban on genetic insurance discrimination, an inherited condition would be covered under another provision of the law that limits the length of time insurers may refuse coverage for preexisting conditions to a single one-year period, to run without interruption across all sequential insurance policies. Even so, in that dementia is a disease that generally arises after retirement or that forces retirement, a genetic prediction of future AD would be of little relevance to the pricing of health insurance for current employees, and, therefore, there is little need of the protection contained in this law.

The complex issues of fair insurance coverage in relation to the information yielded by genetic testing for AD can be illuminated by considering five hypothetical cases:

1. a person with a reliable gene-test-based strong predisposition to dementia (e.g., a sixty-year-old person with normal mental function but with a family history of dementia, abnormal cerebral glucose metabolism [as is often seen in cases of dementia], and two APOE ε4 alleles [Reiman, Caselli, and Lans 1996; Small et al. 1995])
2. a person with gene-confirmed diagnosis of dementia (e.g., a fifty-year-old person with diffuse, progressive cognitive decline and a chromosome 14 dementia-predictive mutation)
3. a person with a reliable clinical diagnosis or prognostication of dementia based on gene products but not on detection of some as-yet presumptively present but unidentified gene
4. a person with a clinical diagnosis or prognostication of dementia that is not known to be gene based either on the basis of a family history, clinical exam, or genetic testing (e.g., a person with early signs of Creutzfeld-Jacob disease, for which there is no genetic marker)
5. a person with a clinical diagnosis or prognostication of an untreatable progressive disease that is comparable to dementia in terms of disability and health care costs (e.g., amyotrophic lateral sclerosis)

It is difficult to see how a law could fairly neglect to protect persons in all five cases if it barred insurance discrimination in any one case. However, the Health Insurance Portability and Accountability Act's restrictions on insurers would bar discrimination for case 1 but not for case 2 when a disease is diagnosed. It thus gives insurers an incentive to endorse scientific work revising diagnostic criteria for early-stage dementia. For example, a genetic test combined with adult or even adolescent biometric or psychometric tests (Reiman, Caselli, and Lans 1996; Small et al. 1995) could lead to redefining case 1 as early-stage Alzheimer disease. If so, the Health Insurance Portability and Accountability Act's protection for the person in case 1 would be void, because the genetic test would be diagnostic. Aside from laboratory technique, diagnostic or prognostic information from genetic tests does not differ from the kind of information obtained from other kinds of clinical tests to diagnose or prognosticate other degenerative diseases (cases 4 or 5) that occasion discrimination in the access to insured health care. It would be unfortunate if a legal protection against misused genetic tests initially made persons with AD (case 1) unfairly privileged relative to persons with case 2 dementia or case 5 disease and then spurred diagnostic revisions that moved persons encompassed by its limited protections against those with inherited disorders by revising the definition of early-stage disease.

The federal protection for case 1 health insurance protection is more like states' idiosyncratic insurance mandates than a profound political endorsement of the duty to equitably insure people. Various state laws require insurers to pay for experimental bone marrow transplants, prostate antigen screening, treatment of temporal mandibular joint disease, or wigs for persons who have lost hair from chemotherapy without enacting universal access to health insurance as a fundamental priority before interest group-sponsored mandates that too often promote therapies of marginal effectiveness. As a stab at a policy to prevent insurance abuses of persons with heritable conditions, federal protection against genetic discrimination seems to reflect a faith that genes are the most fundamental determinant of health and merit morally protected access to health care (Lewontin 1992; Wolf 1995), rather than one that defends a sound biological distinction between heritable disease and conditions that are a result of accident, injustice, or personal responsibility. Even if one could reliably make such a distinction (and reject the intricate synergy between nature, nurture, choice, and circumstance that modulates the expression of disease and disability), one would still need to justify prioritizing health insurance for genetic disease before one could defend the insurance privileges based on "genetic information."

Genetic Screening

In my view, it is unlikely that health insurers will screen potential policyholders for AD. First, the cost-benefit ratio for screening is very low (Glazner et al. 1995). Assuming $500 for testing and counseling and a case prevalence of four thousand cases per million (Medical and Scientific Advisory Committee 1995), the cost of identifying one person at high risk for APOE late-onset dementia would be $125,000, or perhaps half as much if a family history of dementia was used to prescreen those who were tested, though this would decrease the sensitivity of the testing. The fact that for thirty years insurers have not seized the opportunity to screen for a genetic predisposition to a common form of emphysema supports this analysis (Wulfsberg, Hoffman, and Cohen 1994).

Second, screening far in advance of the actual generation of health care costs does not generate savings to insurers, because of the movement of persons between insurance plans (Van Vliet and van de Ven 1992). Third, the consolidation of managed care systems into plans that insure millions of persons dilutes the impact of discovered cases of dementia (Robinson and Gardner 1995).

Fourth, the trend of having managed care plans insure both privately covered and publicly financed persons means that plans have no place to dump people with genetically high risk. Notwithstanding the low likelihood of health insurers undertaking widespread screening for the genetic risk of AD, it is possible that they would discriminate if genetic information about an individual applicant became known to them. Discrimination by health and life insurers with regard to a variety of genetic diseases has been reported by 22–25 percent of persons in genetic support groups (Hudson et al. 1995; Lapham, Kozma, and Weiss 1996), even when the condition poses no significant relation to health care costs or excess morbidity or mortality (Billings et al. 1992).

There are two situations where health insurance screening for AD may be more likely. (1) preretirement evaluation of workers for postretirement health insurance benefits and (2) nursing home insurance. Pension benefits are insured or bonded years in advance of actual need. It is possible that genetic screening followed by requirements for higher employee contributions or more aggressive policies to limit benefits relative to expected medical needs might be applied to the pension benefits of persons with genetic markers for dementing disorders. Nursing home insurance is purchased late in life with the intent of continuing with a single insurer throughout one's life. Dementia is the most common reason for prolonged nursing home care, and persons who know they are at high risk may be inclined to seek insurance. This poses the problem of adverse selection into insurer pools of nursing home policyholders. Given this possibility, insurers are likely to argue that testing and premium adjustment for the nonrandom nature of their members is fair and necessary.

Safeguarding Consent to Genetic Testing

Existing proposals for protecting the interests of persons from the unwanted use of genetic information begin with informed consent. Traditionally, such consent means that the person is told of the ability of the test to predict and fail to predict the risk of disease, of risks for offspring, of how intervening chronic disease would affect the likelihood that dementia would be expressed, and so on. A good genetic counselor would also describe the potential for explicit or attempted discrimination by employers, long-term-care insurers, or health care insurers (Juengst 1995; Li et al. 1992; National Institutes of Health 1990).

The special feature of genetic testing for AD is the long latency, perhaps decades, between testing and the clinical expression of disease, application to a retirement community, or a decision to purchase long-term-care insurance (Post 1994). Contrary to optimistic assessments of personal control over electronic data records (Lennox and Toronto "3" Study Group 1994), a person's ability to delete a test from electronic databases, given the widespread blanket releases, the multiple storage of data in various databases, and automatic data sharing between managed care plans as employers select plans, is nearly nil. Persons who are mildly or moderately cognitively impaired from dementia will be less able to enforce or appeal original understandings of the implications of testing. Finally, the risk of harm accrues more to tested persons than to future pension managers, retirement community admissions committees, or vendors of nursing home insurance. These reasons contradict those who argue that patients should not be told of the risk of insurance discrimination in the future merely because there is little evidence at this time of genetic discrimination in insurance or retirement policies (Ostrer et al. 1993).

Some propose that society promote anonymous testing for genetic markers for AD to enable individuals to preserve their privacy and to avoid potential discrimination (Mehlman et al. 1996). In anonymous testing, the test results are given to the individual tested; neither the testing agency nor the insurer knows the results (somewhat revealing of the possibility of discrimination because of an increased-risk result) or even the fact that a test has been done. People who have experienced, or who fear, genetic discrimination by insurers are more reluctant to seek genetic testing and prefer to do so in a way that preserves privacy from potential insurers.

Though anonymous, self-pay testing will be available for those who are wealthy and motivated to seek it, the case for anonymous genetic testing for dementia markers is not as strong as the case was for fostering access to anonymous HIV testing in the pretreatment phase of that epidemic. Alzheimer disease does not pose a public health threat. It is not concentrated in ethnic groups or subcultures that are especially prone to stigmatization for other reasons. The health insurance consequences of bearing a gene for AD are not likely to be severe, for reasons discussed previously. A public policy to foster anonymous genetic testing for AD would undermine private insurance for nursing home policies and pension health care policies because persons who found themselves to be at low risk would have an incentive to disclose their test results to bargain for better prices for nursing home insurance or pension benefits. The resulting higher-risk pool of untested persons and persons who know that they are at risk for dementing disorders would be more likely to face higher insurance premiums or lower benefits.

Public policy must do more than simply provide a format for informed consent at the time of testing. It should secure robust protections for persons undergoing testing. Perhaps a law could assure that, so long as a person is continuously insured, there will be "temporal portability" of the understandings made at the time of testing with regard to insurability, retirement community admissions, and so on. Such a policy would make it easier to use testing as part of the workup of early dementia, for family planning counseling, and for clinical research of early-stage interventions by creating a durable informed consent based on a societal conclusion that the choice to undergo genetic testing for dementia was of sufficient value that safeguarding consent to testing was a priority.

Insurers and the Population Genetics of Alzheimer Disease

Insurers have an incentive to use genetic information in their competition to insure a disproportionately healthy population. Alzheimer disease is a very costly disease. If future genetic epidemiologic research shows that subpopulations substantially vary in their average risk of dementia, insurers could use such information for discriminatory population-based marketing or to design premiums to decrease the number of members from high-risk populations. This practice would be especially regressive if populations with a higher prevalence of dementia also had a diminished ability to buy insurance. For example, women are poorer than men and are more likely to become demented because of their greater longevity (Miles and Parker 1997). Long-term-care insurance that charges women more because of their greater risk of acquiring dementia are financially regressive.

Meanwhile, Medicare or Medicaid administrators who dispense funds through private managed care systems must assure that public resources are efficiently and equitably used. They want to avoid paying managed care systems an "average" amount for a healthier than average subpopulation. To this end, they are trying to develop risk-adjusted payment mechanisms to correct for variations in the severity of illness of populations that are enrolled in different managed care system (Gicomini, Luft, and Robinson 1995; Kronick, Zhou, and Dreyfus 1995; Polzer 1994). Such risk adjustments pay insurers more for insuring sick persons, such as those requiring dialysis. These risk-adjusted payments must be accompanied by robust ways to prevent insurers from churning policy members after a risk adjustment is calculated (Bowen 1995). Some suggest combining prospective risk-adjusted payments to health plans with retrospective readjustments if evidence of overpayment is found or if the insured group turns out to be unusually healthy and use relatively little health care (Bowen 1995; Gicomini, Luft, and Robinson 1995; Luft 1995; Newhouse 1994; Polzer 1994).

Knowledge of significant variations within subpopulations of the genetic predisposition for AD could affect such risk-adjusting contests. It may be that electronic genetic databases (perhaps partly constructed for public health surveys or longitudinal large-scale health services research like the Framingham study [Myers et al. 1996]) may enable an insurer to identify regional or ethnic subpopulations in which a high degree of kinship affects the prevalence of genetic risks for AD and to whom marketing health or long-term-care insurance would be relatively more or less disadvantageous. Twenty-two states now permit using labeled genetic data for epidemiologic research (Gostin et al. 1996). Government risk payments that are risk adjusted for genetic profiles of populations, coupled with oversight of insurance sales and premium strategies, may be needed.

In addition, a governmental policy to prevent actuarial misuse of electronic medical records for costly and prevalent genetic disorders may be required if there are commercially valuable demographic variations in APOE. Such a public policy differs from customarily recommended laws to protect the personal confidentiality of electronic medical records (Clayton 1995; Clayton et al. 1995). This duel between public payers and private insurers will add to the large share of the U.S. health care budget that is spent on administering the health care system.

The potential problems if managed care plans are able to enroll a demographically advantaged population is compounded if private managed care plans compete with a public Medicare system. Demographic marketing, gender or age preferences by private plans, or different premium structures between public and private plans could create a better demographic mix in private plans that would allow them to offer better services and lower out-of-pocket costs to persons at lower risk of dementia who enroll in private plans. More constricted services would be necessary for the higher-risk demographic group enrolled in public plans. Capitated Medicare HMOs do selectively enroll younger, healthier, and more financially well-off members, leaving a more costly group of persons to public plans (Dowd, Moscovice, and Feldman 1994; Lichenstein et al. 1992).

Genetic Testing and the Allocation of Resources to Persons with Dementia

The perception of fair allocation of resources by managed care systems is a Gordian knot. Some will evaluate managed care according to a high social value placed on rescue of identified persons facing premature death. The recent charge by some "pro-life" groups that any event in managed care that accidentally, negligently, or systematically limits access to potentially life-prolonging interventions is a form of involuntary euthanasia is one example of this phenomenon. The plea of family to do anything, regardless of the cost or efficacy of the therapy, is another. Many people underestimate the high costs of caring for the increasing number of elderly persons with dementia, while others see those high costs as fueling the dehumanizing stigmatization of persons with dementia. These forces for and against the care or treatment of persons with AD occur as more and more costly medical technologies are being demanded of managed care system budgets by entrepreneurial forces, political interests, and patient demand.

The conundrum of how to allocate health care resources to persons with Alzheimer disease is made even more complex because this nation has used private insurance to spread the risk for assuring coverage of acute medical catastrophes. Chronic disease and its consequent long-term care have been financed by private impoverishment and state and federal entitlement programs. It is difficult to see how the cost of health care that is born by entitlement programs could be folded into an insurance pool for resource allocation. To do so, the high costs for medical, nursing, rehabilitative, and community-based services for persons with severe chronic disease would have to be absorbed in health insurance premiums that have been designed for acute care of low prevalence and limited duration. In addition, a way would have to be found to manage, finance, and perhaps redefine "medically necessary" care so as to assure that the sustained provision of health services that enables persons with dementing illnesses to remain in the community could continue.

Concluding Comments

Genetic tests for dementias do not resolve the problem of fair allocation of resources between generations; nor do they balance acute care with chronic care or answer the ironic fact that living well too often sets the stage for the most protracted senescent decline. They may, however, offer something more than the irresistible appeal of a new diagnostic technique of almost quasi-religious insight. They may offer a renewed sense of community as the breadth and limits of information contained in genomic sequences help us see that life's fortunes and misfortunes are not as simple as sin and disease, nature and nurture.

In some way, at some time in each person's life span, his or her genetic heritage predisposes: some to despair and some to a sunny disposition, some to health and some to disease, some to longevity and some to death. In this sense, the DNA icon is not just the "ultimate diagnosis"; it also reveals the deep genesis of fortune, vulnerability, and dependence. This constructive insight into how members of the human community are related points away from the false, inhumane science of race hygiene. The fact that we all have genes for health and disease is why we must create a health care-financing commons that insures all persons and is governed by respect for individual life and a sense of equitable stewardship of the available resources as a durable way to meet our health care needs in a costly, technology-dependent health care system in an aging society.

References

Alper, J. S., Geller, L. N., and Barashi, C. I. 1994. Genetic discrimination and screening for hemochromatosis. *Journal of Public Health Policy* 15:345–48.

Annas, G. J., Glantz, L. H., and Roche, P. A. 1995. *The Genetic Privacy Act and commentary.* Boston: Boston University School of Public Health.

Billings, P. R., Kohn, M. A., deCuevas, M., Beckwith, J., Alper, J. S., Natowiez, M. R. 1992. Discrimination as a consequence of genetic testing. *American Journal of Human Genetics* 50:476–82.

Bowen, B. 1995. The practice of risk adjustment. *Inquiry* 32:33–44.

Clayton, E. W. 1995. Why the use of anonymous samples for research matters. *Journal of Law, Medicine, and Ethics* 23:375–77.

Clayton, E. W., Steinberg, K. K., Khoury, M. J., and Thomson, E. 1995. Informed consent for genetic research on stored tissue samples. *JAMA* 274:1786–92.

Dowd, B., Moscovice, I., and Feldman, R. 1994. Health plan choice in the Twin Cities Medicare market. *Medical Care* 32:1019–39.

Gicomini, M., Luft, H. S., and Robinson, J. C. 1995. Risk adjusting community health plan premiums: A survey of risk assessment literature and policy applications. *Annual Review of Public Health* 17:401–30.

Glazner, J., Braithwaite, W. R., Hull, S., and Lezotte, D. C. 1995. The questionable value of medical screening in the small group insurance market. *Health Affairs* 14:224–34.

Gostin, L. O., Lazzarinia, Z., Neslund, V. S., and Osterholm, M. T. 1996. The public health information infrastructure: A national review of the law on health information. *JAMA* 275:1921–27.

Hudson, K. L., Rothenberg, K. H., Andrews, L. B., Kahn, M. J., and Collins, F. S. 1995. Genetic discrimination and health care insurance: An urgent need for reform. *Science* 270:391–93.

Juengst, E. T. 1995. The ethics of prediction: Genetic risks and the physician-patient relationship. *Genome Science and Technology* 1:21–36.

Kronick, R., Zhou, Z., and Dreyfus, T. 1995. Making risk adjustments work for everyone. *Inquiry* 32:41–55.

Lapham, E. V., Kozma, C., and Weiss, J. O. 1996. Genetic discrimination: Perspectives of consumers. *Science* 274:621-24.

Lennox, A., and Toronto "3" Study Group. 1994. Molecular genetic predictive testing for Alzheimer disease: Deliberations and preliminary recommendations. *Alzheimer Disease and Associated Disorders* 8:126–47.

Lewontin, R. C. 1992. The dream of the human genome. *New York Review of Books* 39 (May 28): 31–34.

Li, P. F., Garber, J. E., Friend, S. H., and Strong, L. C. 1992. Recommendations on predictive testing for germ line p53 mutations among cancer prone individuals. *Journal of the National Cancer Institute* 84:1156–60.

Lichenstein, R., Thomas, J. W., Watkins, B., and Puto, C. 1992. HMO marketing and selection bias: Are TEFRA HMOs skimming? *Medical Care* 30:329–46.

Light, D. 1992. The practice and ethics of risk-related health insurance. *JAMA* 267:2503–8.

Luft, H. S. 1995. Potential methods to reduce risk selection. *Inquiry* 32:23–32.

Medical and Scientific Advisory Committee, Alzheimer's Disease International. 1995. Consensus statement on predictive testing for Alzheimer disease. *Alzheimer Disease and Associated Disorders* 9:182–87.

Mehlman, M. J., Kodish, E. D., Whitehouse, P. H., Zinn, A. B., Sollito, S., Beyer, J., Chiao, E. J., Dosik, M. S., and Cassidy, S. B. 1996. The need for anonymous genetic counseling and testing. *American Journal of Human Genetics* 58:393–97.

Miles, S. H., and Parker, K. 1997. Men, women, and health insurance. *New England Journal of Medicine* 336:218–21.

Myers, R. H., Schaefer, E. J., Wilson, P. W., D'Agostino, R., Ordovas, J. M., Espino, A., Au, R., White, R. F., Knoefel, J. E., Cobb, J. L., McNulty, K. A., Beiser, A., and Wolf, P. A. 1996. Apolipoprotein E epsilon-4 association with dementia in a population-based study: The Framingham study. *Neurology* 46:673–77.

National Institutes of Health. 1990. Workshop on population screening for the cystic fibrosis gene. *Statement* 323:70–71.

Newhouse, J. P. 1994. Patients at risk: Health reform and risk adjustment. *Health Affairs* 13:132–46.

Ostrer, H., Allen, W., Crandall, L. A., Mosely, R. E., Dewar, M. A., Nye, O., and McCrary, S. V. 1993. Insurance and genetic testing: Where are we now. *American Journal of Human Genetics* 52:565–77.

Polzer, K. 1994. The role of risk adjustment in national health reform. *Academic Medicine* 69:445–51.

Post, S. G. 1994. Genetics, ethics, and Alzheimer disease. *Journal of the American Geriatrics Society* 42:782–86.

Reilly, P. R. 1995. The impact of the Genetic Privacy Act on medicine. *Journal of Law, Medicine, and Ethics* 23:378-81.

Reiman, E. M., Caselli, R. J., and Lans, S. Y. 1996. Preclinical evidence of Alzheimer disease in persons homozygous for the ε4 allele for apolipoprotein E. *New England Journal of Medicine* 334:752-58.

Robinson, J. C., and Gardner, L. B. 1995. Adverse selection among multiple competing health maintenance organizations. *Medical Care* 33:1161-75.

Rothenberg, K. H. 1995. Genetic information and health insurance: State legislative approaches. *Journal of Law, Medicine, and Ethics* 23:312-19.

Small, G. W., Mazzotta, J. C., Collins, M. T., and Baxter, L. R. 1995. Apolipoprotein E type 4 allele and cerebral glucose metabolism in relatives at risk for familial Alzheimer disease. *JAMA* 273:942-47.

Van Vliet, R. C., and van de Ven, W. P. 1992. Towards a capitation formula for competing health insurers: An empirical analysis. *Social Science and Medicine* 34:1035-48.

Welch, W. P. 1996. Growth in the HMO share of the Medicare market, 1989-1994. *Health Affairs* 15:201-14.

Wolf, S. 1995. Beyond "genetic discrimination": Toward the broader harm of geneticism. *Journal of Law, Medicine, and Ethics* 23:345-54.

Wulfsberg, E. A., Hoffman, D. E., and Cohen, M. M. 1994. Alpha 1-antitrypsin deficiency: Impact of genetic discovery on medicine and society. *JAMA* 271:217-22.

PART FOUR

Educational Issues

Education for a Too-Hopeful Public

14

STEPHEN G. POST, PH.D.

A general concern in the application of genetic technology is the premature introduction of testing into the asymptomatic population for either predictive purposes (i.e., clearly foretelling disease) or risk analysis (i.e., establishing the extent of susceptibility to disease) or into the symptomatic population for diagnostic confirmation. To avoid this problem, the genotype to be detected by a genetic test must be clearly related to the occurrence of a disease. This requires firm scientific evidence and data replication. In addition, the benefits and risks that accrue from both positive and negative results in these populations must be understood, along with their implications for ethical practice.

The problem of introducing genetic testing before these criteria are met is significant. One way in which potential victims of the premature introduction of testing can avoid this burden is through clear public education. At focus groups I led or attended in 1995-96 involving those who are caregivers for people with Alzheimer disease (AD), the assumption was that a new predictive and broadly applicable genetic test already exists for AD. Family members of AD patients are usually quite surprised to hear that the genetic test is, with respect to predictive purposes, a myth except for those very few families (an estimated 2-5% of all AD) with clearly defined early-onset autosomal-dominant forms of the disease (in order of frequency, chromosomes 14, 1, and 21).

This confusion can be explained. In the summer of 1995, news articles suggested that large numbers of people were affected by new findings in AD genetics focusing on the chromosome 14 discovery (PS1). Many people in our focus groups, concerned with the typical late-onset form of AD, did not realize that PS1 involves only a very few families with early-onset disease. Anecdotally, genetic testing centers around the country reported increased requests for the AD test, which were often referred to the AD clinics for clarification of the limited relevance of PS1 for almost all affected families. Fortunately, as a result of educational programs, this confusion seems to have ended.

The current debate regarding APOE is over its use as a possible diagnostic adjunct in patients who have the symptoms of dementia. In the future, if more susceptibility genes are clarified allowing for better risk analysis in asymptomatic individuals, there may be renewed debate over susceptibility testing.

The public has placed such hope in genetic progress that prematurity is invited, even if researchers remain highly circumspect about the clinical application of their findings. Nevertheless, the researchers must resist premature introduction of genetic testing or of emerging therapies, lest their social covenant with the affected population be broken. Long-term progress in the struggle against many diseases can be seriously undermined by public distrust and resentment toward researchers who indulge irrational hopes. Furthermore, should the public perceive that researchers, clinicians, and pharmaceutical companies are making financial gains based on excessive claims for the benefits of new genetic breakthroughs or on less than clear and precise statements about the currently limited clinical usefulness of such breakthroughs, the long-term damage to scientific progress could be profound.

With regard to presymptomatic APOE genotyping in AD, many observers believe that genetic testing was prematurely introduced in January 1994. With only the most preliminary data, Genica Pharmaceuticals Corporation mailed to physicians across the United States a full packet detailing the $195 APOE test for susceptibility to AD. A sticker on the packet envelope reads, "Rush! Here's the Genica Information You Requested." A cover letter to physicians from Genica's reimbursement manager indicated that, while Medicare classifies APOE genotyping as investigational, the provider is "free to seek payment directly from the patient." The genotyping required 2.5 milliliters of whole blood. Full payment was required with each shipment. While Genica marketed the APOE genotyping as a susceptibility test, it vaguely qualified this with the statement that the test should be interpreted in the light of other "clinical diagnostic information" in people with suspected AD.

Among the critics of this introduction of AD genetic testing was Robert N. Butler, editor of *Geriatrics,* who emphasized that the testing was not yet established as a diagnostic or predictive marker, that people should avoid the emotional toll of thinking that they are doomed on the basis of APOE genotype and minor forgetfulness, and that discrimination in employment and insurance was likely (Butler 1994). Genica withdrew its APOE testing initiative within several months. Although no exact figures are available, Genica representatives at various conferences indicated that an estimated three hundred people had been tested.

Given the power of the hope that is often vested in genetics, commercial interests are never far away. The fact that so many people are affected by AD (an estimated four million in the United States alone) and the prediction that the numbers of affected people will escalate as the population ages indicate that the financial stakes are huge.

In this chapter I encourage serious critical thinking in the general population with respect to AD genetic testing. Potential consumers must have a critical perspective on the pressures — cultural, economic, and therapeutic — for premature introduction of AD genetic testing. I also encourage reflection on the bias against forgetfulness that test results can unleash and on its adverse social implications.

Consumer Education in Critical Thinking

Alzheimer Disease Genes and Cultural Pressures

While cautionary statements against the premature introduction of genetic testing can be effective, geneticists nevertheless find themselves in the whirlwind of public interest. Such statements, therefore, must be strong and vivid. The gene has been described as "a cultural icon, a symbol, almost a magical force" and as the secular equivalent of the soul: "Fundamental to identity, DNA seems to explain individual differences, moral order, and human fate" (Nelkin and Lindee 1995, 2). Sociologist Marque-Luisa Miringoff describes genetic welfare as a distinctive worldview that is gradually emerging, somewhat to the detriment of the social welfare orientation that stresses environment and social intervention (1991). The public follows genetic discoveries with an avid eye and with the feel of progress that these prestigious "breakthrough" discoveries create. People begin to see the world differently. "The emergence of Genetic Welfare," writes Miringoff, "unlike the 'passionate movements' of the past, is a quiet revolution insinuating itself into everyday life in incremental fashion" (1991, 24). The clinical benefits of genetic findings are often extremely limited or virtually nonexistent, although one hopes they will indicate useful directions for researchers. But because they are mediated through the institution of medicine, "each progression has been viewed as palliative or ameliorative, preventive or curative, as beneficent as penicillin or the polio vaccine" (30). While some of the above statements may exaggerate, Miringoff has captured the remarkable hope associated with genetic findings in American culture.

Researchers, clinicians, and the media must not feed this sometimes irrational hope by overstating the predictive powers of genetic testing. Filtered through mass culture, genetics is construed as providing more certainty, predictability, and control than the data indicate. The word *suggested*, as it appears in a flood of news articles on genetic bases for everything from smoking to schizophrenia (disproved for the time being), is dangerous these days.

The first social and ethical duty of all professionals in genetic research, application, and reporting is to be accurate and circumspect with data. Many people may be adversely affected by claims to utility and predictive accuracy that the data do not fully support. For example, a person with the APOE susceptibility gene might unnecessarily retire early from a creative career in order to spend his or her remaining lucid years pursuing other matters. There is a need for education in genetics to avoid attributing a misleading status and certainty to many genetic tests (Knoppers 1991, 46).

Alzheimer Disease Genes and Economic Pressures

The institution of medicine bestows an aura of beneficence on genetics, while business ensures anticipated profits; the two contribute to the accretive nature of the ideology of genetic welfare. There is financial pressure to move directly from the laboratory bench to profit-making venture with little applied research. It has been stated that "a new industry is being built on hopes of better living through genetics" (Hubbard and Wald 1993, 2). It also has been pointed out that numerous new biotechnology companies, their scientist directors and consultants, as well as their shareholders, have a vested interest in creating a genetics market replete with glowing promises. However, "evidence to support such promises is often slight or even nonexistent, but since most of the medical and scientific experts in the field are also connected with the industry they are inclined to be optimistic" (Hubbard and Wald 1993, 2). While many AD researchers are not connected with industry, and while those who are may have the highest integrity, nevertheless the suspicions expressed in the above statement deserve attention. Gone are many of the historical moral restrictions that the medical profession imposed on itself with regard to financial conflicts of interest (Rodwin 1993). It is now only an issue that such conflicts be publicly disclosed—a rule that all AD researchers should follow. As chapter 6 of this volume indicates, however, AD genetics and research is replete with such conflicts.

Conflict of interest has been defined thus: "A conflict of interest is a set of conditions in which professional judgment concerning a primary interest (such as a patient's welfare or the validity of research) tends to be unduly influenced by a secondary interest (such as financial gain)" (Thompson 1993,

573). Rules against conflict of interest exist to maintain professional judgment and confidence in professionals. While academic-industry relationships carry benefits, there is need for enhanced vigilance due to the risk of damage to public support for research (Blumenthal 1992). The nature of the medical profession as a vocation or calling to benefit the sick, classically ensconced in solemn oaths and priestly images, may appear compromised by economic self-interest (Blumenthal 1994).

An Institute of Medicine committee reviewed the policy implications of genetic assessment for adult-onset diseases and offered this caution: "Because of their wide applicability, it is likely that there will be strong commercial interests in the introduction of genetic tests for common, high-profile complex disorders. Strict guidelines for efficacy therefore will be necessary to prevent premature introduction of this technology" (Andrews et al. 1994, 10).

Alzheimer Disease Genes and Therapeutic or Preventive Pressure

Therapeutics. If a cholinergic therapy is of benefit to patients with particular APOE genotypes, then beneficence, "the patient's good," would indicate that genotyping should be widely implemented. However, the benefits of any emergent therapies should not be exaggerated, and the connection between genotype and therapeutic efficacy needs to be very clearly demonstrated.

It seems that cholinergic therapies such as tacrine (Cognex) or donepezil hydrochloride (Aricept) may increase attentiveness in some patients. Aricept was approved in January 1997 for marketing in the United States. Anecdotal reports indicate that it may be somewhat successful in alleviating symptoms for a period of time in some mildly or moderately demented patients. It is also free of adverse side effects, in contrast to tacrine. On the other hand, as Joseph M. Foley has written regarding tacrine, "If vitamin Be in pernicious anemia or insulin in diabetes were to be given a 9.5–9.9 on a scale of 10, tacrine would seem to rate a 0.1 to 0.5" (Foley 1993, 1). So, adds Foley, "Parturient montes, nascitur musculus" (The mountains are in labor, and a little mouse is born).

Even if it is found that responsivity to such cholinesterase inhibitors is determined in part by APOE genotype, this will be of no clinical relevance now that an inhibitor free of side effects is available. Clinicians will prescribe widely in the hope that the particular patient, regardless of genotype, will respond. Thus, genotyping in the context of cholinesterase inhibitors is now both unnecessary and clinically irrelevant.

The remaining question is how to use inhibitors in a humane way. For example, if symptoms can be pushed back to some degree, will this simply recover a patient's insight into the loss of capacity and result in renewed anxiety?

Even if such compounds can keep a patient out of a nursing home for a period of six months to a year, is this good for patients and caregivers?

Preventive Efforts. While the development of new cholinesterase inhibitors sets aside the old tacrine-related question of genotyping as an indicator for prescription, there is still the strong possibility that genetic susceptibility testing could define at-risk populations for whom ibuprofen, estrogen, and other emerging substances that delay or prevent symptoms would be recommended. These substances may have some adverse side effects and would not be recommended for populations with low probability of eventually manifesting AD. The success of such a strategy depends on much more refinement of genetic risk analysis and will surely require the discovery of susceptibility genes in addition to APOE (e.g., there may be another such gene on chromosome 12).

In the absence of a cure for AD, prevention or delay of onset is the most laudable research goal. By delaying onset, many more of the oldest-old (eighty-five years or older) will die of age-related illnesses before the onset of AD. This should relieve caregiver burden, cost, and anxiety.

Consumer Education in Discrimination

In addition to developing the sort of critical thinking about premature use of genetic technologies that is outlined in the above section, consumers need to think through the problem of discrimination based on accurate (and inaccurate) genetic tests. Discrimination based on predisposition to a condition as serious as AD is not unusual.

Workplace Discrimination

It is easy to discriminate against people at risk for AD, especially in the workplace, where interests in both health insurance and in employee productivity collaborate against hiring a person with either a susceptibility gene or a predictive one. Although AD usually manifests after age sixty-five, many believe that deterioration may begin years earlier; moreover, employees frequently work until the age of seventy and beyond. The workplace is inevitably opposed to forgetfulness and possibly opposed as well to those who will in the future surely or possibly lose their cognitive capacities. In the workplace, productivity is the central value. People who will become too forgetful may be treated precedently as mere "throw-outs" (de Beauvoir 1972, 6).

Perhaps the first context in which AD genetic testing will be required is in the workplace. This idea, sometimes designated as "employment screening" or "workplace testing," originated with the British biologist J. B. S. Haldane in his publication *Heredity and Politics* (1938). The idea became influential in the 1960s, as professionals in occupational safety and health began to seriously consider the benefits of testing for adult-onset diseases (Stokinger and Mountain 1963). Today, some American companies are doing genetic testing, and more plan to do so.

Elevated medical costs associated with diabetes, various cancers, heart disease, high blood pressure, and other diseases increasingly encourage employers to test. As yet, workplace genetic testing is rare, but a U.S. survey conducted in 1990 indicates that if affordable testing for common adult- and late-onset diseases becomes easily available, some companies are inclined to implement it (Gostin 1991; Office of Technology Assessment 1991).

Societal Discrimination

The potential for discrimination against people who carry a predictive or a risk gene for AD is most obvious in the workplace. But there are wider possibilities for discrimination of a more general nature. Our culture values rationality and memory, the cardinal values of modern technological societies. People with dementia are easily excluded from the sphere of human dignity and respect (both in their own self-perception, if competent, and in societal perception).

Older people have already been stripped of their classic generative teaching roles in modern industrialized societies, where we tend to look for wisdom in the latest computer software (Bianchi 1990). When theologian Jonathan Swift described the demented "struldbrugs" in *Gulliver's Travels,* people with "no remembrance of anything but what they learned and observed in their youth and middle age, and even that is very imperfect," he indicated that "they are despised and hated by all sorts of people" (Swift 1945, 214-16). Swift was a strong advocate for people with dementia, and he insisted on their proper care despite the fact that many people are repelled by old age to begin with and utterly horrified at the degeneration of the person with AD from some ideal image of human fulfillment.

Exactly what forms this repulsion might take in the lives of those who carry a gene for AD is hard to predict; it is to be hoped that it will have no social manifestation at all. We need to recognize that we are all to some greater or lesser extent demented from the point in young adulthood when the human brain reaches its highest power. Moreover, we will all become somewhat demented because memory normally declines with aging, so the line between "them," who are demented, and "us," who are not, blurs.

Nevertheless, people with AD have been treated as social "throw-outs." For example, between 1940 and 1945 an inconspicuous agency in Nazi Germany operated from offices in Berlin at Tiergartenstrasse 4. The T-4 Project, begun in 1939 and concluded in 1941, was directed by the Wurzburg professor of psychiatry Werner Heyde. An estimated ninety-four thousand psychiatric patients were killed, some in gas chambers, others in psychiatric hospitals and sanatoriums with overdoses of sedatives. A considerable number of those killed were demented, although the exact proportion is unknown (Muller-Hill 1988). People with dementia were dubbed "useless eaters" who wasted precious national resources.

While human experimentation is clearly not the most important area where people with dementia are being harmed, it can be mentioned that Jay Katz devoted the first chapter of his classic *Experimentation with Human Beings* (1972) to the Jewish Chronic Disease Hospital case. In July 1963, three physician researchers from Sloan Kettering injected live cancer cells subcutaneously into twenty-two chronically ill and senile patients at Brooklyn's Jewish Chronic Disease Hospital. The physicians did not inform these human guinea pigs that live cancer cells—potentially deadly material—were being used. A number of these subjects were obviously demented. The purpose of the experiment was to measure immune response and see if the cells would take hold and grow or would be rejected, which was more likely.

Carrying a gene for AD will surely not enable discrimination to the same degree that the vulnerable condition of severe dementia can and does. Yet it is important for consumers to be aware that a genetic marker for AD may elicit some of the same social scorn as the disease condition itself. As chapter 10 in this volume indicates, there is every reason to think that discrimination will occur in the context of private long-term-care insurance and actuarial assessment more broadly.

Would not the value of the person with dementia be interpreted differently in a culture that could see worth in things other than purposeful rational activity? As Michel Foucault argues, before the seventeenth century unreason was considered not a menace but a part of everyday medieval life, as "fools" walked the streets and were even considered holy recipients of a special grace liberating them from the pains of the world and from unhappiness. But unreason became a scandal and a threat in the age of reason, allowing a sharp segregation between "them" and "us" (Foucault 1965).

Self-Discrimination

But even with such a realization in society, people who carry an AD gene may discriminate against their own continued existence through preemptive suicide based on a genetic test. They may fear dementia as much as or more than cancer (in cancer, self-identity is usually not at stake, and physical pain can in most cases be controlled without seriously compromising mental lucidity). On the other hand, people with AD reach a point where they "forget that they forget" and are then free at least from the anxiety of self-perceived loss of capacities. Nevertheless, those with a diagnosis of AD who are competent and insightful will sometimes indicate that pride in one's identity and capacities permits preemptive or surcease suicide before the onset of incompetence (Rhode, Peskind, and Raskind 1995).

Familial Discrimination

In families, memory is power. A remarkable amount of elder abuse and neglect falls upon people with dementia, not just because family caregivers are exhausted or ignorant but also because these people are easily victimized (Lucas 1991). In many focus groups I have attended, mildly affected AD patients indicate some concerns with the label "Alzheimer disease," because this categorizes them in a way that may limit their autonomy in relation to other family members. (Nevertheless, I strongly support diagnostic truth telling and the use of the AD label.)

People with dementia are a vulnerable population in some families and are in need of special protection from those without dementia who are capable of myriad abuses of power. There is in human nature what Nietzsche termed the "will to power," and this will on the part of the strong and rational to dominate and even harm weak and less rational people displays itself regularly. As Nietzsche wrote in 1888, combining elements of rationalism, social Darwinism, and eugenics, "the weak and ill-constituted shall perish: [it is the] first principle of our philosophy, and one shall help them to do so" (1968, 116).

People with dementia do not enjoy the privileged position that comes with being wiser and more experienced They have little or no knowledge left to convey to their children and grandchildren; they no longer are as intertwined with the familial community but rather have lost the memory of relationships, and they are, therefore, easily transgressed and abandoned.

Metaphors commonly heard in discussions of people with dementia by family members reveal values, for they capture our propensity to exclude from moral standing those who are below cognitive standards. Is the patient only a "shell" of his or her former self, a mere "husk"? Is the glass "half empty" (Howell 1984)? Ethically, there is much at stake in the family's metaphorical images of the experience of dementia, for these images will surely shape our response to this growing moral challenge. Shall we nurture the well-being of people with dementia, shall we give them a disrespectful and insensitive pseudocare, shall we efficiently dispatch them to a prompt death? Again, while family members with an AD gene are not vulnerable because of incapacitation, it is still important to underscore the possibility that predisposing genetic information may be used negatively in the political balance of familial power.

Summarizing the Problem of Discrimination

Regarding the possibilities for discrimination in the workplace, in society, and in the family, these warnings are an echo of those by the Institute of Medicine, which stated the following:

> The committee therefore recommends caution in the use and interpretation of presymptomatic or predictive tests. The nature of these predictions will usually be probabilistic (i.e., with a certain degree of likelihood of occurrence) and not deterministic (not definite, settled, or without doubt). The dangers of stigmatization and discrimination are areas of concern, as is the potential for harm due to inappropriate preventive or therapeutic measures. (Andrews et al. 1994, 9)

Clear prediction is rare, and much education is necessary: "The benefits of the various presymptomatic interventions must be weighed against the potential anxiety, stigmatization, and other possible harms to individuals who are informed that they are at increased risk of developing future disease" (ibid).

Genetic findings are particularly sensitive because they often reveal wider information than other medical tests, impose the sometimes unwelcome disclosure of the individual's medical future and that of family members, and can result in serious potential adverse consequences affecting employment and insurability (Powers 1994). Ultimately, such information has the potential of creating a social stratification dividing those relatively free from genetic predispositions to disease from those who are burdened by unemployment as the result of susceptibilities that are perceived to have an impact on job performance and safety.

Before genetic therapies are achieved, and before other interventions are developed based on insights gained from the detection of disease-related genes, the current major product of genome mapping is more information about the individual's genetic predispositions. This raises the possibility of preventive measures for some potentially disease-affected families and groups. However, the information could be used to label individuals as susceptible to disease. Without adequate safeguards, the adverse results can include loss of health insurance in jurisdictions without government-supported universal coverage, as well as loss of employment and opportunity.

Genetic information about any individual should always be guarded with strict confidentiality, protecting individual privacy categorically against potential discrimination (Annas 1995). In 1983, a president's commission was formed in the United States to review the ethical and legal aspects of medicine. In a report issued from the commission, three areas of concern are discussed regarding confidentiality: disclosure of information to third parties such as employers and insurers; access to material stored in databases; and disclosure of information to relatives of the tested individual to either advise them of risks or to gain a more accurate diagnosis of the person tested (President's Commission 1983, 42). The report warns that because of potential misuse, "information from genetic testing should be given to people such as insurers or employers only with the explicit consent of the person screened" (ibid., 42).

With regard to relatives, the commission emphasized that the matter of confidentiality becomes more complex if the disease tested for can be prevented. Then, genetic counselors or medical geneticists would have strong grounds to inform the counselee's family members. Most counselees would readily consent to having relatives contacted or would do this themselves. But this is not always the case. The grounds for setting aside confidentiality are weak when the disorder cannot be treated but compelling when symptoms can be significantly reduced or perhaps, in future years, even prevented.

Lowering Demand: Consumer Education in Limited Benefits

Family members of people with AD place considerable hope in genetic testing. From the context of direct predictive genetic testing for Huntington disease (HD), an unpreventable and fatal disease, it was learned that "most individuals at risk in the general population will not participate in predictive testing for an untreatable late-onset genetic disorder if the cloning of the gene has no immediate impact on approaches to therapy" (Babul, Adam, and Kremer 1993, 2324). In Canada, for example, fewer than 20 percent of persons at risk for HD entered the predictive linkage testing program (ibid.). In the absence of preventive therapies, the only use for testing is in life planning, and this is not enough of a rationale for many. Not only is the actual interest in HD testing quite limited, but also the benefits of it are questionable, although some genetic counselors have attempted to make a case for enhanced psychological well-being, whatever the test results (Wiggins et al. 1992). The study suggests that knowing the result of predictive testing, even if risk is decreased, "reduces uncertainty and provides an opportunity for appropriate planning" (ibid., 1404). Testing, then, supposedly frees people from the anxiety of uncertainty.

Nontesters such as Nancy Wexler are committed to having the option of testing available. Wexler, a psychologist at risk for HD, was instrumental in identifying the genetic marker for the disease through organizing studies of a large Venezuelan pedigree. Yet Wexler herself, after years of scientific leadership and public statements about the anxiety attached to every simple clumsy act as though it were the beginning of disease, has not been linkage tested; neither has she requested direct testing. Wexler's father, a psychoanalyst, believes that it is inhumane to tell someone that he or she will die an early and terrible death when there is no treatment available (Pence 1990, 310).

In AD genetic testing, the demand in presymptomatic individuals in the early-onset families (chromosomes 1, 14, and 21) may be much lower than anticipated. It is too early to predict whether, and to what extent, the members of the autosomal-dominant early-onset families will pursue genetic testing. Many individuals in these families are aware of the specific inheritance pattern that applies to their families. The relief of knowing that one will be spared the disease may be substantial. As with HD, the majority of persons at risk may not want testing in the absence of cure or prevention.

As an example of low demand, sixty individuals in an early-onset (autosomal-dominant) AD family in Sweden were informed of the presymptomatic testing option; only three of them wished to pursue testing. The one subject found to have the mutation reacted with depressive feelings and suicidal ideation after learning his status. The other two subjects were free of the disease-causing mutation and expressed relief. The authors concluded that testing must be handled cautiously (Lannfelt et al. 1995).

Consumers from the Cleveland Area Alzheimer's Association focus groups were not at all interested in testing that could not provide them with a reasonably clear prediction of the onset of AD at a certain stage of their lives, since otherwise no revision of life plans would make sense (e.g., retiring early to travel widely before the onset of AD). One adult woman with considerable late-onset AD in her family stated, "I have accepted that AD may well affect me. There isn't much that can change that. You prepare for your children's future anyway with this possibility in mind, so a vague genetic test wouldn't make any difference to me. Everyone has a fifty-fifty chance of getting AD if they live long enough. What good would come from testing when it can't really help you to make plans and when there are no preventions?" A man in his late sixties stated that he had asked for "the genetic test" when he was having concentration problems and couldn't read well. However, he realized that what he really needed was a general diagnostic workup.

Predictive testing for those very few people with early-onset AD (these families are extremely rare and are well aware of the prevalence of AD in their families in middle age or even earlier) does give clear information and is beneficial in both diminishing the fear of AD in those who do not carry the gene (chromosome 1, 14, or 19) and allowing reliable life planning to occur. But this testing is irrelevant to people concerned with AD in its usual (99% of cases) late-onset form.

Conclusions

The physician's lament over the public's misunderstanding of the role of genetic testing for AD is, at its core, a concern about public trust in medical science and the prevention of considerable harm (Turney 1996). Our focus groups representing the AD-affected population and our physician colleagues indicate that further educational efforts are imperative, particularly because so much misinformation in AD genetics has been disseminated.

References

Andrews, L. B., Fullarton, J. E., Holtzman, N. A., and Motulsky, A. G. 1994. *Assessing genetic risks: Implications for health and social policy.* Washington, D.C.: National Academy Press.

Annas, G. J. 1995. Genetic prophecy and genetic privacy: Can we prevent the dream from becoming a nightmare? *American Journal of Public Health* 85:1196–97.

Babul, R., Adam, S., and Kremer, B. 1993. Attitudes toward direct predictive testing for the Huntington disease gene. *JAMA* 270:2321–25.

Bianchi, E. C. 1990. *Aging as a spiritual journey.* New York: Crossroad.

Blumenthal, D. 1992. Academic-industry relationships in the life sciences: Extent, consequences, and management. *JAMA* 268:3344–49.

———. 1994. Growing pains for new academic/industry relationships. *Health Affairs* 13:176–93.

Butler, R. N. 1994. ApoE: New risk factor for Alzheimer's: Potential is real for abuse in genetic testing for susceptibility to dementia. *Geriatrics* 49:10–11.

de Beauvoir, S. 1972. *Old age.* London: Andre Deutsch.

Foley, J. M. 1993. Marginal to useless medications. *Centerviews* 7 (2): 1, 4.

Foucault, M. 1965. *Madness and civilization: A history of insanity in the Age of Reason.* Trans. R. Howard. New York: Vintage Books.

Gostin, L. 1991. Genetic discrimination: The use of genetically based diagnostic and prognostic tests by employers and insurers. *American Journal of Law and Medicine* 17:109–144.

Haldane, J. B. S. 1938. *Heredity and politics.* New York: W. W. Norton.

Howell, M. 1984. Caretakers' views on responsibilities for the care of the demented elderly. *Journal of the American Geriatrics Society* 32:657–60.

Hubbard, R., and Wald, E. 1993. *Exploding the gene myth.* Boston: Beacon Press.

Katz, J. 1972. *Experimentation with human beings.* New York: Russell Sage Foundation.

Knoppers, B. M. 1991. Human dignity and genetic heritage. Paper prepared for the Law Reform Commission of Canada, Ottawa.

Lannfelt, L., Axelman, K., Lilius, L., and Bason, H. 1995. Genetic counseling of a Swedish Alzheimer family with amyloid precursor protein mutation. *American Journal of Human Genetics* 56:332–35.

Lucas, E. T. 1991. *Elder abuse and its recognition among health service professionals.* New York: Garland.

Miringoff, M.-L. 1991. *The social costs of genetic welfare.* New Brunswick: Rutgers University Press.

Muller-Hill, B. 1988. *Murderous science: Elimination by scientific selection of Jews, Gypsies, and others: Germany, 1933–1945.* Trans. G. R. Fraser. New York: Oxford University Press.

Nelkin, D., and Lindee, M. S. 1995. *The DNA mystique: The gene as a cultural icon.* New York: W. H. Freeman.

Nietzsche, F. 1968. *Twilight of the idols/The Anti-Christ.* Trans. R. J. Hollingdale. New York: Penguin Books.

Office of Technology Assessment. 1991. *Medical monitoring and screening in the workplace: Result of a survey.* Washington, D.C.: U.S. Government Printing Office.

Pence, G. 1990. *Classic cases in medical ethics.* New York: McGraw-Hill.

Powers, M. 1994. Privacy and the control of genetic information. In *The genetic frontier: Ethics, law, and policy,* ed. M. S. Frankel and A. Teich, 77–100. Washington, D.C.: American Association for the Advancement of Science.

President's Commission for the Study of Ethical Problems in Medicine and Biomedical and Behavioral Research. 1983. *Screening and counseling for genetic conditions: A report on the ethical, social, and legal implications of genetic screening, counseling, and education programs.* Washington, D.C.: U.S. Government Printing Office.

Rhode, K., Peskind, E. R., and Raskind, M. A. 1995. Suicide in two patients with Alzheimer's disease. *Journal of the American Geriatrics Society* 43:187–89.

Rodwin, M. A. 1993. *Medicine, money, and morals.* New York: Oxford University Press.

Stokinger, H. E., and Mountain, J. T. 1963. Tests for hypersusceptibility to hemolytic chemicals. *Archives of Environmental Health* 6:57–64.

Swift, J. [1727] 1945. *Gulliver's travels.* Garden City, N.Y.: Doubleday.

Thompson, D. F. 1993. Understanding financial conflicts of interest. *New England Journal of Medicine* 329:573–76.

Turney J. 1996. Public understanding of science. *Lancet* 347:1087–90.

Wiggins, S., Whyte, P., Huggins, M., Shelin, A., Theilmann, J., Bloch, M., Sheps, S. B., Schechter, M. T., and Hayden, M. R. 1992. The psychological consequences of predictive testing for Huntington's disease. *New England Journal of Medicine* 327:1401–5.

Alzheimer Genetics and the Primary Care Physician

GREG A. SACHS, M.D.

In recent decades, genetic information within medicine has primarily been the province of a small group of specially trained professionals whose careers have been devoted to medical genetics or genetic counseling. Indeed, most individuals or families receiving genetics services until now have probably interacted with a team of professionals in a genetics center. Most genetic counselors have entered the field since 1970 and have been trained by programs granting master's degrees. These genetic counselors receive training not only in the science of genetics but also in disciplines such as communication, psychology, and education, enabling genetic counselors to be the primary professionals communicating with patients and families about genetics. Genetic counseling has been defined as

> a communication process which deals with the human problems associated with the occurrence, or the risk of occurrence, of a genetic disorder in a family. This process involves an attempt by one or more appropriately trained persons to help the individual or family to (1) comprehend the medical facts, including the diagnosis, probable course of the disorder, and the available management; (2) appreciate the way heredity contributes to the disorder, and the risk of recurrence in specified relatives; (3) understand the alternatives for dealing with the risk of recurrence; (4) choose the course of action which seems to them appropriate in view of their risk, their family goals, and their ethical and religious standards, and to act in accordance with that decision; and (5) to make the best possible adjustment to the disorder in an affected family member and/or to the risk of recurrence of that disorder. (American Society of Human Genetics 1975, 240-41)

In this model of genetic counseling, there is an emphasis on education of the client, nondirectiveness (i.e., avoiding influencing any specific course of action), and reproductive decision making. Until now, most of the disorders discussed with genetic counselors have been relatively rare diseases with catastrophic impact on affected children. This kind of genetic counseling is a time and labor intensive endeavor, often with multiple counseling sessions both before and after genetic information is obtained.

Genetics Moving into Primary Care

It is clear that this classic model of genetic counseling will not remain the primary way in which people receive genetic health information, for several reasons. First, the number of people at risk for illnesses that we now know to have genetic influences, and to be potentially in need of counseling, far exceeds the capacity of genetic counselors. Even before the Human Genome Project began uncovering large numbers of disease-associated genes in the early 1990s, concerns had been expressed about the adequacy of the supply of genetics professionals in the United States. It has been estimated that it would take all of the genetic counselors in the United States seventeen weeks of their time each year just to do the counseling necessary for population screening for cystic fibrosis of about six million to eight million potential child-bearing couples (Wilfond and Fost 1990). If there are four million people affected by Alzheimer disease in the United States, each with multiple relatives, one can see how classic genetic counselors would have to do AD genetic counseling, and nothing but that, all year round.

Second, the genetic tests themselves have changed greatly. Early genetic testing and counseling often involved detailed pedigree mapping, laborious linkage analysis with samples obtained from multiple relatives, and technically difficult assays. Today, many genetic tests look directly for specific alleles or mutations, can be done on a single individual's blood sample, and may be relatively easy and inexpensive to perform. Apolipoprotein E (APOE) typing, for example, can be carried out for only a few dollars by most laboratories that do lipid analysis. Indeed, automation of tests raises the possibility that several genetic tests might be conducted on a single blood sample, so-called multiplex testing, much in the same way that physicians order a battery of chemistry tests now.

Third, once diagnostic and therapeutic products are available, clinicians tend to use them. This is seen in the common practice of physicians prescribing approved medications for new indications that have not been officially sanctioned, and a similar pattern has emerged in the use of many genetic tests. A combination of consumer demand, economic forces, and professional concerns often leads to the use of a genetic test even when uncertainty exists about the appropriate use of the test. Wilfond and Nolan (1993) describe the efforts of multiple professional organizations and governmental bodies to prevent widespread testing for cystic fibrosis carrier status once it became technically feasible to do the test. Apolipoprotein E testing is already available in the marketplace as an aid in confirming the diagnosis of AD in patients with dementia, so it would not be surprising if practicing clinicians were to be found ordering this test either as a diagnostic tool or as a predictive test in an asymptomatic person despite the caveats about such use.

Fourth, rare diseases affecting children and reproductive decision making were the mainstay of early genetic counseling, and pediatricians and obstetricians were the clinicians most likely to need to work with geneticists and genetic counselors. Today, the genes being identified are associated with adult-onset diseases, such as diabetes, cancer, and AD, that are the province of primary care physicians such as general internists and family practitioners. Finally, the movement within American medicine favoring generalism over specialty care, the rise of managed care, and efforts to decrease costs all further increase the likelihood that primary care physicians will be the professionals expected to provide genetic testing and related services to patients. (One wonders if most patients with AD with a typical course will, in the future, be evaluated by neurologists in managed care practices.) Thus, it is reasonable to assume that primary care physicians will need to know how to handle AD genetic testing in their offices or clinics. The next question is, how prepared are primary care physicians to handle this responsibility?

Genetic Preparedness of Primary Care Physicians

It turns out that only a small amount of empirical information is available on the current state of the genetic knowledge and skills of primary care physicians. Only a few studies have been conducted in the last two decades on primary care physician knowledge of genetics (Firth and Lindenbaum 1992; Hofman et al. 1993; Kapur et al. 1983; Lemkus, Van der Merwe, and Opt Hof 1978). Most of these have looked at physicians' knowledge of principles of genetics or at specific illnesses, such as cystic fibrosis. The most comprehensive of these, by Hofman and colleagues, found general internists and family physicians least knowledgeable of the physicians surveyed, though there was a tendency for the most recently educated physicians, who were more likely to have been required to take a genetics course in medical school, to be the most knowledgeable (Hofman et al. 1993). One survey of neurologists, geriatricians, and other physicians caring for patients with AD (a total of 125 physicians) found a minority of respondents (42%) were able to accurately estimate the lifetime risk of AD for a typical individual, and even fewer could accurately estimate the affect of having an APOE ε4 allele on that lifetime risk (Seshadri, Drachman, and Lippa 1995).

We know even less about primary care physicians' skills in interacting with patients and families around genetic testing for any disease, let alone for AD. Holtzman and colleagues did use vignettes and questions to examine primary care physicians' attitudes toward confidentiality and other issues (Geller, Tambor, Bernhardt, et al. 1993; Geller, Tambor, Chase, et al. 1993). Their results raised interesting and important concerns about such things as physicians' comfort with doing genetic counseling themselves, their willingness to provide genetic information to third parties or family members, and their tendency to be more directive in counseling than genetics professionals.

It is easy to understand why primary care physicians would appear to be ill prepared today to take on the responsibility of AD genetic testing. Genetics has not been a major part of undergraduate medical education. While surveys of medical schools have looked at and expressed concern about the amount of genetics present in curricula since at least 1975, there have not been dramatic improvements. Riccardi and Schmickel (1988) found little change in genetics content of medical school curricula between 1975 and 1985. A review of the American Association of Medical Colleges database in 1991 suggests there has been more genetics teaching in the most recent years (AAMC 1991).

The typical genetics course in medical school, however, remains something that is taught in the first or second (preclinical) year of medical, is most likely to be taught by pediatricians, and averages only thirty hours in length. Genetics is not typically integrated into the clinical training years of medical students. On the graduate education or residency training level, genetics is not even a minor part of training in the primary care disciplines of medicine and family medicine. (The field of obstetrics and gynecology has the most developed standards, with a core curriculum of educational objectives for its trainees.) In the case of practicing primary care physicians, one also must keep in mind that they are attempting to keep up with the burgeoning wealth of information on all of primary care medicine, with genetics and AD only a fraction of what they must try to incorporate. Indeed, because few fields are moving faster than AD genetics—in 1990 no genes had been identified; by 1995 there were three genes linked to familial forms of AD and APOE linked to sporadic AD susceptibility—keeping up with AD alone is a substantial task. In addition, the frontline medical literature focuses mostly on new techniques, identification of new genes, and prospects for treatment. Little is mentioned about the complex ethical, legal, and social aspects of genetic testing or the practical aspects of speaking with individuals and families about genetics.

From examining the standards of classic genetic counseling and the current state of affairs with primary care physicians and genetics, it is clear that preparing physicians to handle AD genetic testing in practice will be quite a challenge. In what follows I outline in more detail some of the critical challenges for preparing primary care physicians for genetic testing in general, as well as the specific challenges represented by AD genetic testing above and beyond that.

General Challenges for Genetics in Primary Care

Several challenges relating to any genetic testing within primary care are likely to be present with AD genetic testing, too. These can be divided into the broad areas of scientific knowledge or content, counseling skills, and the time pressures of primary care practice.

As described briefly above, what is known scientifically about genetics is growing rapidly, and it is crucial that physicians keep up with the latest information. This includes physicians developing or refining their abilities to critically appraise the literature. "The truth" about AD genetic testing is not something that is published in one journal article and then set in stone. Developments have moved in fits and starts, and there is often considerable controversy within the field of experts on "the facts." For example, depending on what articles a physician reads and when he or she reads them, a clinician might conclude that an APOE ϵ4 allele substantially increases the lifetime risk of AD, although in fact that risk remains less than 30 percent (Seshadri, Drachman, and Lippa 1995), or that someone with an ϵ4 allele has more than a 50 percent chance of developing AD. Continuing and critical self-education will be essential.

There are several things that physicians can learn from the classic genetic counseling model in developing their own skills for counseling. The principle of nondirectiveness in genetic counseling is something that physicians most need to learn about. Nondirectiveness refers to the way in which a genetic counselor deliberately avoids telling the client that one option for action is preferred. This is evident in the American Society of Human Genetics' description of genetic counseling, quoted in part at the beginning of this chapter, indicating that the course of action will depend on the client's views of risk, his or her goals, and his or her ethical and religious beliefs. Even today, physicians are most often in a directive mode of interaction with patients, telling patients not to smoke, to lose weight, to take a medicine, or to undergo a test (e.g., "You need a mammogram"). Geller and colleagues found in their survey that primary care physicians were much more likely than geneticists or genetic counselors to advise a family to pursue a specific action in response to a genetic testing and reproductive decision-making scenario (Geller, Tambor, Chase, et al. 1993). It seems likely that the emotionally charged issue of abortion, and the discomfort created by putting a health professional in the position of saying that an abortion should or should not be done, helped emphasize nondirectiveness in genetics counseling.

Some commentators have argued that the notion of nondirectiveness has been exaggerated or overplayed in the genetics counseling field, that either counselors are more directive than they think or claim to be or counselors should be more willing to be directive (Kessler 1992; Yarborough, Scott, and Dixon 1989). Importantly, physicians are already learning to be less directive in other arenas where the values and beliefs of patients are the critical factors in medical decision making, such as decisions to limit life-sustaining treatment near the end of life. In addition, it may turn out that for the right kind of genetic screening, where preventive treatments or increased surveillance would greatly benefit patients with a certain genotype, one might desire a physician who aggressively advocates genetic screening. Mammograms are generally considered a good thing by most people because they are effective screening tools, helping reduce mortality from breast cancer. The single most-often-cited variable in studies examining factors influencing the likelihood of a woman's getting a mammogram is having a physician recommend the test (Fox, Murata, and Stein 1991). The general challenge for physicians, as well as for genetic counselors, will be determining when it becomes appropriate to be more directive.

Another area in which physicians can face a general challenge regarding genetic testing is the communication of risk. In particular, many physicians appear to have considerable difficulty with quantifying risk and with sharing uncertainty in their conversations with patients (Katz 1984; MacKay 1991). Physicians often use vague terms, such as "often," "infrequent," or "rare," when quantifying risk for patients. These terms imply different frequencies of occurrence to different physicians, and this is compounded by patients, likewise, interpreting these phrases to indicate a broad range of numbers. Physicians have been criticized for this practice and could learn something from genetic counselors here, too. Genetic counselors tend to express the risk of a condition in more precise numerical terms, such as one in twenty-five hundred for the risk of a genetic illness or one in two hundred for the risk of a bad outcome for a procedure. Physicians also have been criticized for being unwilling to appear uncertain, to share with patients the uncertainty that is as much a part of medical practice as of any other human endeavor. (On the other hand, even genetic counselors, if they wanted to be totally forthcoming about uncertainty, would have to disclose that all of the point estimates given for occurrences or events have a confidence interval around them or a range of values based on several studies.)

The debates around the use of genetic screening for cystic fibrosis and BRCA1 for breast cancer suggest that, as with AD, there may be a difference of opinion as to how to deal with uncertainty in the early stages of a genetic test becoming available. One can argue that the uncertainty is so great that the genetic test should not be made available or that testing should be provided but accompanied by a great deal of counseling and education and a great number of caveats. While this may sound like the kind of decision that has to be made on the public policy level, it really can be a decision for an individual primary care physician, as with individual physicians offering BRCA1 testing for breast cancer before a consensus is reached that enough is known to counsel patients about its use (Kolata 1996).

Another aspect of genetic testing related to sharing uncertainty is the complexity of diseases that have their onset well into adult life. Most adult-onset disorders such as type II diabetes, cancer, and heart disease simply do not fit the "Gene for Disease X Found" headlines that typify the American public's understanding of genetics. These late-onset diseases are likely to be influenced by multiple genes and multiple environmental factors. The genes being discovered for these diseases affect the probability that an individual will get the diseases, but it is a probability that is likely to be modified by the presence or absence of other genes, exposure to environmental toxins (including cigarette smoking), diet, exercise, other illnesses, and medications.

In fact, an environmental factor like cigarette smoking may prove to be more influential than any gene in determining whether or not lung cancer develops, for example. Many commentators have raised this concern about excessive attention being paid to genetics, along with the warning about genetic determinism or even "the gene as a cultural icon" (Nelkin and Lindee 1995). For genetic testing to become part of the practice of primary care physicians, the complexity of late-onset disorders and the simplistic level of public understanding will be a major challenge. In addition, this state of affairs reminds one that many practicing physicians who completed their training before genetics had even begun to be taught in medical schools may have an understanding of genetics that is not that much more sophisticated than that of the general public.

Many ethical challenges discussed at length in the literature represent challenges to primary care physicians taking on genetic testing. These include topics such as privacy and confidentiality and discrimination. To some extent, primary care physicians are well versed in the strict confidentiality of the doctor-patient relationship. Rarely would a physician breach that confidentiality, and then only for extenuating circumstances involving potential harm to other identified parties (Bayer and Toomey 1992; Tarasoff v. Regents of the University of California [1976], 17 Cal. 3d 334).

Genetic testing, however, brings up new dilemmas with respect to privacy and confidentiality, especially for primary care physicians, such as family practitioners, who may care for multiple individuals within a single family. When a genetic test provides information about one individual in the family, it simultaneously provides information about that person's parents, siblings, children, and other blood relatives. This information is then known to the primary care physician, even if it has not been disclosed to the other pertinent parties. If, for example, a forty-five-year old woman with a family history of breast cancer (mother and maternal aunt both have the disease) undergoes testing for BRCA1 and is found to have the gene, that woman's family physician now knows something new and important about the risk of breast cancer in that woman's eighteen-year-old daughter and her forty-one-year-old sister, both of whom are patients of the same physician. Genetic counselors routinely face such issues of confidentiality, but they do so without the fiduciary responsibility that the physician has to the other family members. Some physicians confront similar issues (the psychiatrist seeing a patient who threatens another individual or the internist seeing an HIV-infected individual who refuses to disclose that status to a partner), but genetic testing will make these issues commonplace for many physicians who have not struggled regularly with confidentiality dilemmas before.

Finally, another challenge to primary care physicians that will affect all genetic testing, and essentially all of medical care, is the demand on physicians' time, the pressure to see more and more patients in less and less time. One can imagine that physicians and patients alike will function in more of a triage mode, attending to acute complaints, potentially life-threatening or serious problems, and cost-effective preventive measures in the limited time available for a visit. Little time will be left over for genetic testing, let alone the kind of detailed and lengthy discussions that make up traditional genetic counseling sessions.

This very practical consideration has led, in part, two leading figures in the field of genetics policy to propose that primary care physicians obtain a "generic consent" for genetic screening, allowing patients to give a single permission to a battery of genetic tests for related diseases after hearing a brief description of the nature of that battery (Elias and Annas 1994). These authors made the analogy to the permission that a patient gives for a physical exam, allowing the physician to do a number of discrete examinations that have varying test performances, without hearing about each maneuver. Physicians do not tell patients about the sensitivity, specificity, and positive and negative predictive values of the cardiac exam for coronary disease and congestive heart failure, the lung exam for obstructive lung disease, the thyroid exam for thyroid nodules, and so on. (I suspect patients would either refuse to be examined or have no time left for an examination after such a lengthy disclosure.) An Institute of Medicine committee, on the other hand, urged caution regarding such "multiplex testing" for multifactorial illnesses with onset in adult life (Andrews et al. 1994, 275–76). It remains to be seen how genetic testing and counseling of any degree can fit into a busy primary care practice.

Special Challenges for Alzheimer Disease Genetics: The Complexities

Regarding scientific knowledge, Alzheimer disease presents one of the clearest examples of how much education a primary care physician will need in order to facilitate informed decision making around genetic testing. The first issue that a primary care physician needs to understand concerns the heterogeneity of Alzheimer disease genetics and the nonexistence of an "Alzheimer gene" for which patients can be tested. As described elsewhere in this text, several genes are linked to Alzheimer disease, and they can be grossly separated into those implicated in cases of familial Alzheimer disease, with early onset and an autosomal-dominant pattern of inheritance, and the APOE gene, which confers an increased susceptibility to the more common, later-onset Alzheimer disease. Thus, the physician needs to know which test or tests even to consider ordering when dealing with a particular patient or family. Clearly, it would not make much sense to consider tests for presenilin 1, presenilin 2, and amyloid precursor protein mutations in a patient who has no family history of Alzheimer disease and is presenting for evaluation at age eighty. Conversely, although the test for APOE is the only AD genetic test on the market at the time of this writing, it would be inappropriate to order this test and not the other tests for a patient with symptoms of dementia at age forty-five and with multiple family members with onset before age sixty. As in most areas in medicine, one cannot simply order tests; there is no substitute for taking a complete history, and this includes a good family history.

Alzheimer disease differs from most other illnesses because of the way in which the timing or context of the test has become a controversial and important consideration. By this, I am referring to the distinction between Alzheimer disease genetic testing as predictive testing and as diagnostic testing (Bird 1995; Roses 1995). Before discussing this further, it is worth noting that this distinction simply does not arise for many diseases, because genetic testing does not play a role in arriving at a diagnosis. The diagnosis of cancer is determined by the presence of certain characteristics on a biopsy specimen, the diagnosis of diabetes is determined by the presence of an elevated serum glucose, the diagnosis of coronary artery disease by blockages seen on a coronary angiogram, and so on. A diagnosis of AD is based on the presence of multiple historical and clinical features and the absence of others — almost a diagnosis by exclusion.

Indeed, the diagnosis that physicians are giving to patients in practice when they diagnose Alzheimer disease is called either "probable AD" or "possible AD" by research criteria. The diagnostic label of probable AD is also only about 85 to 90 percent accurate when the definitive diagnosis is confirmed at autopsy. This is a whole additional level of uncertainty surrounding AD, and I am not aware of any information as to how well this uncertainty is communicated to patients and families. Thus, Alzheimer disease is in the minority of diseases in which current methods for diagnosis are sufficiently uncertain or imprecise that consideration is given to whether or not genetic testing improves diagnostic accuracy. Genetic testing for most other diseases focuses on predictive testing, whether it is for genes that determine that a patient will definitely get the disease or for genes that confer an increased risk for the disease.

For many primary care physicians, understanding the sometimes subtle differences between the use of the identical genetic test in predictive testing versus diagnostic testing will be quite a challenge. When the situation involves a clinically unaffected person in a family thought to be harboring one of the early-onset, familial forms of Alzheimer disease, the primary care physician will need to be able to operate in a counseling mode that most resembles what is done now for Huntington disease, the kind of classic counseling for an autosomal-dominant disease that cannot be treated. In evaluating a seventy-five-year-old patient with no known family history who satisfies clinical criteria for the diagnosis of dementia, the clinician will have to function more in the mode of a diagnostician who understands Bayes's theorem, pretest and posttest probabilities for a test in different settings, and the incremental diagnostic value of a genetic test, something quite different from classic genetic counseling. To see how challenging this can be, one need only look at the overlapping and confusing language used to describe diagnostic testing and genetic testing. A recent report focusing on the use of APOE in diagnosing AD in someone with dementia correctly describes the *positive predictive value* of this *diagnostic* test (Saunders et al. 1996).

While none of the major groups making position statements on the use of APOE testing has supported using it as a predictive test in asymptomatic individuals, once more complete and reliable data are available, such a use will be considered more closely. In the case of a healthy individual asking for APOE screening as a predictive test, the primary care physician will have to shift into yet another mode of discussing AD genetic testing. Here, the clinician will have to understand and be able to discuss the notion of a gene that confers increased susceptibility, including the concept that having this gene is neither sufficient nor necessary to cause the disease. This susceptibility will have to be understood and communicated as something that even varies with the age at which someone has the test done. The physician and patient will have to know that whether they test for them or not, the patient is probably carrying other genes that put him or her at risk for various kinds of cancer, heart disease, or other illnesses that may act as a competing cause of morbidity or mortality. That is, the patient who comes concerned about AD may die from something else before reaching the age at which he or she is likely to develop AD. In properly discussing a susceptibility gene, appropriate attention must be given to interactions with other genes (Kamboh et al. 1995) and the environment (Andersen, Launer, and Ott 1995; Birge 1996; Stern et al. 1994), areas that are just beginning to be explored in AD.

For the time being, in addition to handling the complexities of multiple AD genes, predictive versus diagnostic testing, and determinative versus susceptibility genes, primary care physicians must become adept at communicating with patients and families about a disease that cannot be effectively treated (Quill and Townsend 1991). Delivering bad news to patients and families is a task that physicians do not always handle well, and AD, whether the risk of it in the future or the diagnosis of it now, remains very bad news. Unlike screening for genetic susceptibility for some kinds of cancer, there is no diet, drug, or other preventive intervention available or increased surveillance that will benefit someone found to carry the offending gene. And while many are hopeful about the future for therapy against AD, the only approved drugs in the United States provide only small benefits for most patients.

Thus, even the interested physician who masters the aspects of genetic counseling needed for AD genetic testing must still become expert at giving the diagnosis for a condition that is progressive, devastating for families as well as patients, and eventually fatal. Importantly, this is where primary care physicians who will follow the patient and the family over the long haul of the illness are the most appropriate people to be involved in giving the diagnosis. The clinician can be sure to offer the patient and family ongoing care for symptoms and complications, help plan for the future, refer to support services, arrange for enrollment in research if that is desired, and ensure that no one feels abandoned.

Another complexity that is specific to AD genetic testing (and genetic testing for some other mental illnesses) is the impact of the disease on the consent process and confidentiality. The model of classic genetic counseling assumes a competent, cognitively intact client who consents to the testing. Certainly in the diagnostic setting for AD, depending on the severity of the dementia at the time, the patient for whom one may be asked to do the test may lack decision making capacity. This creates problems concerning who consents to the test, who is given the results of the test, how counseling is conducted with a person suffering from dementia, and even at what point genetic counseling is no longer feasible for the patient but still crucial for the family.

In addition, there is some evidence that APOE genotype may influence how a patient responds to drug therapy, with certain genotypes being more likely to benefit from a drug or more likely to develop adverse effects to a medication (Poirier et al. 1995). If these kinds of findings are replicated with tacrine, and other drugs as they become available, then genotyping will be done in the clinical setting to help physicians select a treatment for the patient. While this information may not have been obtained for a predictive purpose, the physician will nonetheless be in possession of information about susceptibility to AD of the patient's family members. Will physicians withhold this genetic information and simply tell family members that they are prescribing a particular drug because it will work best for that patient, or will they enter into discussions about predictive testing and all of its pitfalls?

Finally, another complexity of Alzheimer disease genetic testing arises from the potential availability of information on patients' APOE status from other sources. Most genes found to be associated with adult-onset illnesses have been newly identified, their location, structure, and function all unknown before their being found because of an association with a particular disease. Apolipoprotein E has the distinction of having been a known entity at the time that its association with AD was discovered, being one of many lipoproteins previously studied for its potential role in lipid metabolism and the development of coronary artery disease. Thus, a substantial number of people already had their APOE status determined before the scientific community knew about its link to AD. Some of these patients may now know their APOE status but not know how to interpret the rapidly advancing knowledge regarding its implications for their risk of AD. Since APOE has been used predominantly in research settings, unlike cholesterol testing, it has not proven useful enough to enter clinical practice. It is more likely that people who have had APOE testing for other reasons do not know their APOE status, although it is recorded somewhere in their medical record or separate research records held by investigators. Primary care physicians and investigators who come across the APOE test results face the difficult question of whether or not these individuals should be contacted and given the information.

Hope in Medical Education

At this point, I would expect that one would be convinced that preparing primary care physicians to incorporate genetic testing and counseling services into their practices is a fairly daunting task. Clearly, the educational effort needed to meet this challenge will have to occur at multiple levels of training, incorporate teaching about counseling skills as well as teaching the science of genetics, and address the complexities presented by AD genetics that add to the general difficulties surrounding all genetic testing for late-onset disorders. The Institute of Medicine's Committee on Assessing Genetic Risks provided an excellent series of recommendations on professional education in genetics, including the importance of developing continuing medical education programs in clinical genetics for primary care providers already out in practice (Andrews et al. 1994, 202–33).

Although I earlier cited studies that suggest the medical profession is currently ill prepared for this challenge, other studies are more hopeful. A study of medical students use of MEDLINE to search the medical literature demonstrates how new learning methods using computers can be used effectively in teaching clinical genetics (Proud, Johnson, and Mitchell 1993). A study of residents in obstetrics and gynecology found superior genetics test scores by those residents trained at institutions with a specific program in obstetrics-gynecology-genetics run by faculty board certified in clinical genetics (Kershner, Hammond, and Donnenfeld 1993). A pilot training program involving physicians who provide prenatal care (obstetricians and family practitioners) found that primary care providers completing the training counseled patients with hemoglobinopathies at the same rate, and with the same knowledge, as a tertiary care provider group (Rowley et al. 1995). A study in the United Kingdom demonstrated the feasibility of having general practitioners incorporate into their practices genetic counseling for cystic fibrosis at the first prenatal visit (Harris et al. 1993).

Finally, while skeptics might point out that most of the studies just cited focused on reproductive decision making and counseling and not the primary care physicians who see patients with AD, the body of literature on continuing medical education (CME) in general still suggests that these kinds of efforts can be successful. A review of fifty randomized controlled trials of CME interventions found that the majority of studies showed positive results (Davis et al. 1992). Importantly, the trials that focused on improving counseling and primary prevention practices all improved physician performance. Additional take-home points from this review of CME trials include the correlation between the intensity of the educational effort and the likelihood of success and the greater effectiveness of workshops (printed materials alone have a weak effect) and other methods that involve discussion and rehearsal of desired behaviors when compared with more traditional didactic programs. Interestingly, some of these trials involved reminders or other measures directed at patients. Indeed, some of the most effective CME trials combined interventions directed at both patients and doctors. This should emphasize the important role that public education on genetics can play in improving our ability to wisely handle genetic testing.

Conclusions

I would like to close this examination of the prospects for genetic testing for Alzheimer disease in the primary care setting with four observations or conclusions. First, it is highly likely that genetic testing for Alzheimer disease, as well as for most other adult-onset diseases, will become the province of primary care physicians such as family physicians and general internists. The combination of technological advances, personnel forces within medicine and genetics, and market forces all conspire in that direction. Second, AD presents some special challenges for any genetic counselor or primary care physician performing testing. These special challenges include the existence of a number of Alzheimer disease-related genes, genes that operate as single-gene disease-causing entities and others that modify susceptibility; the debate over predictive versus diagnostic testing; the lack of effective treatment; the impact of the disease on informed consent and counseling; and the availability of APOE results from testing done for other reasons. Third, at present, primary care physicians are poorly prepared to incorporate Alzheimer disease genetic testing into their practices. Finally, research on genetic training for other kinds of physicians and research on physician education in general both hold out the promise that these challenges can be met if our society chooses to rise to the occasion.

References

AAMC (Association of American Medical Colleges). 1991. *1991–1992 AAMC curriculum directory.* Washington, D.C.: AAMC.

American Society of Human Genetics. 1975. Genetic counseling (Ad Hoc Committee on Genetic Counseling). *American Journal of Human Genetics* 27:240–42.

Andersen, K., Launer, L. J., and Ott, A. 1995. Do nonsteroidal anti-inflammatory drugs decrease the risk for Alzheimer's disease? The Rotterdam study. *Neurology* 45:1441–45.

Andrews, L. B., Fullarton, J. E., Holtzman, N. A., and Motulsky, A. G., eds. 1994. *Assessing genetic risks: Implications for health and social policy.* Washington, D.C.: National Academy Press.

Bayer, R., and Toomey, K. E. 1992. HIV prevention and the two faces of partner notification. *American Journal of Public Health* 82:1158–64.

Bird, T. D. 1995. Apolipoprotein E genotyping in the diagnosis of Alzheimer's disease: A cautionary view. *Annals of Neurology* 38:2–4.

Birge, S. J. 1996. Is there a role for estrogen replacement therapy in the prevention and treatment of dementia? *Journal of the American Geriatric Society* 44:865–70.

Davis, D. A., Thomson, M. A., Oxman, A. D., and Haynes, R. B. 1992. Evidence for the effectiveness of CME: A review of fifty randomized controlled trials. *JAMA* 268:1111–17.

Elias, S., and Annas, G. J. 1994. Generic consent for genetic screening. *New England Journal of Medicine* 330:1611–13.

Firth, H., and Lindenbaum, R. 1992. U.K. clinicians' knowledge of and attitudes to the prenatal diagnosis of single-gene disorders. *Journal of Medical Genetics* 29:20–23.

Fox, S. A., Murata, P. J., and Stein, J. A. 1991. The impact of physician compliance on screening mammography for older women. *Archives of Internal Medicine* 151:50–56.

Geller, G. E., Tambor, E. S., Bernhardt, B. A., Chase, G. A., Hofman, K. J., Faden, R. R., and Holtzman, N. 1993. Physicians' attitudes toward disclosure of genetic information to third parties. *Journal of Law, Medicine, and Ethics* 21:238–40.

Geller, G., Tambor, E. S., Chase, G. A., Hofman, K. J., Faden, R. R., and Holtzman, N. A. 1993. Incorporation of genetics in primary care practice: Will physicians do the counseling and will they be directive? *Archives of Family Medicine* 2:1119–25.

Harris, H., Scotcher, D., Hartley, N., Wallace, A., Craufurd, D., and Harris, R. 1993. Cystic fibrosis carrier testing in early pregnancy by general practitioners. *British Medical Journal* 306:1580–83.

Hofman, K. J., Tambor, E. S., Chase, G. A., Geller, G., Faden, R. R., and Holtzman, N. A. 1993. Physicians' knowledge of genetics and genetic tests. *Academic Medicine* 68:625-32.

Kamboh, M. I., Sanghera, D. K., Ferrell, R. E., and DeKosky, S. T. 1995. APOE*4-associated Alzheimer's disease risk is modified by alpha 1-antichymotrypsin polymorphism. *Nature Genetics* 10:486-88.

Kapur, S., Higgins, J. V., Doughty, A., and Kallen, D. J. 1983. Medical practice and genetics in the mid-Michigan area. *Journal of Medical Education* 58:186-93.

Katz, J. 1984. *The silent world of doctor and patient*. New York: Free Press.

Kershner, M. A., Hammond, E. A., and Donnenfeld, A. E. 1993. Knowledge of genetics among residents in obstetrics and gynecology. *American Journal of Human Genetics* 53:1356-58.

Kessler, S. 1992. Psychological aspects of genetic counseling. Part 7, Thoughts on directiveness. *Journal of Genetic Counseling* 1:9-17.

Kolata, G. 1996. Breaking ranks, lab offers test to assess risk of breast cancer. *New York Times*, April 1.

Lemkus, S. M., Van der Merwe, C. E., and Opt Hof, J. 1978. Genetic and congenital disorders: Knowledge and attitudes of the public, nurses, and medical practitioners in South Africa. *South African Medical Journal* 53:491-94.

MacKay, C. R. 1991. The effects of uncertainty on the physician- patient relationship in predictive genetic testing. *Journal of Clinical Ethics* 2:247-50.

Nelkin, D., and Lindee, M. S. 1995. *The DNA mystique: The gene as cultural icon*. New York: W. H. Freeman.

Poirier, J., Delisle, M.-C., Quirion, R., Aubert, I., Farlow, M., Lankin, D., Hui, S., Bertrand, P., Nalbangtoglu, J., and Gilfix, B. M. 1995. Apolipoprotein E4 allele as a predictor of cholinergic deficits and treatment outcome in Alzheimer disease. *Proceedings of the National Academy of Sciences* 92:12260-64.

Proud, V. K., Johnson, E. D., and Mitchell, J. A. 1993. Students online: Learning medical genetics. *American Journal of Human Genetics* 52:637-42.

Quill, T. E., and Townsend, P. 1991. Bad news: Delivery, dialogue, and dilemmas. *Archives of Internal Medicine* 151:463-68.

Riccardi, V., and Schmickel, R. 1988. Human genetics as a component of medical school curricula: A report of the American Society of Human Genetics. *American Journal of Human Genetics* 42:639-43.

Roses, A. D. 1995. Apolipoprotein E genotyping in the differential diagnosis, not prediction, of Alzheimer's disease. *Annals of Neurology* 38:6-14.

Rowley, P. T., Loader, S., Sutera, C. J., and Kozyra, A. 1995. Prenatal genetic testing for hemoglobinopathy carriers: A comparison of primary providers of prenatal care and professional genetic counselors. *American Journal of Human Genetics* 56:769-76.

Saunders, A. M., Hulette, C., Welsh-Bohmer, K. A., Schmechel, D. E., Crain, B., Burke, J. R., Alberts, M. J., Strittmatter, W. J., Rosenberg, C., Scott, S. V., Gaskell, P. C., Pericak-Vance, M. A., and Roses, A. D. 1996. Sensitivity, specificity, and predictive value apolipoprotein E genotyping for sporadic Alzheimer's disease. *Lancet* 348:90-93.

Seshadri, S., Drachman, D. A., and Lippa, C. F. 1995. Apolipoprotein E e4 allele and the lifetime risk of Alzheimer's disease: What physicians know, and what they should know. *Archives of Neurology* 52:1074-79.

Stern, Y., Gurland, B., Tatemichi, T. K., Tang, M. X., Wildrer, D., and Mayeux, R. 1994. Influence of education and occupation on the incidence of Alzheimer's disease. *JAMA* 271:1004-10.

Wilfond, B. S., and Fost, N. 1990. The cystic fibrosis gene: Medical and social implications for heterozygote detection. *JAMA* 263:2777-83.

Wilfond, B. S., and Nolan, K. 1993. National policy development for the clinical application of genetic diagnostic technologies: Lessons form cystic fibrosis. *JAMA* 270:2948-54.

Yarborough, M., Scott, J. A., and Dixon, L. K. 1989. The role of beneficence in clinical genetics: Non-directive counseling reconsidered. *Theoretical Medicine* 10:139-49.

Culture and Values at the Intersection of Science and Suffering

Encountering Ethics, Genetics, and Alzheimer Disease

ATWOOD D. GAINES,
PH.D., M.P.H.

Genetic research on Alzheimer disease (AD) necessarily intersects with ethics, for it has significant implications for the entire AD-affected and potentially affected population. This represents an intersection of science, suffering, and values that has important implications for clinical and counseling practices, research, social policy, and the lives of those at risk as well as their significant others. This chapter engages the debates generated by this intersection from the vantage points of cultural and medical anthropology and the cultural studies of science.

Genetic research has begun to yield information on the cause of certain of the conditions known as dementia. Specifically, AD has been shown to be, as noted in earlier chapters, divisible into two general types: late-onset sporadic AD and early-onset genetically determined familial AD. Almost all cases of AD are sporadic, with as yet no known genetic cause, although some of these cases are associated with the apolipoprotein E (APOE) susceptibility gene. The much smaller number of cases are "caused" (perhaps an overstatement) by genetic abnormalities in the DNA of three chromosomes (1, 14, and 21).

Genetic discoveries have led to heightened research activity, which in turn has increasingly complicated, rather than simplified, understandings of causation in AD. Certain of the genetic findings have produced sufficient certainty of increased risk that testing for some now looms on the practical landscape of AD. This landscape is enlarged to include genetic counseling as well as some clinical (prophylactic) practices that are new. But problems with the plural nature of society in the United States and with the cultural nature of science need attention in order to avoid complications in later stages.

In this chapter, I analyze two specific areas at the intersection of ethics, genetics, and AD: (1) cultural notions appearing in the science(s) of AD (i.e., the cultural models of kinship and social identity employed in genetics) and

(2) the lay cultural issues relating to AD testing that arise out of the plural nature of United States society. Different ethnic and demographic spheres are seen as being differently involved and influenced by technological and social developments associated with AD. In general, this chapter is intended as a contribution to both the literature on cultural issues related to AD and the cultural studies of science.

Culture in Science

In addition to more obvious cultural issues that are related to ethnicity and religious values, which are considered below, other cultural beliefs appear embedded in the scientific concern with AD. The very assessment of risk itself, it is suggested below, may owe much to geneticists' implicit cultural beliefs about kinship. The often dominant role of nonscientific beliefs in science is well known and documented. Since Thomas Kuhn (1970), few knowledgeable about the philosophy, history, sociology, and anthropology of science would claim that it is acultural and value neutral (Hacking 1983; Longino 1990).

The cultural bases of scientific practice and interpretation have been explored for medical and clinical medical sciences (e.g., Feldman 1995; Foucault 1975; Gaines 1991, 1992, 1995; Gilman 1988; Good 1995; Hahn and Gaines 1985; Kirmayer 1988; Lock and Gordon 1988; Mishler et al. 1981), the social and biological sciences (e.g., Fausto-Sterling 1992; Gould 1981; Harding 1993; Keller 1992; Russet 1989), the natural sciences (e.g., Hacking 1983; Keller 1992; Knorr-Cetina and Mulkay 1983; Kohler 1991; Kuhn 1970; Latour and Woolgar 1979; Longino 1990; Pickering 1992), and the international and public health sciences (e.g., Brandt 1978; Gaines 1997a; Jones 1996; Kleinman 1995; Schiller, Crystal, and Lewellen 1996).

One may specify two levels at which cultural values and beliefs appear in science. First is the "contextual" level (Longino 1983, 1990), where cultural beliefs become part of scientific thinking (e.g., gender or "racial" biases or beliefs in the divine order of nature). The second level is that of the internal norms and values of the scientific communities themselves (Latour and Woolgar 1979; Mulkay 1977; Pickering 1992). Here I explore the first level at which culture and science intersect. In particular, I am concerned with cultural beliefs about kinship, descent, and social identity that appear in modern genetics.

A Problem in Medical Science: Is Alzheimer Disease Real?

Assumptions about kinship, especially descent, that affect science are elements of contextual values, those that derive not from the constitutive values of science but from the culture in which the science is done. In the present discussion, I leave aside concerns about internal values as they form research itself within the scientific community (see Longino 1990; Mulkay 1977).

To begin the discussion of the influence of cultural beliefs in the dementia-related sciences, one may raise the issue of the very reality of AD. Indeed, AD researchers sometimes refer to the development of their focal concern as a time during which "we made up AD" or when "we created AD" (the "we" apparently referring to various combinations of geneticists, psychiatrists, advocacy groups, patients, the government, and the public at large). That is, at least some important figures see AD as a creation, what interpretive anthropologists refer to as a "cultural construction" (Gaines 1992).

Such a conception is not unusual, for in the cultural studies of science, we see myriad examples of precisely such constitutive activity through which medical and other scientific "realities" have been observed to be created rather than "discovered" (e.g., Foucault 1975; Gaines 1992, 1995; Gilman 1988; Hacking 1995; Latour and Woolgar 1979; Lock and Gordon 1988; Pickering 1992; Young 1995).

While doubting Thomases may be found in the United States, it is important to note that certain medical traditions or members thereof, such as some in Germany, consider the behavioral and pathophysiological symptoms of AD to be nothing more or less than universal manifestations of aging; such manifestations may occur earlier or later in life but do not constitute disease. As such, in the view of some in that medical tradition, AD's plaques and tangles constitute not a disease but rather the normative, though problematic, processes of aging.

In Japan, the study of and concern for dementia has a very recent history; its originator-founder is still active as dean of a medical school. Japan's concern with AD may be more an example of emulation or cultural diffusion than the internal development of a locally "discovered," focal illness reality.

Differing conceptions of disease are not unusual in professional biomedicines. Biomedical traditions of specific countries exhibit different diseases and therapies; they also have different therapies for the same diseases and very large differences in therapies for the same disorders. What is considered a disease condition in one biomedical tradition may not exist at all in others, as appears to be the case with AD. Others include post-traumatic stress disorder (PTSD) and premenstrual syndrome (PMS) in the United States, dropped stomach and *shinkieshitsu* in Japan, neurasthenia in China, *triste tout le temps* and *crise de fois* (liver crisis) in France, and heart insufficiency in Germany (Gaines 1992; Hahn and Gaines 1985; Kleinman 1986; Lindenbaum and Lock 1993; Lock and Gordon 1988; Payer 1989; Wright and Treacher 1982; Young 1995).

Likewise, specific life stages said to be generative of, or characterized by, specific disturbances appear in one medical tradition but not in others (Gaines 1991, 1992). The life course is not everywhere divisible in the same way, even over time in a single culture (e.g., the creation of "childhood" and "adolescence" in U.S. medicine and psychiatry [Gaines 1992] or babyhood-infancy in England at the turn of the century [Wright 1988]).

Genethics

We now live in a period some call "the age of the gene." Although some may see genetics as the Holy Grail, as the ultimate answer to questions of being and doing, disease and health, the field's findings and interpretations are seen as highly problematic to some and totally unacceptable to others. In general, it appears that for all that is seen as negative or unwanted in the dominant culture (which, I might add, is the culture of a relatively small minority group), explanations are sought in biology, the sine qua non of which is now genetics. However, the same cultural view applies; it is the case that the atomistic and reductionist tendency of U.S. science and medicine has pushed us to ever lower levels of explanation, just as in physics, researchers seek ever smaller, more "basic" and "elemental" particles as the basic units of matter and of nature (Gaines 1991, 1995; Gordon 1988; Keller 1992).

The genetic work on AD produces ethical issues and challenges, for the encounter is one between views of determined behavior and behavior that is a result of human agency (Kirmayer 1988). While some seek to reduce disease, and even human behavior, to genetics, there remain human relations, experiences, and constructions far too complicated and too varied across cultures to be determined simply by a few genes. Genetics research does not produce a guide to action; rather, the field calls forth the need for one, or many, guides, for there are many cultural worlds into which genetic information may be interjected and many ways such information may be construed.

Culture and Research

The nature of scientific research itself is not acultural; rather, it is greatly influenced and, often, externally determined. The nature and direction of medical and scientific research is often, if not always, determined by wider cultural interests and values. These interests determine what research is encouraged and funded by the government, patrons, and corporations (pharmaceutical, medical, manufacturers of consumer products, etc.) (see Kohler 1991), which results are disseminated and which are lauded as important and significant (Longino 1990). As Kohler has pointed out, "The importance of patronage in modern science is almost too obvious to dwell upon" (1991, 1). And, of course, the interests and agendas of extramural funding entities are never quite the same as those of their researchers, who regularly bend their research to fit funding guidelines.

The sort of research and the subjects used is determined by cultural contextual ideas, as well; for example, the Tuskegee syphilis experiment was not considered ethically (or legally) problematic in medicine from 1930 until the 1970s (Brandt 1978; Jones 1996). Today, we see and have seen similar "constructions" of at-risk or vulnerable groups that owe far more to United States "racial" and gender biases than to value-neutral scientific reasoning (Fausto-Sterling 1992; Gaines 1995; Gilman 1988; Harding 1993; Jones 1996; Longino 1990; Russet 1989).

In addition, what issues are important to address, such as specific diseases, is determined outside of the field of science, as in the case of AD, where popular pressure led to increased activity, then funding, resulting in findings of interest to many and helping to constitute a community of concerned persons organized around a specific disease. However, the research that concerns the genetics of AD is in fact pointing to a wide variety of illnesses now labeled AD. That is, much like the history of diabetes mellitus, one disease may turn out to be many.

From Unity to Diversity: A Model

In our area of interest, Alzheimer disease, we see the construction of a "genetic disease" long before there was any evidence that the disorder might have a genetic basis. Now that we have discerned some genetic involvement in some cases of AD, we assume that more data and a firmer grasp of the genetics of AD are just around the next polymerase chain reaction. That is, while we have some evidence that rare cases have clearly a genetic component—though what that component is varies for each problem mutation discerned—most cases do not have a known genetic component. However, many accept on faith, which is ideally not an element of science, that further research will lead to the discernment of the essential genetic basis of AD or, what is more likely to be the case, the genetic *bases*.

There is here implicated a model, what George Devereux (1978) called a "cultural thought model," wherein past cultural experience serves as a model for future action. The past experience, the model in this case, is Huntington disease (HD). Huntington disease is the classic autosomal-dominant disorder. It is associated with severe neurological pathology and dementia with onset typically postreproductive, in the fifth decade of life. It was the first Mendelian disorder mapped by linkage to DNA markers, in 1983 (Thompson, McInnes, and Willard 1991).

Conversations with geneticists participating in this volume clearly reveal the conscious presence of an HD model of AD, but its implications for research remain unexplored and can be but noted here. The important cultural issue is that although there are models of and models for disease entities, they are not views of the actual disease entity. It is in terms of these culturally historically constructed models that scientific action is predicated.

The Forms of Diabetes Mellitus as Countermodels

The development of AD as a focal disease may have a history analogous to that seen with diabetes mellitus (DM). When a disorder known from external signs is investigated, it produces new knowledge, which in turn may indicate that a disorder is not unitary. In the case of DM, heterogeneity emerged from unity in the course of research on "the" disease.

Diabetes mellitus exists in two "forms," it is said: insulin dependent and non-insulin dependent (IDDM and NIDDM, respectively). Insulin dependent diabetes mellitus was diagnosed as a deficiency or absence of the protein insulin caused by a malfunctioning or nonfunctioning region of the pancreas. The problem usually occurs in children, hence the condition's common name, juvenile diabetes.

Insufficient insulin leads to high blood glucose levels, as the body cannot absorb glucose without insulin. The high blood glucose levels cause organ damage over time and in acute cases can cause organ shutdown and even death. Much later research ascertained that many older people, usually in their early forties, may develop diabetes. In those cases, it was called NIDDM. However, a cursory exploration of NIDDM leads to the realization that this disorder is not at all the same as IDDM. We find similarity in result but not in cause.

In NIDDM, we do not find a deficit in insulin production, though we find high blood glucose levels. But, these levels generally do not have nearly the upper range of those found in IDDM, even without the use of insulin (which is used by many people with NIDDM, despite its name) or oral hypoglycemics. Clearly, these are two unrelated conditions: one concerns a failure of insulin production by a specific organ; the other involves a general systemic insensitivity of the body's cells to insulin. The differentiation occurred as a result of research. Still, however, we refer to the two condition as diabetes type I and diabetes type II, as if they are versions of the same disorder. Clearly, they are not. They do not have the same pathophysiology or histopathology nor time and means of onset. The tie that binds the two disorders together is a popular prescientific understanding that yet holds sway in the medical classification of the two diseases, the presence of "high blood sugar." A superficially similar clinical picture derives from empirically different causes and consequences, but a sense of unity is maintained.

A similar model of a unitary disease, AD appears to be crumbling with increased research in genetics. Two types, early-onset familial AD (FAD) and the later-onset sporadic AD (SAD) are already identified. Research indicates differences in the risk of affliction in SAD based on APOE genotype, as Allen Roses and others note elsewhere in this volume. Thus, there appear to be three classes of AD.

Genetic research, and that of the Human Genome Project, is "producing immediate and recurrent consequences concerning the localization and identification of medically interesting genes" (Juengst 1995, 21). But, "most often, genetics will not reveal our precise, unalterable fate" (Yesley 1995, 21). Indeed, Juengst argues that genetics' predictive power is more akin to that of a meteorology than fortune-telling. The former predicts the circumstances clients will face as they go about their lives but not how the clients will experience that environment. By contrast, fortune tellers are expected to predict the course of their clients' future life experiences (Juengst 1995, 22–23).

Spheres of Society and Alzheimer Disease

From interpretive cultural anthropology we draw an important notion, that of "local knowledge" (Geertz 1983). With this notion we understand reality to be relative and everywhere a local construct, based on local principles, values, and assumptions. Crimes in one place are heroic deeds in another; blameless accident in one area is dastardly culpability in another; natural disaster in one area is spiritual retribution in another; spiritual communication in one area is psychotic ideation in another; psychiatric disease identified in one culture is unremarkable behavior or ideation in another; medical disease in one culture is a quaint foreign practice in another (e.g., France's *crise de foie*); "genetic disease" in one culture is a curse of an ancestral shade in another.

As all cultures are constantly changing, it is possible for a single culture to show the development over time of such antitheses. As such, the meaning of things generated in one area may be nonexistent or very different in another. History and context give meaning to process or entity and in so doing confer their moral dimensions (e.g., "It is a good thing [to do]" or "It is a bad thing [to do]").

Most important for our considerations here is the fact that cultures are made up of many different sectors or spheres, each with moral specificity. Anthropologists say that there are many distinct niches or vantage points from which people may speak. In cultures and societies, such as those in the West, where there is considerable inequality, some people, such as stigmatized ethnic groups, are heard far less than others, if they are heard at all. Some, such as women, often remain, or rather are made to be, silent. We may call these voicings a culture's "vocal geography" (Gaines 1997a), the loci from and on which one or one group may or may not speak.

Different domains of a society exist and have different levels of worth conferred on them; some practices, institutions, and events are more important than others in a particular culture. In complex modern societies, many different domains of human action exist, some cultural (ethnic groups), some economic (social classes), some regional, some occupational, some educational (levels of literacy), some interactional (levels of social integration or connectedness), and some are certainly gendered (male and female worlds, psychologies, roles, etc.).

A central problem, then, for any sophisticated cultural considerations of genetics and AD is that practices and beliefs, significance and value, vary from one cultural or social domain to another within a single complex, plural society. The United States is certainly such a society. It exhibits complex, differentiated ethnic and social prestige, economic and political structures often conceptually organized as a single system. As such, we cannot hope to produce anything concerning social or medical actions, ethical or otherwise, that can be universally understood, let alone accepted and acted on in each of the identifiable spheres.

In a plural society such as the United States, and most other Western nations, knowledge and practice related to genetics of disease and to AD in particular may be conceived of as goods to be distributed. But what shall be the principles of distribution? the mechanisms? the agents? Furthermore, that which is distributed by whomever, for whatever reason, by whatever means, becomes something other than what it was in terms of its original discursive construction in its original cultural locus (e.g., "science," "genetics," "medicine," "academic community," etc.) (e.g., Gaines 1989). It is, of course, true that each one of these loci is a world a bit unto itself in both local and national senses.

The implications of the genetic tests indicating various levels of risk for the development of AD are great. But such implications are not everywhere the same; the same news is not good in all cultural spaces. Depending on the cultural context, testing, the divulging of results, the receipt of results, and the clinical activities based on them may be accepted or rejected by concerned individuals, kin, or community. There are complex issues related to this point that concern the individual and community authority and decision making. Ultimately, these issues relate morality to the nature of the individual, the self, and her or his kinship system.

Kinship, Science, and Person

Though seen as "natural," kinship systems are always and everywhere symbolic systems (Geertz and Geertz 1975). Kinship is one institution that, in less complex cultures, determines most social relationships. Kinship systems represent cultural values projected onto the local human family. To assume that pedigrees and family trees constitute an accurate retelling of biological familial history is a potentially large mistake. It is not just that there are reporting errors or issues of "who the real father is" (note the implicit gender bias of that notion); it is rather a matter of fundamentally different systems of descent and affinity.

Geneticists in their work assume a northern European bilateral kinship system in which unrelated individuals marry into the kindred. But many of the people in the United States come from lineal systems, usually patrilineal (or patrilateral or bilateral with a patrilateral bias). In such systems, people not descended through the male line are not considered relatives. Thus, cousins of any stripe born to women of the mother's family lineage (which is her patrilineage, for she must marry into another patrilineage) would not be considered "relatives." Hence, they are marriageable.

In the Middle East, a preferred, but not the majority, form of marriage is between a man's child and his brother's child ("patrilateral parallel cousin marriage"). Cross-cousin marriage is a form of marriage found among Native Americans and entails the preference for marriage to the offspring of a father's sister or a mother's brother. However, in genetics, such people as cousins are considered relatives. Such marriage partners would appear as unrelated individuals marrying into a line in geneticists' pedigrees, thus masking the fact that the individuals already share genetic heritage.

There is a second large problem with kinship systems. In cases where individuals are descended from groups that practice bilateral descent, a problem of historic proximity exists. Most European Americans came from sedentary peasant communities. Their ancestors lived in small villages and valley communities that had rules determining whom one married. But their rules of exclusion from and inclusion in the marriageable or the unmarriageable group should not be assumed to represent the northern European (Protestant) model of bilateral kinship that geneticists use. That is to say, most of the people whom one might consider as a mate in these peasant worlds are already related to one in a variety of ways, owing to the relatively isolated nature of the communities. If one village married its women to the men of another, in short order in genealogical time, any newlyweds would already be related. In fact, in most remote areas, the ties of kinship are multiple, not single stranded. What all this suggests is that inherited disorders may not be inherited in the way that geneticists now understand. Multiple overlapping ties of kinship and extragenetic material may produce the disorders like AD, not single genes.

Models and Problems

There are several sources of misinformation in kinship models. First, the model that researchers use is a Western model of bilateral descent (with Eskimo terminology). The same descent system can use different terminology, as in the French, which distinguishes cousins by sex (*cousin* versus *cousine*), whereas in English this distinction is not made. They thus make data they receive conform to a cultural model of terminology.

Second, immigrants are aware of the taboo against "inbreeding" in the United States. As a consequence, they may fabricate their family history to make it conform to the model used in the United States. Third, the individuals may not know their family history very well, or they may in fact have been misinformed to conceal certain family secrets. One can say that such secrets are a part of virtually all families in the United States with long histories. This can be highlighted by the fact that, as biological anthropologists have shown, at least 15 percent of the ancestry of Southern "whites" is from West Africa, and another sizable percentage is from native North America (Gaines 1995). The topic of ancestry relates to another issue for geneticists, the nature of social identity in the United States.

Ethnicity and Alzheimer Disease: "Race" As Identity

In the United States, most writers, scientific and popular, assume that there is a single dominant culture, often termed "white." Empirically, however, no such cultural entity can be found in the United States or anywhere else in the world. Those who are classified as white and who are alleged to bear a unitary culture are, in fact, members of a variety of ethnic and religious groups with distinctive cultural backgrounds.

The belief that there is a culture to which a majority of (European-American) *USians** belong, called "white culture," is a local cultural construction, one powerful enough to influence science and society (Gaines, 1989, 1991, 1995; Gilman 1988; Gould 1981) despite its logical implausibility and total lack of empirical foundation (Cyrus 1993; Gaines 1982, 1995; Gould 1981). Where is the source, the ancestral homeland, of "white" culture? Clearly, the cultures of Europe do not form a unity, but in the United States, one constructs them as such. Thus, Bulgarians, Scots, the Swedish, and the French are implicitly asserted to have a common "Western" or "white" culture. However, cultures do not come in colors, nor is culture related to "race" (Gaines 1995; Gould 1981; Harding 1993).

"Racial" ideas are aspects of what may be called "local biology" (Gaines 1992, 1995) in that ethnic differences are constructed differently in different cultures according to local "biological" knowledge. In the United States, cultural differences are often, if not commonly, constructed as biological differences ("race"). The criteria of inclusion and exclusion are not, however, cross-culturally valid. Thus, they represent local constructions of putative biology, or local biology.

This concept, we note, poses a challenge to those who construe biology as the bedrock of reality, of which culture is a mere reflection. As it happens, the biologies of all of the world's professional medicines actually show sharp differences (see Gaines 1992; Leslie and Young 1992; Lindenbaum and Lock 1993; Payer 1989).

The idea of "white culture" appears to be a restating in modern (cultural) terms of racialist notions in U.S. science, society, and history. The racialist notions held that behavior is linked to and even a product of putative "race"; people are said to do things, think things, even get sick, because of their "race." Such "racial" constructions also have serious ethical implications as well as scientific problems (Gaines 1995).

The term *culture,* when used in relation to *race,* is, in such discourse, misused. In the common discourse of science and medicine, the use of this term or old "racial" labels *(white, black, Asian)* conceals logically and empirically indefensible, implicitly "racial" conceptions (Gaines 1982, 1995, 1997a). This use of "racial" terms actually has the effect of masking cultural differences, not revealing them. This masking is most especially noteworthy among immigrants and the elderly in the United States (Gaines et al. 1995).

The problem for genetics research and risk assessment of populations is

---

* The term *Americans* would necessarily include Canadians as well as all Latin Americans.

that U.S. science regularly uses the folk categories of "race," though sometimes called ethnicity, in comparative studies. Comparing populations leads researchers to replicate the past cultural history of social classification, treating social groups as if they are distinct internally homogeneous biological groups.

Ethnicity, Alzheimer Disease, and Ethics

In the United States one sees a collage of cultural spheres. As a nation of immigrants, the United States boasts great cultural heterogeneity, though public discourse often denies this by the use of "racial" terms that efface cultural differences, as noted above. Within our cultural spheres there is variety in terms of class, age, gender, and other features physical or social.

Selves, Autonomy, and Kinship

A host of problems confront us when we look at the issues relating to AD, which include testing, dissemination of test results (seen as property), and advance life planning (Post 1995). With the issue of informed consent, we also confront the cultural problem of autonomy. In most parts of the world, including many parts of the United States, the self is seen as an expression of a larger kinship group, that symbolic system noted above. We find such distinctive self-concepts in Chinese culture, Mediterranean cultures, various African cultures, and Latin American or Native American cultures, among others. In these cultures the self exists as an expression of a larger kindred, usually unilineal (descent traced only through males or only through females). It is not the autonomous, bounded, independent center of thought and action, that self-construct found in the dominant minority culture in the United States (Gaines 1982, 1985; Geertz 1973) and often said to be the "Western" (Shweder and Bourne 1982), even universal, psychological self-construct.

As an expression of a larger whole, the individual is not the arbiter of her or his own destiny; she or he is not the locus of control or decision making. In Zaire, we see a formalized "therapy management group" responsible for care of the sick (Janzen 1987). Composed of relatives and concerned others, the therapy management group makes all decisions regarding a patient's care, including where and when therapy will be sought. The identified patient is not involved in any of these decisions, including those terminating treatment (Janzen 1987). In other culture areas, decisions are made by the descent group, lineage, or clan, as in Native American groups, Africa, and Asia.

In China and Japan, the importance of the family group, and not the individual, is shown in the fact that the identified patient may not appear in the medical context; family members appear in their stead (Kleinman 1980; Ohnuki-Tierney 1984). The autonomous hypercognitive individual with a sense of control over self and destiny (Gaines 1992; Post 1995) is actually a rather rare and strange cultural psychological construct among the world's cultures. Yet much of our discussions of informed consent in bioethics and research and discussions of genetic testing presume this cultural-psychological construct.

In terms of genetic testing, issues may be raised that relate to the authority to request such testing and what to do with results. In much of the world, such requests would come from a senior lineage leader or head, usually male. In addition, if permission were given, the results would be seen as the property of the group, not the individual. One can imagine that in some areas the individual at risk would not be allowed access to such information unless deemed appropriate by the elder(s). In general, in lineage systems found throughout the world, property or possessions or information, such as test results or medical records, are group possessions and are administered by the senior member. As well, such "property" cannot be alienated from the group by individual initiative.

Depending on the context in the United States or elsewhere in the world, such issues as those noted above with respect to group control and ownership may loom large in the responses to ethical policies and procedures, most of which assuredly will be developed based on the implicit notion of the northern European Protestant, autonomous self.

Authority and Medical Knowledge

In many cultures, such as the ethnic groups of Latin America (excluding the Indian cultures), authority figures are assumed to have superior knowledge. It may be seen as inappropriate to "challenge" authority by expecting to be completely informed of procedures or alternatives. It is assumed that the professional will tell the family members (not the individual) what the correct course of action should be. But, neutral genetic counseling following testing is designed with another model in mind, a model in which the self, given all the information available, makes informed decisions. This model emphasizes the acquisition of knowledge, which promotes power in the form of self-directedness and self-control. Education and counseling are seen as empowering, returning control (which could not be returned unless it were thought to be present in the first place) to self.

Thus, the thrust of new education initiatives and counseling philosophies of nondirectiveness may meet formidable opposition from such groups as the Latin ethnics who seek decisive professional action. Many do not seek cultural means of enhancing a sense of control over destiny, which they do not believe is in the hands of individuals. Their beliefs mirror those in the Mediterranean (see, e.g., Gaines and Farmer 1986), which is the Old World source of the Latin traditions. It is also true that in the United States, the "empowering" efforts of education are designed for those cultural groups begotten of the Word (i.e., those northern European Protestant groups whose tradition emphasizes literacy, cognitive functioning, interpretation, and decision making) (Gaines 1982, 1991; Geertz 1983; Post 1995).

Destiny

Another issue of potential import that can be but mentioned here is that of communicating the diagnosis. In many parts of the world, such as Japan, France, and Italy, the telling of a fatal diagnosis is considered improper for a variety of reasons (see Gordon 1991; Zanotti 1995). In Italy, telling the diagnosis of a fatal disorder, a category that would include positive tests for FAD, is considered playing or replacing God, who makes all ultimate decisions about life and death. As well, it is believed there and in Japan that a fatal diagnosis destroys what quality of life is left. While some changes can be seen indicating that these beliefs are no longer universal in Japan or Italy, they are yet dominant and can also be found in the United States among culture mates of these groups.

Clearly, ethical issues with immigrant groups in the United States concern telling the diagnosis. In certain groups diagnoses should be told to a relative, not the patient. How will informed consent work in this context? What is the ethical procedure for obtaining it from a proxy of an incompetent person?

Aging

Special emphasis may be placed on elderly people aside from their increased risk of AD, because many, and in some areas, most, U.S. elderly persons are immigrants or children of immigrants whose primary language and local communities were not English (Gaines et al. 1995; Gaines and MacDonald 1997). The ubiquitous studies using "white" and "black" as cultural designations misrepresent culture in general and in the particulars of the many ethnic groups lumped together as one or the other. Thus, in elderly people who are likely to be afflicted, cultural and ethnic issues may be most germane, especially as they relate to mental disorders or failure of memory (Gaines 1997b).

Gender

Another issue (and sphere) is gender. Findings, policies, and practices related to genetics, as they ripple through other sectors of the cultures of the United States, may have more implications for women than for men; that is, policies and practices are not gender neutral (Murphy 1995; Stoller 1994). This is for the simple reason that for most of the cultures in the United States, women, not men, provide the bulk of the caring and emotional labor (Stoller 1994; Stoller and Cutler 1992). Research shows that what I call the "third shift" (in addition to primary family work and outside job) has negative health consequences for women (Brody 1985), as well as occupational consequences (Scharlach and Boyd 1989). With genetic testing, preparing to care for the afflicted may be a psychological burden occurring before women are saddled with subsequent social, financial, and physical burdens.

Gender inequalities resulting from the intersection of ethics, genetics, and AD may be doubled or trebled when one factors in the vulnerability of stigmatized minority women (i.e., problems of identity and class). Such women already face burdens related to social identity and, often as a consequence, to social class (see, e.g., Stoller and Gibson 1994). Thus, there may be new burdens for women, and especially disadvantaged women, as a result of genetic research on AD. In general, I speak here of a potential "feminization of AD."

Conclusions

We may say that knowledge is local in the United States. It is generated in particular spheres or sectors of society such as the scientific. It is received in other spheres but transformed by their contextual redefinition into something else, sometimes something altogether different. But, as noted above, ideas in science are themselves amenable to cultural deconstruction. They exhibit and embody particular cultural values and beliefs (of kinship and identity) in ostensibly acultural scientific discourse.

Ideas generated in one sphere of U.S. culture may be constructed as very different entities with different meanings, values, impact, and significance in other cultural spheres, such as those of stigmatized ethnicities, elder age groups, and women. Complex issues of disclosure, privacy, authority, caring, affliction, and experience become even more complex as we view them through cultural lenses that impress us with their plurality. Universal rules, policies, and practices appear quite unattainable and, in light of an understanding of culture and context, quite inappropriate for a plural society such as the United States. It would appear that we need to consider a plural approach to education, values, and ethics to accommodate culturally diverse worlds of suffering.

References

Brandt, A. 1978. Racism and research: The case of the Tuskegee syphilis study. *Hastings Center Report* 8:21–29.

Brody, E. 1985. Parent care as normative stress. *Gerontologist* 25:19–29.

Cyrus, V., ed. 1993. *Experiencing race, class, and gender in the United States*. Mountain View, Calif.: Mayfield Publishing.

Devereux, G. 1978. Cultural thought models in primitive and modern psychiatric theories. In *Ethnopsychoanalysis: Psychoanalysis and anthropology as complementary frames of reference*, 265–96. Berkeley: University of California Press.

Fausto-Sterling, A. 1992. *Myths of gender: Biological theories about women and men*. 2d ed. New York: Basic Books.

Feldman, J. 1995. *Plague doctors: Responding to AIDS in France and America*. Westport, Conn.: Bergin and Garvey.

Foucault, M. 1975. *The birth of the clinic*. New York: Vintage Books.

Gaines, A. D. 1982. Cultural definitions, behavior, and the person in American psychiatry. In *Cultural conceptions of mental health and therapy*, ed. A. Marsella and G. White, 167–92. Dordrecht: D. Reidel Publishing.

———. 1985. The once- and the twice-born: Self and practice among psychiatrists and Christian psychiatrists. In *Physicians of Western medicine: Anthropological approaches to theory and practice*, ed. R. A. Hahn and A. D. Gaines, 223–43. Dordrecht: D. Reidel Publishing.

———. 1989. Alzheimer's disease in the context of black (Southern) culture. *Health Matrix* 6 (4): 33–38.

———. 1991. From DSM I to III-R, voices of self, mastery and the other: A cultural constructivist reading of U.S. psychiatric classification. *Social Science and Medicine* 35:3–24.

———. 1995. Race and racism. In *The encyclopedia of bioethics*, ed. W. T. Reich, 2189–2201. 2d ed. New York: Macmillan.

———. 1997a. Medicine and personal reason. *Anthropology and Medicine* (in press).

———. 1997b. Mental illness and immigration. In *Handbook of immigration health*, ed. Sana Loue. New York: Plenum.

———, ed. 1992. *Ethnopsychiatry: The cultural construction of professional and folk psychiatries*. Albany: State University of New York Press.

Gaines, A. D., and Farmer, P. A. 1986. Visible saints: Social cynosures and dysphoria in the Mediterranean tradition. *Culture, Medicine, and Psychiatry* 10:295–330.

Gaines, A. D., and MacDonald, P. E., with Wykle, M. L. 1997. Aging and immigration: Who are the elderly? *Journal of Immigration and Health* (in press).

Gaines, A. D., Stange, K., Ford, A., Haug, M., Noelker, L., Mafrouche, Z., and Jones, P. 1995. Numbers and narratives. Paper presented at the Gerontological Society of America Meeting, Nov. 14, Los Angeles, Calif.

Geertz, C. 1973. Thick description: Toward an interpretive theory of culture. In *The interpretation of cultures*, 3–30. New York: Basic Books.

———. 1983. "From the native's point of view": On the nature of anthropological understanding. In *Local knowledge*, 55–70. New York: Basic Books.

Geertz, H., and Geertz, C. 1975. *Kinship in Bali*. Chicago: University of Chicago Press.

Gilman, S. L. 1988. *Disease and representation: Images of illness from madness to AIDS*. Ithaca: Cornell University Press.

Good, B. J. 1995. *Medicine, rationality, and experience*. Cambridge: Cambridge University Press.

Gordon, D. 1988. Tenacious assumptions in Western medicine. In *Biomedicine examined*, ed. M. Lock and D. Gordon, 19–56. Dordrecht: Kluwer Academic Publishers.

———. 1991. Culture, cancer, and communication. In *Anthropologies of medicine*, ed. B. Pfleiderer and G. Bibeau. Wiesbaden: Vieweg Verlag.

Gould, S. J. 1981. *The mismeasure of man*. New York: W. W. Norton.

Hacking, I. 1983. *Representing and intervening: Introductory topics in the philosophy of natural science*. Cambridge: Cambridge University Press.

———. 1995. *Rewriting the soul: Multiple personality and the sciences of memory*. Princeton: Princeton University Press.

Hahn, R. A., and Gaines, A. D., eds. 1985. *Physicians of Western medicine: Anthropological approaches to theory and practice*. Dordrecht: D. Reidel Publishing.

Harding, S. 1993. *The "racial" economy of science: Toward a democratic future*. Bloomington: University of Indiana Press.

Janzen, J. 1987. Therapy management: Concept, reality, process. *Medical Anthropology Quarterly* 1 (1): 68–84.

Jones, J. 1996. The Tuskegee syphilis experiment. In *Perspectives in medical sociology*, ed. P. Brown, 386–98. Prospect Heights, Ill.: Waveland Press.

Juengst, E. 1995. The ethics of prediction: Genetic risk and the physician-patient relationship. *Genome Science and Technology* 1:21–36.

Keller, E. F. 1992. *Secrets of life, secrets of death: Essays on language, gender, and science*. New York: Routledge.

Kirmayer, L. J. 1988. Mind and body as metaphors: Hidden values in biomedicine. In *Biomedicine examined*, ed. M. Lock and D. Gordon, 57–93. Dordrecht: D. Reidel Publishing.

Kleinman, A. 1980. *Patients and healers in the context of culture*. Berkeley: University of California Press.

———. 1986. *Social origins of distress and disease: Depression, neurasthenia, and pain in modern China*. New Haven: Yale University Press.

———. 1995. *Writing at the margins: Discourse between anthropology and medicine*. Berkeley: University of California Press.

Knorr-Cetina, K., and Mulkay, M., eds. 1983. *Science observed*. London: Sage Publications.

Kohler, R. E. 1991. *Partners in science: Foundations and national scientists, 1900–1945.* Chicago: University of Chicago Press.

Kuhn, T. 1970. *The structure of scientific revolutions.* Chicago: University of Chicago Press.

Latour, B., and Woolgar, S. 1979. *Laboratory life: The social construction of scientific facts.* Beverly Hills, Calif.: Sage Publications.

Leslie, C., and Young, A., eds. 1992. *Paths to Asian medical knowledge.* Berkeley: University of California Press.

Lindenbaum, S., and Lock, M., eds. 1993. *Knowledge, power, and practice: The anthropology of medicine and everyday life.* Berkeley: University of California Press.

Lock, M., and Gordon, D., eds. 1988. *Biomedicine examined.* Dordrecht: Kluwer Academic Publishers.

Longino, H. E. 1983. Beyond bad science: Skeptical reflections on value freedom of scientific inquiry. *Science, Technology, and Human Values* 8 (1): 7–17.

———. 1990. *Science as social knowledge: Values and objectivity in scientific inquiry.* Princeton: Princeton University Press.

Mishler, E., Amara Singham, L. R., Hauser, S., Liem, R., Osherson, S., and Waxler, N. 1981. *Social contexts of health, illness, and patient care.* Cambridge: Cambridge University Press.

Mulkay, M. 1977. Sociology of the scientific research community. In *Science, technology, and society,* ed. I. Spiegel-Rosing and D. de Solla Price, 93–148. Beverly Hills, Calif.: Sage Publications.

Murphy, J. 1995. *The constructed body: AIDS, reproductive technology, and ethics.* Albany: State University of New York Press.

Ohnuki-Tierney, E. 1984. *Health and illness in contemporary Japan.* Cambridge: Cambridge University Press.

Payer, L. 1989. *Medicine and culture.* New York: Penguin.

Pfleiderer, B., and Bibeau, G., eds. 1991. *Anthropologies of medicine: A colloquium on West European and North American perspectives.* Wiesbaden: Vieweg Verlag.

Pickering, A., ed. 1992. *Science as practice and culture.* Chicago: University of Chicago Press.

Post, S. G. 1995. *The moral challenge of Alzheimer disease.* Baltimore: Johns Hopkins University Press.

Russett, C. E. 1989. *Sexual science: The Victorian construction of womanhood.* Cambridge: Harvard University Press.

Scharlach, A., and Boyd, S. 1989. Caregiving and employment: Results of an employee survey. *Gerontologist* 27:627–31.

Schiller, N. G., Crystal, S., and Lewellen, D. 1996. Risky business: The cultural construction of AIDS risk groups. In *Perspectives in medical sociology,* ed. P. Brown, 707–27. Prospect Heights, Ill.: Waveland Press.

Shweder, R., and Bourne, P. 1982. Do conceptions of the person vary cross-culturally? In *Cultural conceptions of mental health and therapy,* ed. A. Marsella and G. White, 97–137. Dordrecht: D. Reidel Publishing.

Stoller, E. P. 1994. Why women care: Gender and the organization of lay care. In *Worlds of difference: Inequality in the aging experience,* ed. E. P. Stoller and R. C. Gibson, 187–93. Thousand Oaks, Calif.: Pine Forge/Sage Press.

Stoller, E. P., and Cutler, S. J. 1992. The impact of gender on configurations of care among married elderly couples. *Research on Aging* 14:313–30.

Stoller, E. P., and Gibson, R. C., eds. 1994. *Worlds of difference: Inequality in the aging experience*. Thousand Oaks, Calif.: Pine Forge/Sage Press.

Thompson, M. W., McInnes, R. R., and Willard, H. F. 1991. *Genetics in medicine*. 5th ed. Philadelphia: W. B. Saunders.

Wright, P. 1988. Babyhood: The social construction of infant care as a medical problem in England in the years around 1900. In *Biomedicine examined*, ed. M. Lock and D. Gordon, 299–329. Dordrecht: Kluwer Academic Publishers.

Wright, P., and Treacher, A., eds. 1982. *The problem of medical knowledge: Examining the social construction of medicine*. Edinburgh: University of Edinburgh Press.

Yesley, M. S. 1995. Editor's introduction to *Genome Science and Technology* 1:21.

Young, A. 1995. *The harmony of illusions: Inventing post-traumatic stress disorder*. Princeton: Princeton University Press.

Zanotti, R. 1995. First appraisal of breast cancer risk. Ph.D. diss., Bolton School of Nursing, Case Western Reserve University, Cleveland.

Index

abortion issues, 8, 142–44, 146–47
Adam, S., 121, 122, 235
Adams, E. K., 159
Adler Foundation conference, 43
age of onset, 19, 27, 31, 32, 37, 41, 44–45, 53, 191
Alberts, M. J., 55
Alper, J. S., 210
Altstiel, L., 77
Alzheimer disease (AD), 1, 124; clinical classification of, 37, 40; genes associated with, 2; long-term care and, 155–74; neuropathological criteria for, 40–41; pathogenesis of, 17, 74; prenatal testing for, 8, 109, 121, 133, 140, 141, 147–50, 200, 252; preventive therapy for, 6, 47, 230; slower progression of, 71–72. *See also* early-onset Alzheimer disease; late-onset Alzheimer disease
Alzheimer disease centers (ADCs), 50–51
Alzheimer's Association, 70, 85, 155; Cleveland Area, 2, 236; internet address, 44
Alzheimer's Disease and Related Disorders Association, 5, 6, 9
Alzheimer's Disease Collaborative Group, 30, 43
Alzheimer's Disease Genetics Consortium (UK), 4
Alzheimer's Disease International, 128; Medical and Scientific Advisory Committee of, 4, 65, 127, 128, 129, 131, 180, 192, 213
American Association of Medical Colleges (AAMC), 242

American Association of Retired Persons, 158
American College of Medical Genetics (ACMG), 4, 42, 43, 44, 46, 48, 51, 58, 128
American Historical Society of Germans from Russia (AHSGR), 20–21
American Society of Human Genetics (ASHG), 128, 239, 243; Working Group on ApoE and Alzheimer Disease, 4
amino acids, 18, 26, 29, 44, 73
Amouyel, P., 43, 77
amyloid β-peptide (Aβ), 26
amyloid precursor protein (APP), 20, 26–27, 40, 94, 104, 247. *See also* beta amyloid precursor protein gene
Andersen, K., 249
Andrews, L. B., 229, 234, 247, 251
Annas, G. J., 140, 145, 235, 247
Anwar, N., 43
Aouizerate, A., 43, 45
apolipoprotein E (APOE): age factor and, 206; allele (gene), 44–45, 47, 256; discovery of, 3, 74; education and, 228; genetic test for, 248; genotyping, 6, 43, 45–54, 58, 177, 179, 180–81; primary care physicians and, 250–51; testing and diagnosis and, 241
apolipoprotein E (APOE) ϵ4 allele, 2, 6, 42–44; age of onset and, 25, 45; autopsy results and, 49–50; cardiovascular disease and, 9, 177; genetics of, 44–45; genetic testing and, 123–28; prenatal testing and, 200; as susceptibility locus, 41–42. *See also* late-onset Alzheimer disease

275

apolipoprotein E protein (apoE), 2, 42, 77
APP717 mutations, 47
Arduengo, P. M., 30
artificial hearts, 193–94, 198–99
Assman, G., 177
Athena Neurosciences, 58; Athena Diagnostics (division of), 92, 93, 96
Austin, J. H., 17
autopsy confirmations, 7, 12, 37, 48–49, 75, 248; diagnosis and, 45, 58; Volga Germans and, 20
autosomal-dominant traits: age of onset and, 29–30, 46–47; education and, 225; in families, 11, 25, 32; genetic risk and, 74; genetic testing and, 236; Huntington disease and, 119, 248; mutations and, 41, 43. *See also* families; inheritance patterns
Axelman, K., 26

Babul, R., 235
Baird, P., 178
Barashi, C. I., 210
Bartels, D. M., 132
Basun, H., 43
Bates, M., 119
Bayer, R., 246
beanbag genetics, 178–79
de Beauvoir, S., 230
Beck, A. T., 120
Bekker, H., 126
Bengston, V. L., 161
Bennett, R. L., 22
Berchuck, A., 150
Berkman, B., 121
beta amyloid precursor protein gene (βAPP), 25, 26–27, 30, 31, 73
Bianchi, E. C., 231
Billings, P. R., 166, 181, 214
Binstock, R. H., 9, 155, 158, 170, 171, 173
Biomedical Ethics Advisory Committee, 90
Bird, T. D., 6–7, 48, 104, 248; on Aβ amyloid study, 20; AHSGR and, 21; on apolipoprotein E genotyping, 42, 43; on genetic testing, 22; on Volga German study, 17, 18, 19
Birge, S. J., 249

Black Sea Germans, 17, 20
Bloch, M., 106, 112, 113, 120, 122
Blumenthal, D., 229
Borgaonkar, D. S., 43
Botkin, J. R., 144
Bowen, B., 216
Boyd, S., 270
Brandt, A., 257, 259
Brandt, J., 119, 121
breast cancer, 11, 118, 127, 129–30, 191, 192, 203–4, 244–45
Breitner, J. C. S., 42, 43, 46, 52, 178
Brodaty, H., 4, 128, 129, 131
Brody, B., 195
Brody, E. M., 161, 270
Buchanan, A., 144
Burgess, M., 110–11
Burner, S. T., 159
Burton, L., 161
Burwell, B. O., 159
Butler, R. N., 8–9, 226

Cafferata, G. L., 161
Cai, X. D., 26, 27
Callahan, D., 193, 194
Campion, D., 30
Capitman, J., 157, 164
caregivers, 8, 66–67, 158, 225, 230
Caselli, R. J., 212
Chaliki, H., 130
Chase, G. A., 126
Chellis, R. D., 164
Christine, D., 71
chromosome 1 mutations, 17–22, 29–30, 73, 85, 103, 114, 190, 256
chromosome 12 mutations, 11, 12
chromosome 14 mutations, 18, 29–30, 73, 85, 103, 114, 190, 225, 256
chromosome 19 mutations, 2, 42, 85, 124, 190
chromosome 21 mutations, 6, 26–27, 42, 73, 85, 89–90, 94, 103, 104, 114, 190, 256
Churchill, L. R., 193
Citron, M., 26
Clarke, A., 133
Clayton, E. W., 217

Clifford, K. A., 166
Clinton, Bill, 160, 171
Cluff, L. E., 158, 173
Cockburn, I., 87, 89
Codori, A.-M., 121
cognitive impairment, 66, 68; causes of, 1-2, 74, 114. *See also* dementia
Cohen, J., 88
Cohen, M. A., 164
Cohen, M. M., 214
commercialization of genetic testing, 74-76, 84-98
Congressional Budget Office, 160
Consortium to Establish a Registry for Alzheimer's Disease (CERAD), 50, 54
Cook, R. H., 17
Cook-Deegan, R. M., 84
Cordell, B., 73
Corder, E. H., 42, 44, 45
Couch, F. J., 11
Couderc, R., 48
Cras, P., 26
Craufurd, D., 119, 121
Crawford, F., 26
Crown, W. H., 157, 159, 164
Cruts, M., 30
Crystal, S., 257
cultural issues, 10-11; genetic discoveries and, 227-28; studies of science and, 256-71
Cumming, A. M., 177
Cummings, J. L., 71
Cutler, S. J., 270
Cyrus, V., 266
cystic fibrosis, 89-90, 126-27, 141, 191, 192, 201-5, 245
Czech, C., 43

Daniels, N., 167, 193, 196, 200
Davignon, J., 177
Davis, D. A., 252
dementia, 6, 39, 67, 70-71, 250; causes of, 46, 114; clinical evaluation of, 37-58; cultural beliefs and, 258; managed care and, 209-10, 214; symptoms of, 3, 66, 226
Department of Commerce, 163

Department of Health and Human Services: Agency for Health Care Policy and Research, 70; National Alzheimer's Advisory Board Panel Therapeutic Goals Project of, 66; patents assigned to, 94
Derogatis, L. R., 120
Devereux, G., 259
Devlin, B., 42
diagnostic testing, 1, 4, 48, 74-76, 248; accuracy and, 37; communication of, 66, 249, 269; contradictory opinions and, 42; early-onset AD and, 114-15; life decisions and, 52
discrimination: education and, 230-35; genetic testing and, 3, 9, 211-14, 246
Dixon, L. K., 244
Donnenfeld, A. E., 251
Dowd, B., 217
Drachman, D. A., 42, 43, 242, 243
Dresser, R., 148
Dreyfus, T., 216
drug therapies, 66, 68, 77-78, 114, 250; Aricept, 229; deprenyl, 72; donepezil, 68, 69-70, 229; erythropoietin, 92; estrogen, 71, 72; olanzepine, 71; propentofylline, 72; risperidane, 71; S12024, 74; sertindol, 71; tacrine, 68-70, 74, 76-77, 229; vitamin E, 72; xanomilline, 74, 77
Duke University Medical Center, 48, 58, 96

early-onset Alzheimer disease, 2; autosomal dominance and, 105, 262; family testing and, 7; genetic risk and, 112; molecular genetics of, 25-33; mutation carriers and, 103; similarity to Huntington disease and, 127
economic issues, 67, 86-89; conflict of interest and, 228-29; gene therapy and, 201-2; genetic testing and, 3, 213-14; long-term care and, 157-58
Eddy, D., 194
education issues, 10-11; APOE genotyping and, 3, 182-83; counseling and, 268-69; counselors and, 239-52; genetic research and, 256-71; genetic testing and, 225-37, 245

Eldridge, R., 120
Elias, S., 140, 145, 247
ELSI. *See* Working Group on Ethical, Legal, and Social Implications of Human Genome Research
Elston, R. C., 39
Engelhardt, H. T., 193
ethical issues, 7–8; counseling and, 103–16; cultural studies and, 256–71; insurance coverage and, 75, 211; prenatal testing and, 140–50; susceptibility testing and, 118–34
ethnic factors: APOE allele and, 44; genetic testing and, 267–68; social developments and, 257; stigma and, 263
Evans, D. A., 124
Experimentation with Human Beings (Katz), 232

familial Alzheimer disease (FAD), 17, 25, 191, 262; APOE and, 42; cause of, 6; counseling and, 105–11, 115; research on, 20–22
families: economic issues for, 218; founder effect and, 17–18; genetic counseling and, 75; genetic heritage and, 2, 25, 42, 264–65; genetic testing and, 225; long-term care and, 161–62; primary care physicians and, 246, 249–50; public policies and, 170–71. *See also* autosomal-dominant traits; caregivers
Farlow, M. R., 76
Farmer, P. A., 269
Farrer, L. A., 4, 75, 128
Fausto-Sterling, A., 257, 259
Feinberg, J., 148
Feldman, J., 257
Feldman, R., 217
Fine, B. A., 132
Fineberg, H. V., 75
Firth, H., 241
Fleck, L. M., 10, 190, 193, 195, 197, 198, 206
Fletcher, J. C., 133
Foley, J. M., 229
Folstein, S. E., 119, 121
Foncin, J.-F., 30

Fost, N., 126, 240
Foucault, M., 232, 257, 258
founder effect, 17–18
Fox, P., 85
Fox, S. A., 106, 119, 244
Friedland, R., 157, 164
Frommelt, P., 30

Gaines, A. D., 10–11, 256, 257, 258, 259, 263, 265, 266, 267, 268, 269
Galasko, D., 37
Gambardella, A., 87
Gardner, L. B., 214
Garver, B., 132
Garver, K. L., 132
Geertz, C., 262, 264, 267, 269
Geertz, H., 264
Geldmacher, D. S., 6, 71
Geller, G. E., 242, 244
Geller, L. N., 119, 125, 210
gender factor: cultural issues and, 263, 264, 270; genetic testing and, 77; inheritance patterns and, 25; prenatal testing and, 133, 145–46
General Accounting Office, 155, 158, 160
genethics, 259
genetic counseling, 28–29, 103–16, 239; βAPP mutations and, 27–29; example, 31–32; families and, 75; genetic risk and, 74; genetic testing and, 3; Huntington disease and, 28; pretest, 107–11; of PS2 FAD families, 22. *See also* education issues
genetic counselors, 7–8, 125–26; ethical issues for, 149–50; sensitivity of, 118–23; training for, 132, 239–40, 242, 252
Genetic Information and Health Insurance (NIH/DOE), 164–65
genetic susceptibility, 2, 25, 42
genetic testing, 2, 5–6, 25, 27–29, 58, 125; changing context of, 123; chart, 5; clinical diagnosis and, 38–39; commercialization of, 74–76, 84–98; decisions about, 65; demand for, 129–31; discrimination and, 3, 9, 211–14, 230–35, 246; education issues and, 225–37; impli-

cations of, 8, 74–79, 133–34, 263–64; proliferation of, 191; public perceptions of, 57–58; purpose of, 128–29, 140–42; results disclosure, 111–12; risk assessment and, 3, 25; Volga German families, 19
genetic testing, predictive, 2, 4, 7, 103–5, 120–21, 125, 248; in asymptomatic subjects, 46–48; autopsy confirmations and, 49–50; counseling and, 190–91; justice issues and, 9–10, 52, 190–207
Genica Pharmaceuticals Corp., 8, 226
Geriatrics (Butler, ed.), 8–9, 226
Giardello, F. M., 131
Gibson, R. C., 270
Gicomini, M., 216, 217
Gilbert, F., 126
Gilman, S. L., 257, 258, 259, 266
Glazner, J., 213
Goate, A. M., 26, 53
Golde, T. E., 26, 27
Goldgaber, D., 26
Good, B. J., 257
Gordon, D., 257, 258, 259, 269
Gostin, L. O., 9, 217, 231
Goudsmit, J., 30
Gould, S. J., 257, 266
Graham, D. I., 54–55
Graves, A. B., 124
Grayson, P. J., 164
Greenwald, I., 30
Gregg, R. E., 177
Grundke-Iqbal, I., 73
Gulliver's Travels (Swift), 231
Gusella, J. F., 104, 119

Haass, C., 26
Hacking, I., 257, 258
Hahn, R. A., 257, 258
Haines, J. L., 57
Haldane, J. B. S., 231
Hammond, E. A., 251
Hanley, R. J., 157, 162, 164
Hardewig, A., 177
Harding, S., 257, 259, 266
Harper, P. S., 120
Harris, H., 252

Harris, R., 119
Health Care Financing Administration, 12, 98
health care justice issues, 10, 52, 190–207
health care reform, 122, 160, 171. *See also* insurance issues
Healy, B., 11
Heeren, T. C., 126
Helix, 129, 131
Henderson, R., 87, 89
Hendricks, M., 26
Heredity and Politics (Haldane), 231
Heyde, W., 232
Hoffman, D. E., 214
Hofman, K. J., 131, 241, 242
Holtzman, N. A., 124, 125, 131, 178
Houlden, H., 43
Howard Hughes Medical Institute, 85
Howell, M., 233
Hubbard, R., 228
Hudson, K. L., 214
Huggins, M., 113, 120
Human Genome Project, 3–4, 5, 50, 90, 164, 193, 198, 240, 262
Huntington disease (HD), 7, 22, 32–33, 119, 144–45, 191; autosomal-dominance and, 28, 260–61; counseling for, 43, 248; predictive testing and, 104, 107, 110, 235–36
Huntington's Disease Collaborative Research Group, 104, 121
Huntington's Disease Society of America (HDSA), 120
Hutton, M., 56

Illston, L. H., 157, 158, 162, 163, 164
inheritance patterns, 2, 25, 42
Institute of Medicine (IOM), 90, 251
insurance issues: access to genetic information, 12, 216–17; actuarial discrimination and, 9, 166–70; ethical aspects of, 75, 211; genetic counseling and, 22; genetic testing and, 106, 210–18; long-term care and, 155–74, 209–10, 215; risk assessment and, 47, 169
internet addresses: of Alzheimer's Asso-

internet addresses (*cont.*)
  ciation, 44; for diagnostic test studies (ELSI working group), 50; of Genetic Testing Task Force (NIH), 90
Itabashi, S., 49
Iuculano, R. P., 166

Jaffe, A. B., 87
Janzen, J., 267
Jewish Chronic Disease Hospital, 232
John Douglas French Foundation, 85
Johnson, E. D., 251
Johnson, W. D., 39
Jones, J., 257, 259
Juengst, E. T., 9, 177, 215, 262
justice issues. *See* medical justice issues; social justice issues

Kakulas, B. A., 49
Kamboh, M. I., 56, 249
Kang, J., 26
Kapur, S., 241
Karlinsky, H., 7, 26, 29, 103, 114
karyotyping, 185–86
Kassner, E., 160
Katz, J., 232, 244
Katzman, R., 84
Kaufer, D. I., 71
Kawano, M., 44
Keller, E. F., 257, 259
Kershner, M. A., 251
Kessler, S., 106, 119, 121, 125, 244
Kevorkian, J., 148
Khachaturian, Z. S., 40, 48
kinship, 264–65. *See also* families
Kirmayer, L. J., 257
Kladetzky, R.-G., 177
Kleinman, A., 257, 258, 268
Knopman, D., 70
Knoppers, B. M., 228
Knorr-Cetina, K., 257
Kohler, R. E., 257, 259
Kolata, G., 118, 129, 144, 245
Koop, C. E., 142
Kosunen, O., 177
Kovacs, D. M., 18
Kozma, C., 166, 214

Krainer, M., 11
Kremer, B., 235
Kronick, R., 216
Kuhn, T., 257
Kuhse, H., 141

Lampe, T. H., 19
Lancaster, J., 150
Lander, E. S., 42, 56
Lannfelt, L., 43, 104, 236
Lans, S. Y., 212
Lapham, E. V., 166, 214
late-onset Alzheimer disease, 2, 262; APOE and, 25, 42; missense mutations and, 27
Latour, B., 257, 258
Launer, L. J., 249
Lawton, M. P., 66
Leber, P., 69, 72
legislation, 85, 86–87, 211–13; Bayh-Dole Act (1980), 86–87; Employee Retirement Income Security Act, 209; Health Insurance Portability and Accountability Act, 211–12; long-term care and, 158–60
Lemkus, S. M., 241
Lennox, A., 104, 108, 127, 129, 180, 215
Lerman, C., 130
Lerman, M. I., 26
Lerner, A. J., 71
Leslie, C., 266
Leutz, W. N., 157, 164
Levit, K. R., 157
Levitan, D., 30
Levy, E., 26
Levy-Lahad, E., 18, 20, 29, 46, 53
Lewellen, D., 257
Lewontin, R. C., 213
L'Hernault, S. W. L., 30
Li, P. F., 215
Lichenstein, R., 217
Light, D., 210
Lindee, M. S., 227, 245
Lindenbaum, R., 241
Lindenbaum, S., 258, 266
Lippa, C. F., 42, 43, 242, 243
Liu, B. M., 161
Liu, K., 161
Lock, M., 257, 258, 266

Longino, H. E., 257, 258, 259
Lovestone, S., 181
Lucas, E. T., 233
Lucotte, G., 43, 45, 77
Luft, H. S., 216, 217

MacDonald, P. E., 269
MacGowan, S. H., 77
MacKay, C. R., 244
Maestre, G., 44
managed care issues, 9–10, 122, 207, 209–19
Mann, D. M. A., 26
Mansfield, E., 89
Manton, K. M., 161
Marcyniuk, B., 26
Markel, D. S., 121
Marks, J. H., 132
Martin, J. B., 43
Martin, J.-J., 30
Marx, J., 42
Maslow, K., 70
Mastromauro, C., 121
Mattson, M. P., 71
Mayeux, R., 12, 43, 54, 65, 124, 125
Mayieux, F., 48
Mayr, E., 178–79
McBride, O. W., 26
McClamrock, R., 141
McGeer, E. G., 71
McGeer, P. L., 71
McInnes, R. R., 260
McKay, C. R., 125, 127
McKhann, G., 37, 48
McKusick, D. R., 159
Medicaid, 172, 191
medical justice issues, 9–10, 52, 190–207
Medicare, 98, 158–60, 191, 194, 207
medications. *See* drug therapies
MEDLINE, 251
Mehlman, M. J., 215
Meiners, M. R., 159, 172, 173
Meissen, G. J., 28, 105, 119
Mendelian inheritance, 91, 96–97, 178
Menzel, H.-J., 177
MetLife Foundation, 85
Michel, B. F., 77
Miles, S. H., 10, 216

Miller, N. A., 159
Miringoff, M.-L., 227
Mirra, S. S., 40, 48
Mishler, E., 257
missense mutations, 26–32
Mitchell, J. A., 251
Morris, M., 108, 121
Mortimer, J. A., 124
Moscovice, I., 217
Moseley, R., 184
Mountain, J. T., 231
Mulkay, M., 257, 258
Mullan, M. J., 26
Muller-Hill, B., 232
Murakami, K., 43
Murata, P. J., 244
Murphy, J., 270
Murray, T. H., 9, 155, 167
Murrell, J., 26
mutations: genetic, 2, 25, 26, 27–29; missense, 26–32; presenilin genes and, 12, 18, 19, 22, 29–30, 31–32; protein function and, 20. *See also specific chromosome mutations*
Myers, R. H., 47, 121, 217

Nacmias, B., 27
Nalbantoglu, J., 48
Narin, F., 89
National Academy of Engineering, 88
National Academy on Aging, 161
National Center for Human Genome Research, 90
National Human Genome Research Institute, National Study Group, 3–4, 5
National Institute on Aging, 5, 12
National Institute on Aging/Alzheimer's Association Working Group, 42, 43, 46, 58, 65, 124, 128, 149, 181–83
National Institutes of Health (NIH), 85, 89, 215; Genetic Testing Task Force, 90. *See also* Working Group on Ethical, Legal, and Social Implications of Human Genome Research
National Society of Genetic Counselors (NSGC) Code of Ethics, 131–32
National Study Group, 3–4, 5

Nee, L., 30
Nelkin, D., 227, 245
Newhouse, J. P., 217
Newman, M. F., 55
Nicoll, J. A., 54–55
Nietzsche, F., 233
NINDS-ADRDA classification of AD, 37
Noguchi, S., 43
Nolan, K., 241
nondirective counseling, 243–44
Nordberg, A., 72

Oddoze, C., 77
Office of Technology Assessment, 85, 87, 88, 155, 156, 231
Ohnuki-Tierney, E., 268
Okuizumi, K., 45, 56
Olivastro, D., 89
Opt Hof, J., 241
Ostrer, H., 215
Ott, A., 249
ovarian cancer, 130

Parker, K., 216
Partnership for Long-Term Care Program, 172
patents, 88–89, 92–97
paternalism in medicine, 44, 51, 126–27
Patterson, M. B., 66
Payami, H., 43
Payer, L., 258, 266
Pelias, M. Z., 133, 180
Pence, G., 236
Penney, J. B., 121
Pericak-Vance, M. A., 37, 39, 42, 57
Peskind, E. R., 233
Pharmaceutical Research and Manufacturers Association (PhRMA), 87–88, 93
Pickering, A., 257, 258
Poirier, J., 43, 44, 46, 53, 76, 77, 250
Pokorski, R. J., 9, 168
Pollen, D. A., 30, 85, 95
Polvikoski, T., 41
Polzer, K., 216, 217
Post, S. G., 5, 10, 144, 148, 215, 225, 267, 268, 269; on moral basis for limiting treatment, 67; on public interest in AD ethics, 1; on testing and ethical issues, 65
Powers, M., 9, 234
prenatal testing, 121, 133, 140, 150, 252; abortion and, 8, 109, 142–44, 146–47
presenilin 1 gene (PS1): discovery of, 225; missense mutations and, 30, 31–32; mutations and, 2, 6, 12, 18, 25, 247; mutations table, 18; prenatal testing and, 8
presenilin 2 gene (PS2): composition of, 18; discovery of, 19; missense mutations and, 30; mutations and, 2, 6, 22, 47, 247; mutations table, 18; nonpenetrance of, 19–20; prenatal testing and, 8
President's Commission for the Study of Ethical Problems in Medicine and Biomedical and Behavioral Research, 89, 185–86, 235
primary care physicians, 10, 239–53
Pritchard, M. L., 57
privacy issues, 109
Proud, V. K., 251
public perceptions, 1–4, 57–58, 225–37, 245

Quaid, K. A., 8, 22, 108, 118, 119, 120, 121, 125, 133
Quill, T. E., 249

Rabins, P. V., 66
racial factor, 44, 265–67
Raskind, M. A., 233
Ratzan, R., 184
Rawls, J., 196
Rebeck, G. W., 43
Reilly, P., 147, 184
Reiman, E. M., 51, 212
Relkin, N. R., 5, 42, 43, 46, 58, 124, 128, 181, 182, 183
research and development, 20–22, 46, 56–57, 87–89, 259–60
respite care, described, 156
Rhode, K., 233
Rhoden, N. K., 148
Riccardi, V., 242
risk assessment: as actuarial tool, 98; APOE and, 45, 74–76; APOE genotyping and,

46, 52, 180–81; genetic markers and, 74; genetic tests and, 2; spoiler association and, 187–88; treatment decisions and, 47–48
Ritchie, K., 77
Rivlin, A. M., 157, 164
Roberts, G. W., 54–55
Robertson, F., 177
Robertson, J. A., 141, 148
Robert Wood Johnson Foundation, 85, 172
Robinson, J. C., 214, 216, 217
Rodwin, M. A., 228
Rogaev, E. I., 18, 29, 30, 53
Rogers, C. R., 132
Rosenthal, C., 161
Roses, A. D., 6, 11, 37, 41, 43, 45, 46–47, 48, 53, 65, 74, 96, 248; on AD, 39; on amyloid and AD, 54–55; on APOE genotyping in diagnosis, 180, 206–7; on beta amyloid dependence, 44, 53; on genetic prediction, 2; on late-onset AD, 42
Rossor, M. N., 72
Rothenberg, K. H., 211
Rothman, R. K., 142–43
Rowley, P. T., 252
Rozek, R. P., 89
Rudolphi, K. A., 71
Russet, C. E., 257, 259

Sachs, G. A., 10, 239
Sangl, J., 161
Sano, M., 72
Sarah Lawrence genetic counseling degree program, 132
Sato, S., 30
Saunders, A. M., 12, 124, 249; on amyloid and AD, 54–55; on APOE ε4 testing and, 76; on APOE genotyping, 39, 48, 49, 53, 58; on late-onset AD, 42, 43, 44
Scharlach, A., 270
Schellenberg, G. D., 17–18, 95
Scheuner, D., 20, 30
Schiller, N. G., 257
Schmickel, R., 242
Schneider, L., 78
Schork, N. J., 42, 56

Schulman, J. D., 118, 129
Schulzer, M., 71
Schupf, N., 65, 125
science and culture, 256–71
Scott, J. A., 244
Selkoe, D. J., 30, 40, 53, 65, 73
Seshadri, S., 42, 43, 242, 243
Sharpe, N. F., 133
Shea, S., 12
Sherrington, R., 18, 29, 30, 53
Shoji, M., 26
Sing, C. F., 177
Singer, G. G. S., 132, 133
Singer, P., 141
Small, G. W., 51, 212
Smith, A. D., 49
Smith, M. A., 71
Snyder, L., 126
social justice issues, 8–10, 172–74, 190–207; APOE genotyping and, 177–88; managed care and, 209–18
Sorbi, S., 47
Sorenson, J. R., 126
St. George-Hyslop, P. H., 6, 21, 30, 103; on βAPP gene mutations, 26; on chromosome 21, 42; on early-onset AD, 27; on gene interaction, 47; on missense mutations, 27; on susceptibility loci claims, 12
"Statement on the Use of APOE Testing" (*JAMA*), 58
Stein, J. A., 244
Steinbock, B., 8, 140, 141
Stern, R., 120
Stern, Y., 249
Stokinger, H. E., 231
Stoller, E. P., 270
Stone, D. A., 168
Stone, R., 161
Strittmatter, W. J., 42, 43
Struewing, J. P., 11
Susuki, N., 27
Swift, J., 231

Tabira, R., 30
Talbot, C., 56
Tamaoka, A., 27

Tarasoff v. Regents of the University of California (1976), 246
Tardiff, B., 55
Tay-Sachs disease, 141, 144, 191
Teachers Insurance and Annuity Association (TIAA), 162–63
Tell, E. J., 164
Temkin-Greener, H., 164
Teri, L., 22
Terry, R. D., 41
Therapeutic Goals Project, 66
therapeutic interventions, 66–73, 87, 93, 229–30; in clinical research, 46; genetic advances and, 65–80; misinterpretation of, 52–54. *See also* drug therapies
Thompson, D. F., 228
Thompson, M. W., 260
Tibben, A., 120
Toomey, K. E., 246
Toronto "3" Study Group, 215
Townsend, P., 249
Trajtenberg, M., 87
Treacher, A., 250
Turek-Brezina J., 9
Turney, J., 237
Tyler, A., 120

Ueda, K., 43
Ueki, A., 44
Utermann, G., 177

Val717Ile missense mutation, 26, 27–28, 32
Van Broeckhoven, C., 30
Van der Merwe, C. E., 241
van de Ven, W. P., 214
van Duijn, C. M., 26, 45
Van Vliet, R. C., 214
Volga German family studies, 6, 20–22
von Mering, O., 158, 173

Wachbroit, R., 132, 177, 180
Wald, E., 228
Waldo, D. R., 159
Walkington, R. A., 85
Wallack, S. S., 164
Walters, L., 133
Walzer, M., 167, 173
Ward, B. E., 17

Wasserman, D., 132
Weinstein, M. C., 75
Weiss, J. O., 166, 214
Weissert, W. G., 158
Welch, W. P., 209
Welsh-Bohmer, K. A., 49, 50, 54
Went, L., 120, 127
Wertz, D. C., 126, 133
Wesson, M. K., 119, 121, 125
Wexler, N., 236
Whitehouse, P. J., 1, 6, 65, 66, 68, 69, 70, 72, 78, 144; on moral basis for limiting treatment, 67; on pharmacotherapy, 71; on quality of life, 66
Wiener, J. M., 157, 158, 162, 163, 164
Wiggins, S., 109, 120, 129, 235
Wilcock, G. K., 77
Wilfond, B. S., 126, 240, 241
Willard, H. F., 260
Williams, T. F., 164
Wilson, P. W. F., 47
Wilton, S. D., 49
Wiseman, R., 150
Wolf, S., 213
Woolgar, S., 257, 258
Working Group on Ethical, Legal, and Social Implications of Human Genome Research (ELSI), 3–4, 5, 90, 164, 193, 198, 240, 262; internet address, 50
World Federation of Neurology, 104, 112, 120, 127
Wragg, M., 56
Wright, P., 258, 259
Wulfsberg, E. A., 214

Yamada, N., 43
Yarborough, M., 244
Yates, P. O., 26
Yesley, M. S., 262
Yoshizawa, T., 45
Young, A. B., 121, 258, 266
Younkin, S. G., 26, 27, 73

Zanotti, R., 269
Zhou, Z., 216
Zimmer, F., 177
Zinn, A. B., 1

Library of Congress Cataloging-in-Publication Data

Genetic testing for Alzheimer Disease : ethical and clinical issues / edited by Stephen G. Post and Peter J. Whitehouse.
    p.   cm.
    Includes bibliographical references and index.
    ISBN 0-8018-5840-2 (alk. paper)
    1. Alzheimer's disease—Genetic aspects. 2. Alzheimer's disease—Diagnosis—Moral and ethical aspects.   3. Alzheimer's disease—Diagnosis—Social aspects. 4. Human chromosome abnormalities—Diagnosis—Moral and ethical aspects.
    I. Post, Stephen Garrard, 1951–
    II. Whitehouse, Peter J.
    [DNLM: 1. Alzheimer's Disease—genetics. WT 155 G328 1998]
RC523.G45   1998
616.8'31042—dc21
DNLM/DLC
for Library of Congress   97-42661
                                          CIP